Acne Vulgaris

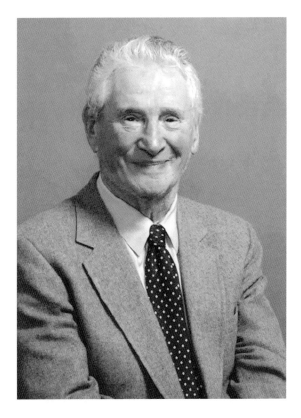

In memory of Albert M. Kligman, MD, PhD
teacher, scientist, clinician, mentor, and friend to us all

Photograph by courtesy of Skin & Aging (www.skinandaging.com).

Acne Vulgaris

Edited by

Alan R. Shalita, MD
Department of Dermatology
SUNY Downstate Medical Center
Brooklyn, New York, U.S.A.

James Q. Del Rosso, DO
Division of Dermatology
Valley Hospital Medical Center
Las Vegas, Nevada, U.S.A.

Guy F. Webster, MD, PhD
Department of Dermatology
Jefferson Medical College
Hockessin, Delaware, U.S.A.

Published in association with the American Acne & Rosacea Society

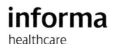

informa
healthcare

First published in 2011 by Informa Healthcare, Telephone House, 69-77 Paul Street, London EC2A 4LQ, UK.

Simultaneously published in the USA by Informa Healthcare, 52 Vanderbilt Avenue, 7th Floor, New York, NY 10017, USA.

Informa Healthcare is a trading division of Informa UK Ltd. Registered Office: 37–41 Mortimer Street, London W1T 3JH, UK. Registered in England and Wales number 1072954.

A CIP record for this book is available from the British Library.

ISBN-13: 978-1-84184-707-8

Orders may be sent to: Informa Healthcare, Sheepen Place, Colchester, Essex CO3 3LP, UK
Telephone: +44 (0)20 7017 5540
Email: CSDhealthcarebooks@informa.com
Website: http://informahealthcarebooks.com/

For corporate sales please contact: CorporateBooksIHC@informa.com
For foreign rights please contact: RightsIHC@informa.com
For reprint permissions please contact: PermissionsIHC@informa.com

Typeset by MPS Limited, a Macmillan Company
Printed and bound in the United Kingdom

Library of Congress Cataloging-in-Publication Data

Acne vulgaris / edited by Alan R. Shalita, James Q. Del Rosso, Guy F. Webster.
   p. ; cm.
   ''Published in association with the American Acne & Rosacea Society.''
   Includes bibliographical references and index.
   ISBN 978-1-84184-707-8 (hb : alk. paper)   1. Acne. I. Shalita, Alan R. II. Del Rosso, James Q. III. Webster, Guy F. IV. American Acne & Rosacea Society.
   [DNLM: 1. Acne Vulgaris--therapy. WR 430]
RL131.A265 2011
616.5'3--dc22   2011000367

Contents

Contributors . . . . *ix*

Preface . . . . *xii*

Part 1: Social and Scientific Aspects of Acne

1.1 Introduction: epidemiology, cost, and psychosocial implications *1*
Whitney P. Bowe and Alan R. Shalita

1.2 Sebum *3*
Amanda M. Nelson and Diane M. Thiboutot

1.3 Innate immunity in the pathogenesis of acne vulgaris *12*
Sheila Krishna, Christina Kim, and Jenny Kim

1.4 Comedogenesis *28*
Carol Heughebaert and Alan R. Shalita

1.5 Scarring *43*
Thy Thy Do, Manisha Patel, and Sewon Kang

Part 2: Overview of Treatment Principles

2.1 Enhancing the success of acne therapy *55*
Alan R. Shalita

2.2 The relationship between acne and diet *57*
Whitney P. Bowe, Maria C. Kessides, and Alan R. Shalita

2.3 Overview of treatment principles for skin of color *70*
Marcelyn K. Coley, Diane S. Berson, and Valerie D. Callender

Part 3: Topical Therapy

3.1 Topical retinoids *86*
Andrea M. Hui and Alan R. Shalita

3.2 Topical antibiotics *95*
James Q. Del Rosso

3.3 Combination therapy *105*
Jennifer Villasenor, Diane S. Berson, and Daniela Kroshinsky

Part 4: Systemic Therapy

4.1 Oral antibiotics *113*
James Q. Del Rosso

4.2 Clinical implications of antibiotic resistance: risk of systemic
infection from *Staphylococcus* and *Streptococcus* *125*
Whitney P. Bowe and James J. Leyden

Part 5: Isotretinoin

5.1 Isotretinoin *134*
Michael G. Osofsky and John S. Strauss

Part 6: Hormonal Treatment

6.1 Hormonal treatment of acne in women *146*
Jonette Keri, Diane S. Berson, and Diane M. Thiboutot

Part 7: Variants and Special Situations

7.1 Gram-negative folliculitis *156*
Elizabeth Gaines, Alan R. Shalita, and Guy F. Webster

7.2 Acne fulminans *161*
Morgan Rabach and Guy F. Webster

7.3 Drug and acneiform eruptions *166*
Deeptej Singh, Alan R. Shalita, and Guy F. Webster

7.4 Acne in pregnancy *177*
Tobechi L. Ebede and Diane S. Berson

Part 8: AARS Acne Treatment Guidelines

8.1 Acne in children *182*
Caroline D. S. Piggott, Lawrence F. Eichenfield, and Anne W. Lucky

8.2 Treatment guidelines in adult women *198*
Jennifer Villasenor, Diane S. Berson, and Daniela Kroshinsky

Part 9: Physical Modalities in Acne Treatment

9.1 Procedural treatments for acne *208*
Whitney P. Bowe and Alan R. Shalita

Index *218*

Contributors

Diane S. Berson   Department of Dermatology, Weill Cornell Medical College, New York, New York, U.S.A.

Whitney P. Bowe   Department of Dermatology, SUNY Downstate Medical Center, Brooklyn, New York, U.S.A.

Valerie D. Callender   Department of Dermatology, Howard University, Washington D.C., U.S.A.

Marcelyn K. Coley   Department of Dermatology, SUNY Downstate Medical Center, Brooklyn, New York, U.S.A.

James Q. Del Rosso   Division of Dermatology, Valley Hospital Medical Center, Las Vegas, Nevada, U.S.A.

Thy Thy Do   Department of Dermatology, University of Michigan, Ann Arbor, Michigan, U.S.A.

Tobechi L. Ebede   Department of Dermatology, Weill Cornell Medical College, New York, New York, U.S.A.

Lawrence F. Eichenfield   Pediatric and Adolescent Dermatology, Rady Children's Hospital, University of California, San Diego School of Medicine, San Diego, California, U.S.A.

Elizabeth Gaines   Department of Dermatology, SUNY Downstate Medical Center, Brooklyn, New York, U.S.A.

Carol Heughebaert   Department of Dermatology, SUNY Downstate Medical Center, Brooklyn, New York, U.S.A.

Andrea M. Hui   Department of Dermatology, SUNY Downstate Medical Center, Brooklyn, New York, U.S.A.

Sewon Kang Department of Dermatology, Johns Hopkins University School of Medicine, Baltimore, Maryland, U.S.A.

Jonette Keri Department of Dermatology and Cutaneous Surgery, University of Miami, and Dermatology Service, Miami VA Hospital, Miami, Florida, U.S.A.

Maria C. Kessides Department of Dermatology, SUNY Downstate Medical Center, Brooklyn, New York, U.S.A.

Christina Kim Division of Dermatology, University of California Los Angeles, Center for Health Sciences, Los Angeles, California, U.S.A.

Jenny Kim Division of Dermatology, University of California Los Angeles, Center for Health Sciences, Los Angeles, California, U.S.A.

Sheila Krishna Division of Dermatology, University of California Los Angeles, Center for Health Sciences, Los Angeles, California, U.S.A.

Daniela Kroshinsky Department of Dermatology, Massachusetts General Hospital, Harvard Medical School, Boston, Massachusetts, U.S.A.

James J. Leyden Department of Dermatology, University of Pennsylvania, Philadelphia, Pennsylvania, U.S.A.

Anne W. Lucky Division of Pediatric Dermatology, Cincinnati Children's Hospital, Cincinnati, Ohio, U.S.A.

Amanda M. Nelson The Jake Gittlen Cancer Research Foundation, Pennsylvania State University College of Medicine, Hershey, Pennsylvania, U.S.A.

Michael G. Osofsky Department of Dermatology, Roy J. and Lucille A. Carver College of Medicine, University of Iowa, Iowa City, Iowa, U.S.A.

Manisha Patel Department of Dermatology, Johns Hopkins University School of Medicine, Baltimore, Maryland, U.S.A.

Caroline D. S. Piggott Division of Dermatology, Department of Medicine, University of California, San Diego, California, U.S.A.

Morgan Rabach Department of Dermatology, SUNY Downstate Medical Center, Brooklyn, New York, U.S.A.

Alan R. Shalita Department of Dermatology, SUNY Downstate Medical Center, Brooklyn, New York, U.S.A.

Deeptej Singh Department of Dermatology, SUNY Downstate Medical Center, Brooklyn, New York, U.S.A.

John S. Strauss Department of Dermatology, Roy J. and Lucille A. Carver College of Medicine, University of Iowa, Iowa City, Iowa, U.S.A.

Diane M. Thiboutot Department of Dermatology, Pennsylvania State University College of Medicine, Hershey, Pennsylvania, U.S.A.

Jennifer Villasenor Harvard Medical School, Boston, Massachusetts, U.S.A.

Guy F. Webster Department of Dermatology, Jefferson Medical College, Hockessin, Delaware, U.S.A.

Preface

The concept of this book comes from the American Acne and Rosacea Society, an organization dedicated to advancing the science related to acne and rosacea and enhancing communication between those interested in these diseases. The book is not meant to be a comprehensive treatise on all aspects of acne, but rather to address major points of interest by acknowledged thought leaders in the field assisted by residents in training at their affiliated institutions. It is the hope of the editors that this book will lead to further research, discussion, and refinement of our concepts of both the pathogenesis and treatment of acne and, as such, should be considered more of a work in progress than the definitive work on acne.

Alan R. Shalita
James Q. Del Rosso
Guy F. Webster

1.1

Introduction: epidemiology, cost, and psychosocial implications

Whitney P. Bowe and Alan R. Shalita

Acne vulgaris is a ubiquitous, multifactorial disorder of the pilosebaceous unit. The source of the word acne is controversial. It may be derived from the Greek *achne*, a word meaning efflorescence, or the Greek *acme* (Latin acme), which implies a summit or peak. Others have pointed to a hieroglyphic for the word AKU-T as the first written record referring to acne, a symbol interpreted to mean "boils," "pustules," or "a painful swelling" (1). The clinical picture can range from mild comedonal acne to a fulminant, scarring, and systemic condition. Approximately 95% to 100% of adolescent boys and 83% to 85% of adolescent girls aged 16 to 17 years are afflicted (2). Although acne tends to resolve in many cases following adolescence, 42.5% of men and 50.9% of women continue to suffer from this disease into their twenties (3). At 40 years of age, 1% of men and 5% of women still have acne lesions (4). Acne remains the leading cause for visits to a dermatologist (5), and the average total cost per episode of care for an acne patient is estimated at $689.06 (6).

Although many dermatological diseases are not life threatening, they pose a unique challenge to the human psyche. Cutaneous disease carries a distinctive psychosocial burden in that patients who suffer from these diseases display the stigma on their skin for the world to see and criticize on a daily basis. Specifically, acne has a known potential to cause significant psychological distress. Between 30% and 50% of adolescents experience psychological difficulties associated with acne, including body image concerns, embarrassment, social impairment, anxiety, frustration, anger, depression, and poor self-esteem (7). Additionally, suicidal ideation and suicide attempts related to the negative psychosocial impacts of acne have also been documented (8,9). The prevalence of body dysmorphic disorder among acne patients has been measured to be as high as 21% in some office settings (10), and these patients are more likely to report dissatisfaction with dermatologic treatment, attempt suicide, and threaten health care providers both legally and physically (11,12). Not only does acne result in emotional distress, but also the anxiety evoked by having acne can aggravate the skin condition itself, thereby creating a vicious cycle (13).

The purpose of this book is to provide a comprehensive and up-to-date review of acne vulgaris. It was written to serve as a resource for students, researchers, and clinicians alike. Pathophysiology, management, and treatment options will be discussed along with novel discoveries, cutting edge therapeutic approaches, and areas in which further research is needed.

REFERENCES

1. Blau S, Kanof NB. Acne: from pimple to pit. N Y J Med 1965; 65:417–424.
2. Burton JL, Cunliffe WJ, Stafford I, et al. The prevalence of acne vulgaris in adolescence. Br J Dermatol 1971; 85(2):119–126.
3. Collier CN, Harper JC, Cafardi JA, et al. The prevalence of acne in adults 20 years and older. J Am Acad Dermatol 2008; 58(1):56–59.
4. Cunliffe WJ, Gould DJ. Prevalence of facial acne vulgaris in late adolescence and in adults. Br Med J 1979; 1(6171):1109–1110.
5. Pawin H, Chivot M, Beylot C, et al. Living with acne. A study of adolescents' personal experiences. Dermatology 2007; 215(4):308–314.
6. Yentzer BA, Hick J, Reese EL, et al. Acne vulgaris in the United States: a descriptive epidemiology. Cutis 2010; 86(2):94–99.
7. Baldwin HE. The interaction between acne vulgaris and the psyche. Cutis 2002; 70(2):133–139.
8. Cotterill JA, Cunliffe WJ. Suicide in dermatological patients. Br J Dermatol 1997; 137(2):246–250.
9. Gupta MA, Gupta AK. Depression and suicidal ideation in dermatology patients with acne, alopecia areata, atopic dermatitis and psoriasis. Br J Dermatol 1998; 139(5):846–850.
10. Bowe WP, Leyden JJ, Crerand CE, et al. Body dysmorphic disorder symptoms among patients with acne vulgaris. J Am Acad Dermatol 2007; 57(2):222–230.
11. Mackley CL. Body dysmorphic disorder. Dermatol Surg 2005; 31(5):553–558.
12. Veale D, Boocock A, Gournay K, et al. Body dysmorphic disorder. A survey of fifty cases. Br J Psychiatry 1996; 169(2):196–201.
13. Koblenzer CS. Psychodermatology of women. Clin Dermatol 1997; 15(1):127–141.

1.2

Sebum

Amanda M. Nelson and Diane M. Thiboutot

HOLOCRINE SECRETION

The sebaceous glands exude lipids by disintegration of entire cells, a process known as *holocrine secretion*. The life span of a sebocyte from cell division to holocrine secretion is approximately 21 to 25 days (1). Because of the constant state of renewal and secretion of the sebaceous gland, individual cells within the same gland are engaged in different metabolic activities dependent on their differentiation state (2). The stages of this process are evident in the histology of the gland (3). The outermost cells, basal cell layer membrane, are small, nucleated, and devoid of lipid droplets. This layer contains the dividing cells that replenish the gland as cells are lost in the process of lipid excretion. As cells are displaced into the center of the gland, they begin to produce lipid, which accumulates in droplets. Eventually, the cells become greatly distended with lipid droplets with the nuclei and other subcellular structures disappearing. As the cells approach the sebaceous duct, they disintegrate and release their contents. Only neutral lipids reach the skin surface. Proteins, nucleic acids, and the membrane phospholipids are digested and most likely recycled during the disintegration of the cells.

LIPID COMPOSITION OF SEBUM

Human sebum, as it leaves the sebaceous gland, contains squalene, cholesterol, cholesterol esters, wax esters, and triglycerides (Table 1.2.1). During passage of sebum through the hair canal, bacterial lipases from *Propionibacterium acnes* hydrolyze some of the triglycerides, so that the lipid mixture reaching the skin surface contains free fatty acids (FFA) and small proportions of mono- and diglycerides in addition to the original components. The wax esters and squalene

3

Table 1.2.1 Composition of Sebum and Epidermal Lipids

Lipid	Sebum weight (%)	Epidermal surface lipid weight (%)
Triglycerides, diglycerides, and free fatty acids	57	65
Wax esters	26	NA
Squalene	12	NA
Cholesterol	2	20

Source: From Ref. 5.

distinguish sebum from the lipids of human internal organs, which contain no wax esters and little squalene. Human sebaceous glands, however, appear to be unable to cyclize squalene to sterols such as cholesterol. The unsaturation patterns of the fatty acids in the triglycerides, wax esters, and cholesterol esters also distinguish human sebum from the lipids of other organs. The "normal" mammalian pathway of desaturation involves inserting a double bond between the ninth and tenth carbons of stearic acid (18:0) to form oleic acid (18:1Δ9). However, in human sebaceous glands, the predominant pattern is the insertion of a Δ6 double bond into palmitic acid (16:0). The resulting sapienic acid (16:1Δ6) is the major fatty acid of adult human sebum. Elongation of the chain by two carbons and insertion of another double bond gives sebaleic acid (18:2Δ5,8), a fatty acid thought to be unique to human sebum (4).

Sebaceous fatty acids and alcohols are also distinguished by chain branching. Methyl branches can occur on the next to last (penultimate) carbon of a fatty acid chain (iso branching), on the third from the last (antepenultimate) carbon (anteiso branching), or on any even-numbered carbon (internal branching).

FUNCTION OF SEBUM

The precise function of sebum in humans is unknown. Cunliffe and Shuster proposed that sebum's solitary role is to cause acne (6). Another theory suggests that sebum reduces water loss from the skin's surface and functions to keep skin soft and smooth. The sebaceous gland-deficient mouse (Asebia) model provides evidence that glycerol derived from triglyceride hydrolysis in sebum is critical for maintaining stratum corneum hydration (7), but there is no evidence for this in humans as stratum corneum hydration is normal during periods, such as, childhood when the gland is fairly quiescent. Similarly, vitamin E delivery to the upper layers of the skin protects the skin and its surface lipids from oxidation;

thus, sebum flow to the surface of the skin may provide the transit mechanism necessary for vitamin E to function (8).

Recent evidence suggests that sebaceous glands and sebum play a role in the skin's innate immune defense mechanism. Initial investigations showed that sebum has mild antibacterial action, presumably due to the presence of immunoglobulin A, which is secreted from most exocrine glands (9). Recent studies show that FFA in human sebum is bactericidal against gram-positive organisms as a result of its ability to increase antimicrobial peptide, β-defensin 2 (HBD2) expression (10). Additional antimicrobial peptides including cathelicidin, psoriasin, β-defensin 1, and β-defensin 2 are expressed within the sebaceous gland. Functional cathelicidin peptides have direct antimicrobial activity against *P. acnes* but also initiate cytokine production and inflammation in the host organism (11,12). Innate immune Toll-like receptors 2 and 4 (TLR2, TLR4) and CD1d and CD14 molecules are also expressed in sebaceous glands and immortalized human sebocytes (13). The antibacterial activities of sebum itself and the expression of innate immune receptors and antibacterial peptides within the sebaceous gland provide compelling evidence that the sebaceous gland may play an important role in pathogen recognition and protection of the skin surface.

FACTORS REGULATING SEBUM PRODUCTION

The exact mechanisms underlying the regulation of human sebum production are not fully defined. A variety of experimental models are used to study the factors involved in sebaceous gland regulation including cell culture of isolated human sebaceous glands, primary sebocytes, and immortalized sebocyte cell lines; as well as mouse and hamster animal models. Results from these investigations clearly indicate that sebaceous glands are regulated by androgens and retinoids. Recent evidence suggests that peroxisome proliferator–activated receptors, melanocortins, corticotropin-releasing hormone, and fibroblast growth factor receptors play a role as well.

Androgens

Androgen receptors are located in both the keratinocytes of the outer root sheath of hair follicles as well as the basal layer of the sebaceous gland (14). Individuals with a genetic deficiency of androgen receptors (complete androgen insensitivity) have no detectable sebum secretion and do not develop acne (15). Conversely, addition of testosterone and dihydroepiandrosterone increases the size and secretion of sebaceous glands (16), although which androgen is physiologically significant is still debated. The most potent androgens are testosterone and dihydrotestosterone (DHT); however, levels of testosterone do not parallel the patterns of sebaceous gland activity. Sebum secretion starts to increase in children (5–6 years of age) during adrenarche, although the levels of androgens are very low at this time (17). Testosterone levels are significantly higher in males than in females, with no overlap between the sexes. However, the average rates of sebum secretion are only slightly higher in males than in females, with considerable overlap between the sexes (18,19). The majority of females with acne have serum androgen levels that, although higher, are within normal limits, and it has been hypothesized that locally produced androgens within the sebaceous gland may contribute to acne (20,21). The weak adrenal androgen, dehydroepiandrosterone sulfate (DHEAS), may regulate sebaceous gland activity through its conversion to testosterone and DHT within the sebaceous gland. The enzymes required to convert DHEAS to more potent androgens are present within sebaceous glands (22). The predominant isozymes in the sebaceous gland include the type 1 3β-hydroxysteroid dehydrogenase (3β-HSD), the type 2 17β-HSD, and the type 1 5α-reductase (23–25). Investigations into the influence of locally produced androgens indicated that the activities of 5α-reductase and 17β-HSD enzymes within the sebaceous gland are not higher in male or female patients with acne compared with patient controls with no acne. Because of the small sample size, the influence of local androgen synthesis cannot be ruled out (19). Clearly, androgens influence sebaceous glands and sebum production, although which androgens are important and the mechanism of their influence are not known.

Retinoids

Isotretinoin [13-*cis* retinoic acid (13-*cis* RA), Accutane®] is the most potent pharmacologic inhibitor of sebum secretion. Significant reductions in sebum production can be observed as early as two weeks after use (26). Histologically, sebaceous glands are markedly reduced in size, and individual sebocytes appear undifferentiated, lacking the characteristic cytoplasmic accumulation of sebaceous lipids.

Isotretinoin does not interact with any of the known retinoid receptors. It may serve as a prodrug for the synthesis of all-*trans* RA or 9-*cis* RA, which does interact with retinoid receptors; however, it has greater sebosuppressive action than do all-*trans* or 9-*cis* RA (27). The mechanism by which 13-*cis* RA lowers sebum secretion is currently under investigation. Experimental evidence shows that 13-*cis* RA inhibits the 3α-hydroxysteroid activity of retinol dehydrogenase leading to decreased androgen synthesis (28). In addition, isotretinoin triggers cell cycle arrest in human sebocytes and immortalized cell culture models of human sebocytes (SZ95 and SEB-1), as well as induces apoptosis in SEB-1 sebocytes in part due to an increase in the neutrophil gelatinase–associated lipocalin (NGAL) (29–32). Inhibition of androgen synthesis, cell cycle arrest, and apoptosis by 13-*cis* RA may explain the reduction of sebaceous gland size after treatment.

Peroxisome Proliferator–Activated Receptors

Peroxisome proliferator–activated receptors (PPARs) are orphan nuclear receptors that are similar to retinoid receptors in many ways. Each of these receptors forms heterodimers with retinoid X receptors to regulate the transcription of genes involved in a variety of processes, including lipid metabolism and cellular proliferation and differentiation (33–36). Rat preputial cells serve as a model for human sebocytes in the laboratory (37). In rat preputial cells, agonists of the PPAR-α and PPAR-γ receptors induced lipid droplet formation in preputial sebocytes but not in epidermal cells, while linoleic acid (PPAR-β/δ agonist) induced lipid formation in both preputial sebocytes and epidermal cells (38). On the basis of the results from their studies, Rosenfield et al. propose that PPAR-α activation plays a role in the beginning stages of lipogenesis, PPAR-β/δ activation enhances the lipogenesis, and PPAR-γ activation controls the transition to a more differentiated state complete with more lipid droplets within the cells, clearly identifying PPARs as a key player in sebocyte differentiation (38). Within human sebocytes, PPAR-α, -β/δ, and -γ receptor subtypes are expressed in basal sebocytes. PPAR-γ is also present in differentiated sebocytes (39–41). In patients receiving fibrates (PPAR-α agonists) for hyperlipidemia or thiazolidinediones (PPAR-γ agonists) for diabetes, sebum secretion rates are increased (41), indicating that PPARs do play a role in sebocyte differentiation and maturation in humans.

Melanocortins

Melanocortins include melanocyte-stimulating hormone (MSH) and adrenocorticotropic hormone (ACTH). In rodents, melanocortins increase sebum production. Human primary sebocyte cultures treated with MSH have increased numbers of cytoplasmic lipid droplets (42). Both melanocortin 1 receptor (MC1R) and melanocortin 5 receptor (MC5R) are expressed within human sebaceous glands (43,44). MC1R expression is increased in sebaceous glands of both noninvolved and involved skin of acne patients when compared with normal patients. MC5R expression is only detectable within differentiated sebocytes, both within human skin biopsies and cell culture models (45). It is currently unknown whether MC1R or MC5R mediates the effects of melanocortins on sebaceous glands, although transgenic mice deficient in MC5R have hypoplastic sebaceous glands and reduced sebum production (46), suggesting that receptor involvement is highly likely.

Corticotropin-Releasing Hormone

Recent evidence suggests that physiological stress plays a role in sebaceous gland regulation. The expression of corticotropin-releasing hormone (CRH), its receptors (CRH-R1, CRH-R2), as well as CRH-binding protein (CRHBP) has been detected within human sebaceous glands by immunohistochemistry (47). Immortalized sebocyte cells (SZ95) also express CRH, CRHBP, and the receptors. Furthermore, treatment with CRH increased lipid synthesis within SZ95 sebocytes (48). The presence and functionality of this pathway in sebaceous glands suggest that sebaceous glands and sebum production may be influenced by neuroendocrine mechanisms.

Fibroblast Growth Factor Receptors

Fibroblast growth factor receptors 1 and 2 (FGFR1 and 2) are expressed in the epidermis and skin appendages. Expression of FGFR3 and FGFR4 is localized to dermal vessels and microvessels and is notably absent in epidermis and appendages (49). FGFR2 plays an important role during embryogenesis in skin formation (50). Germline mutations in FGFR2 lead to Apert's syndrome, which is commonly associated with acne. In addition, somatic mutations in the same location can lead to acne, but how this receptor is involved in sebaceous gland development and how its mutation leads to acne are unknown (51,52).

SEBUM IN THE PATHOGENESIS OF ACNE VULGARIS

The role of sebum in the pathogenesis of acne is closely associated with the activity of *P. acnes*. The microenvironment within the sebaceous gland is anaerobic, therefore favoring the survival of *P. acnes* bacteria over others (i.e., *Staphylococcus epidermidis*). The *P. acnes* bacterium relies on sebaceous lipids as a nutrient source and breaks down triglycerides into FFA (53). FFA within sebum can be irritating and contribute to the inflammatory response (54). Furthermore, experiments demonstrated that *P. acnes* is capable of stimulating the production of both proinflammatory cytokines/chemokines and antimicrobial peptides from keratinocytes and cultured sebocytes (SZ95), indicating that keratinocytes and sebocytes themselves may play a role in the inflammatory aspects of acne (55,56).

REFERENCES

1. Plewig G, Christophers E. Renewal rate of human sebaceous glands. Acta Dermatovener (Stockholm) 1974; 54:177–182.
2. Potter JE, Prutkin L, Wheatley VR. Sebaceous gland differentiation. I. Separation, morphology and lipogenesis of isolated cells from the mouse preputial gland tumor. J Invest Dermatol 1979; 72(3):120–127.
3. Ito M. New findings on the proteins of sebaceous glands. J Invest Dermatol 1984; 82:381.

4. Nicolaides N. Skin lipids: their biochemical uniqueness. Science 1974; 186:19–26.
5. Thiboutot D. Regulation of human sebaceous glands. J Invest Dermatol 2004; 123(1):1–12.
6. Cunliffe WJ, Shuster S. Pathogenesis of acne. Lancet 1969; 1(7597):685–687.
7. Flurh JW, Mao-Qiang M, Brown BE, et al. Glycerol regulates stratum corneum hydration in sebaceous gland deficient (Asebia) mice. J Invest Dermatol 2003; 120(4):728–737.
8. Thiele JJ, Weber SU, Packer L. Sebaceous gland secretion is a major physiologic route of vitamin E delivery to skin. J Invest Dermatol 1999; 113(6):1006–1010.
9. Gebhart W, Metze D, Jurecka W. Identification of secretory immunoglobulin A in human sweat and sweat glands. J Invest Dermatol 1989; 92(4):648.
10. Nakatsuji T, Kao MC, Zhang L, et al. Sebum free fatty acids enhance the innate immune defense of human sebocytes by upregulating beta-defensin-2 expression. J Invest Dermatol 2009; 130(4):985–994; [Epub December 24, 2009].
11. Lee DY, Yamasaki K, Rudsil J, et al. Sebocytes express functional cathelicidin antimicrobial peptides and can act to kill Propionibacterium acnes. J Invest Dermatol 2008; 128(7):1863–1866.
12. Lai Y, Gallo RL. AMPed up immunity: how antimicrobial peptides have multiple roles in immune defense. Trends Immunol 2009; 30(3):131–141.
13. Oeff MK, Seltmann H, Hiroi N, et al. Differential regulation of Toll-like receptor and CD14 pathways by retinoids and corticosteroids in human sebocytes. Dermatology 2006; 213(3):266.
14. Kariya Y, Moriya T, Suzuki T, et al. Sex steroid hormone receptors in human skin appendage and its neoplasms. Endocr J 2005; 52(3):317–325.
15. Imperato-McGinley J, Gautier T, Cai LQ, et al. The androgen control of sebum production. Studies of subjects with dihydrotestosterone deficiency and complete androgen insensitivity. J Clin Endocrinol Metabol 1993; 76(2):524–528.
16. Pochi PE, Strauss JS. Sebaceous gland response in man to the administration of testosterone, delta-4-androstenedione, and dehydroisoandrosterone. J Invest Dermatol 1969; 52(1):32–36.
17. Pochi PE, Strauss JS, Downing DT. Skin surface lipid composition, acne, pubertal development, and urinary excretion of testosterone and 17-ketosteroids in children. J Invest Dermatol 1977; 69(5):485–489.
18. Harris H. Sustainable rates of sebum secretion in acne patients and matched normal control subjects. J Am Acad Dermatol 1983; 8:200.
19. Thiboutot D, Gilliland K, Light J, et al. Androgen metabolism in sebaceous glands from subjects with and without acne. Arch Dermatol 1999; 135(9):1041–1045.
20. Levell MJ, Carwood ML, Burke B, et al. Acne is not associated with abnormal plasma androgens. Br J Dermatol 1989; 120(5):649–654.
21. Lookingbill DP, Horton R, Demers LM, et al. Tissue production of androgens in women with acne. J Am Acad Dermatol 1985; 12(3):481–487.
22. Chen W, Thiboutot D, Zouboulis C. Cutaneous androgen metabolism: basic research and clinical perspectives. J Invest Dermatol 2002; 119:992–1007.
23. Fritsch M, Orfanos CE, Zouboulis CC. Sebocytes are the key regulators of androgen homeostasis in human skin. J Invest Dermatol 2001; 116(5):793–800.

24. Thiboutot D, Harris G, Lles V, et al. Activity of the type 1 5 alpha-reductase exhibits regional differences in isolated sebaceous glands and whole skin. J Invest Dermatol 1995; 105(2):209–214.

25. Thiboutot D, Martin P, Volikos L, et al. Oxidative activity of the type 2 isozyme of 17beta-hydroxysteroid dehydrogenase (17beta-HSD) predominates in human sebaceous glands. J Invest Dermatol 1998; 111(3):390–395.

26. Stewart ME, Benoit AM, Stranieri AM, et al. Effect of oral 13-cis retinoic acid at three dose levels on sustainable rates of sebum secretion and on acne. J Am Acad Dermatol 1983; 8:532–538.

27. Hommel L, Geiger JM, Harms M, et al. Sebum excretion rate in subjects treated with oral all-trans-retinoic acid. Dermatology 1996; 193(2):127–130.

28. Karlsson T, Vahlquist A, Kedishvili N, et al. 13-cis-retinoic acid competitively inhibits 3a-hydroxysteroid oxidation by retinol dehydrogenase RoDH-4: a mechanism for its anti-androgenic effects in sebaceous glands? Biochem Biophys Res Commun 2003; 303:273–278.

29. Zouboulis CC, Korge BB, Akamatsu H, et al. Effects of 13-cis-retinoic acid, all-trans-retinoic acid, and acitretin on the proliferation, lipid synthesis and keratin expression of cultured human sebocytes in vitro. J Invest Dermatol 1991; 96(5):792–797.

30. Zouboulis CC, Seltmann H, Neitzel H, et al. Establishment and characterization of an immortalized human sebaceous gland cell line (SZ95). J Investig Dermatol 1999; 113(6):1011–1020.

31. Nelson A, Gilliland KL, Cong Z, et al. 13-cis retinoic acid induces apoptosis and cell cycle arrest in human SEB-1 sebocytes. J Investig Dermatol 2006; 126(10):2178–2189; [Epub March 30, 2006].

32. Nelson AM, Zhao W, Gilliland KL, et al. Neutrophil gelatinase-associated lipocalin mediates 13-cis retinoic acid-induced apoptosis of human sebaceous gland cells. J Clin Invest 2008; 118(4):1468–1478.

33. Schoonjans K, Staels B, Auwerx J. The peroxisome proliferator activated receptors (PPARs) and their effects on lipid metabolism and adipocyte differentiation. Biochim Biophys Acta 1996; 1302:93–109.

34. Rosen ED, Sarraf P, Troy AE, et al. PPAR gamma is required for the differentiation of adipose tissue in vivo and in vitro. Mol Cell 1999; 4(4):611–617.

35. Spiegelman BM, et al. PPAR gamma and the control of adipogenesis. Biochimie 1997; 79(2–3):111–112.

36. Kim MJ, Deplewski D, Ciletti N, et al. Limited cooperation between peroxisome proliferator-activated receptors and retinoid X receptor agonists in sebocyte growth and development. Mol Genet Metab 2001; 74(3):362–369.

37. Laurent SJ, Mednieks MI, Rosenfield RL. Growth of sebaceous cells in monolayer culture. In vitro Cell Dev Biol 1992; 28A:83–89.

38. Rosenfield RL, Kentsis A, Deplewski D, et al. Rat preputial sebocyte differentiation involves peroxisome proliferator-activated receptors. J Investig Dermatol 1999; 112(2):226–232.

39. Downie MM, Sanders DA, Maier LM, et al. Peroxisome proliferator-activated receptor and farnesoid X receptor ligands differentially regulate sebaceous differentiation in human sebaeous gland organ cultures in vitro. Br J Dermatol 2004; 151:766–775.

40. Chen W, Yang CC, Sheu HM, et al. Expression of peroxisome proliferator-activated receptor and CCAAT/enhancer binding protein transcription factors in cultured human sebocytes. J Invest Dermatol 2003; 121:441–447.

41. Trivedi NR, Cong Z, Nelson AM, et al. Peroxisome proliferator-activated receptors increase human sebum production. J Invest Dermatol 2006; 126(9):2002–2009.

42. Zhang L, Anthonavage M, Huang Q, et al. Proopiomelanocortin peptides and sebogenesis. Ann N Y Acad Sci 2003; 994:154–161.

43. Ganceviciene R, Graziene V, Böhm M, et al. Increased in situ expression of melanocortin-1 receptor in sebaceous glands of lesional skin of patients with acne vulgaris. Exp Dermatol 2007; 16(7):547–552.

44. Thiboutot D, Sivarajah A, Gilliland K, et al. The melanocortin 5 receptor is expressed in human sebaceous glands and rat preputial cells. J Invest Dermatol 2000; 115(4):614–619.

45. Zhang L, Li WH, Anthonavage M, et al. Melanocortin-5 receptor: a marker of human sebocyte differentiation. Peptides 2006; 27(2):413–420.

46. Chen W, Kelly MA, Opitz-Araya X, et al. Exocrine gland dysfunction in MC5-R deficient mice: evidence for coordinated regulation of exocrine gland function by melanocortin peptides. Cell 1997; 91:789–798.

47. Ganceviciene R, Graziene V, Fimmel S, et al. Involvement of the corticotropin-releasing hormone system in the pathogenesis of acne vulgaris. Br J Dermatol 2009; 160(2):345–352.

48. Zouboulis CC, Seltmann H, Hiroi N, et al. Corticotropin-releasing hormone: an autocrine hormone that promotes lipogenesis in human sebocytes. Proc Natl Acad Sci U S A 2002; 99(10):7148–7153.

49. Hughes SE. Differential expression of the fibroblast growth factor receptor (FGFR) multigene family in normal human adult tissues. J Histochem Cytochem 1997; 45(7):1005–1019.

50. Li C, Guo H, Xu X, et al. Fibroblast growth factor receptor 2 (Fgfr2) plays an important role in eyelid and skin formation and patterning. Dev Dyn 2001; 222:471–483.

51. Munro CS, Wilkie AOM. Epidermal mosaicism producing localized acne: somatic mutation in FGFR2. Lancet 1998; 352(9129):704–705.

52. Gilaberte M, Puig L, Alomar A. Isotretinoin treatment of acne in a patient with Apert Syndrome. Pediatr Dermatol 2003; 20(5):443–446.

53. Gribbon EM, Cunliffe WJ, Holland KT. Interaction of Propionibacterium acnes with skin lipids in vitro. J Gen Microbiol 1993; 139(8):1745–1751.

54. Ro BI, Dawson TL. The role of sebaceous gland activity and scalp microfloral metabolism in the etiology of seborrheic dermatitis and dandruff. J Investig Dermatol Symp Proc 2005; 10(3):194–197.

55. Graham GM, Farrar MD, Cruse-Sawyer JE, et al. Proinflammatory cytokine production by human keratinocytes stimulated with Propionibacterium acnes and P. acnes GroEL. Br J Dermatol 2004; 150(3):421–428.

56. Nagy I, Pivarcsi A, Kis K, et al. Propionibacterium acnes and lipopolysaccharide induce the expression of antimicrobial peptides and proinflammatory cytokines/chemokines in human sebocytes. Microbes Infect 2006; 8(8):2195–2205.

1.3

Innate immunity in the pathogenesis of acne vulgaris

Sheila Krishna, Christina Kim, and Jenny Kim

INTRODUCTION

Acne vulgaris is a disease of pilosebaceous units. Major hypotheses on its pathophysiology include the following (1,2):

1. Altered follicular keratinization (hyperkeratinization) of the pilosebaceous unit (3)
2. *Propionibacterium acnes* (*P. acnes*) follicular colonization and activity (4)
3. Hormonal influence (5–7)
4. Sebum production (8)
5. Release of inflammatory mediators (4,9)

These hypotheses have traditionally been viewed as independent factors that, as a whole, contribute to acne pathogenesis. In particular, inflammation has been viewed as a distinct contributor to acne, but the mechanism by which this occurred was not well elucidated. Recent advances in molecular and cellular studies now reveal that inflammation promotes acne via activation of the innate immune system. In addition, studies now show that mechanisms involving the innate immune system could initiate and influence many of the traditionally described factors in acne pathogenesis, as listed above (1,10–12). The importance of the innate immune system in the pathogenesis of acne is a significant advance in our understanding of acne with important implications for treatment. Therefore, this chapter focuses on new and evolving insights into the role of the innate immune system in association with acne, specifically on the manner in which these new findings build upon traditionally known pathogenetic factors and suggest additional hypotheses of acne pathophysiology. These new hypotheses include the following:

1. Inflammatory events mediated by interleukin 1 (IL-1) precede hyperkeratinization (9,13–15).
2. *P. acnes* activates the innate immune system via Toll-like receptors (TLRs) (16,17).
3. *P. acnes* induces matrix metalloproteinase (MMP) (18,19) and antimicrobial peptide (AMP) production (20–22).
4. Sebaceous gland lipids influence the innate immune system (23,24).

CUTANEOUS IMMUNE SYSTEM

The human immune system is comprised of two distinct functional parts: innate and adaptive (25). These two components have different types of recognition receptors and differ in the speed in which they respond to a potential threat to the host. While the innate immune system responds rapidly to commonly shared pathogen structures and lacks memory, the adaptive immune response is delayed to specific antigens and retains memory against the pathogen (25). The specific components of the cutaneous innate immune system include barriers such as the skin and mucosal epithelium (25); soluble factors such as complement, antimicrobial peptides, chemokines, and cytokines (26); cells including keratinocytes, monocytes/macrophages, dendritic cells (DCs), natural killer cells (NK cells) and polymorphonuclear cells (PMNs), or neutrophils. Cells use pattern recognition receptors (PRRs) encoded directly by the germline DNA to respond to specific pathogen-associated molecular patterns (PAMPs) shared by a variety of different pathogens to elicit a rapid response against these pathogens (25).

The skin provides important functions in innate immunity. As the largest organ in the human body, the skin provides a vital and direct barrier from exogenous toxins. The stratum corneum is composed of highly cross-linked proteinaceous cellular envelopes with extracellular lipid lamellae consisting of ceramides, free fatty acids, and cholesterol (27). The free fatty acids create an acidic environment that inhibits colonization by certain bacteria such as *Staphylococcus aureus*, providing further protection (27). Soluble factors such as complement, antimicrobial peptides, chemokines, and cytokines provide an additional critical layer of innate immune defense for those pathogens that overcome the physical barrier (25,26).

Importantly, the cutaneous innate immune system also provides rapid cellular responses enacted by keratinocytes, melanocytes, and Langerhans cells, and by recruitment of DCs, monocytes/macrophages, NK cells, and PMNs to protect a newly infected host (25). These cells express PRRs that mediate responses to PAMPs that are conserved among microorganisms. While there are many families of PRRs, human TLRs are one such family that is capable of initiating innate immune responses and influencing subsequent adaptive immune responses (25).

TLRs were first identified in *Drosophila*, and mammalian homologs have been shown to mediate immune responses to microbial ligands (25,28,29). TLRs are transmembrane proteins capable of mediating responses to PAMPs conserved among microorganisms. The extracellular portion of TLRs is composed of leucine-rich repeats while the intracellular portion shares homology with the cytoplasmic domain of the IL-1 receptor (25,28,29). When TLRs are activated by exposure to microbial ligands, the intracellular domain of certain TLRs trigger a MyD88-dependent pathway, while other pathways are MyD88 independent (Fig. 1.3.1). This leads to the nuclear translocation of the transcription factor nuclear factor κB (NF-κB), which acts to modulate expression of many immune response genes. The activation of these TLRs and their downstream pathways ultimately leads to the release of critical proinflammatory and immunomodulatory cytokines such as IL-1, IL-6, IL-8, IL-10, IL-12, and tumor necrosis factor-alpha (TNF-α) (25,28,29).

Currently, 11 TLR genes have been identified in humans (25,29). The microbial ligands for many of these receptors have been demonstrated and include bacterial cell wall components and genetic material. More specifically, TLR2 mediates responses to peptidoglycan from gram-positive bacteria (30–32); TLR4 mediates host responses to bacterial lipopolysaccharide from gram-negative bacteria (30–32); and TLR5 mediates the host response to bacterial flagellin (33). In addition, TLR9 mediates the response to the unmethylated CpG DNA comprising bacterial genomes; and TLR3 mediates responses to viral double-stranded RNA (34,35). Furthermore, TLR heterodimers have been shown to mediate responses to microbial lipoproteins, with TLR2/1 heterodimers mediating responses to triacylated lipoproteins and TLR2/6 heterodimers mediating responses to diacylated lipoproteins (36,37) (Fig. 1.3.2). *P. acnes* can activate TLR2, but the exact molecular structure of the TLR2 ligand has not been defined (16,17,28).

Taken together, the cutaneous innate immune system comprises a specific immunologic environment in which pathogens that evade the physical and

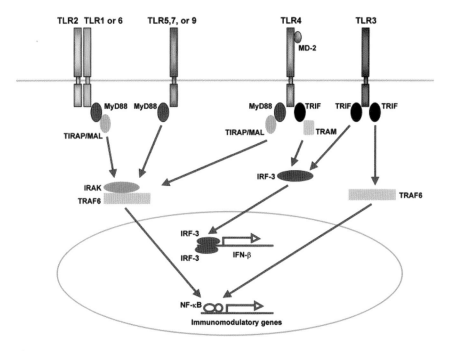

Figure 1.3.1 Human Toll-like receptor activation triggers MyD88-dependent and MyD88-independent signaling pathways resulting in gene transcription. *Abbreviations*: IRAK, Interleukin-1 receptor-associated kinase; IRF-3, Interferon regulatory factor 3; IFN-β, Interferon β; MAL, MyD88 adapterlike; MyD88, Myeloid differentiation response gene 88; NF-κB, Nuclear factor κB; TIRAP, Toll-interleukin 1 receptor domain containing adaptor protein; TLR, Toll like receptor; TRAF6, TNF receptor associated factor 6; TRIF, TIR-domain-containing adaptor-inducing interferon-β; MD-2; TRAM, TRIF-related adaptor molecule. *Source*: From Ref. 29.

chemical barrier of the skin itself are rapidly detected by pathogen receptors such as TLRs and destroyed by effector cells, such as PMNs or NKs, and secreted soluble substances, such as antimicrobial peptides. However, this sequence of events, while acting against a pathogen, can also trigger inflammatory responses that result in tissue injury, alterations in tissue growth cycles, and local changes in the tissue environment that lead to disease states (17). Evidence now suggests that acne lesions express different levels of innate immune system components than normal skin (10) and that upregulation and activation of these components and their downstream pathways in the cutaneous innate immune system result in

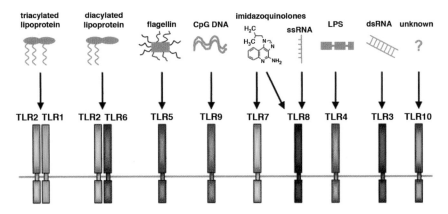

Figure 1.3.2 Human Toll-like receptors display specificity in their recognition of pathogen-associated molecular patterns and/or synthetic compounds. *Abbreviations*: TLR, Toll-like receptors; LPS, Lipopolysaccharide.

the clinical manifestations of acne (1,11,17,28,38,39). Multiple components of the innate immune system contribute to acne pathogenesis, including derangements in barrier function of the skin itself, upregulation of soluble factors such as chemokines, cytokines, and antimicrobial peptides, and alteration of downstream effector pathways activated by pathogen recognition of *P. acnes*. These events precede and promote acne formation and contribute to our current understanding of acne pathogenesis.

INFLAMMATORY EVENTS PRECEDE HYPERKERATINIZATION

Acne develops in the pilosebaceous unit. While the exact sequence and nature of the events that initiate and promote acne are not fully understood, it is generally believed that one of the early events is the obstruction of the pilosebaceous follicles (17). This occurs when the follicular infundibulum becomes occluded by either hyperkeratinization or hyperproliferation of keratinocytes or both. This results in the formation of the microcomedone, which is the earliest subclinical acne lesion, characterized by hyperproliferation of the follicular epithelium (17). Recent evidence suggests that inflammatory events not only precede hyperkeratinization but also initiate and promote hyperkeratinization.

Jeremy et al. demonstrated that early inflamed acne lesions exhibited increased expression of the cytokine IL-1 (14). Their work suggests that upregulation of IL-1 could be initiated by perturbation of the barrier function within an individual follicle due to increased sebum production and a relative deficiency of linoleic acid, which normally acts to preserve the integrity of the follicle (13,40,41). This breakdown of barrier function then triggers the innate immune response resulting in the release of IL-1, a potent proinflammatory cytokine, which stimulates an inflammatory cascade including the activation of local endothelial cells and upregulation of inflammatory vascular markers such as E-selectin, vascular cell adhesion molecule-1 (VCAM-1), intercellular adhesion molecule-1 (ICAM-1), and human leukocyte antigen–DR (HLA-DR) in the vasculature around the pilosebaceous follicle (14). The authors suggest that these immune changes and inflammatory responses occur before hyper-proliferation of keratinocytes in a manner similar to a type IV delayed hyper-sensitivity response (14).

The importance of IL-1 production as a critical initiating event of follicular hyperkeratinization coincides with the concept of the "keratinocyte activation cycle" (42,43). It is proposed that in a number of pathologic conditions, keratinocytes can either undergo activation or differentiation. While differentiation allows the keratinocyte to slowly proliferate in the basal layer and differentiate in the suprabasal layers, activation promotes hyperproliferation, migration, cytoskeletal change, and increased production of signaling molecules (42,43). IL-1 production is initiated by injured keratinocytes and activates paracrine signaling, attracting lymphocytes, stimulating selectins, and signaling migration of fibroblasts. IL-1 also acts in an autocrine fashion, activating keratinocytes to migrate, proliferate, and produce IL-1, granulocyte-macrophage colony stimulating factor (GM-CSF), TNF-α, ICAM-1, and integrins. Together, these further activate and sustain hyper-keratinization (14,42,43).

Thus, it is believed that inflammatory events, specifically the production of IL-1, precede and contribute to hyperkeratinization. While the exact initial event is not known, one hypothesis is that increased sebum production with a relative deficiency of specific fatty acids disrupts the normal lipid layers that protect the skin and allow the skin to act as a barrier to pathogens (14,15). This imbalance, along with physical injury, leads to IL-1 release from keratinocytes resulting in sustained activation of the keratinocyte, which triggers hyperkeratinization and hyperproliferation. Although the full sequence of events that initiate acne are not understood, the role of IL-1 as an early component of hyperkeratinization is an important new concept in our understanding of the innate immune response in the pathogenesis of acne lesions. Furthermore, this evidence that inflammation is the basis of an early acne lesion suggests that therapy should be directed at reducing inflammation, both for treating new acne lesions as well as for maintenance.

PROPIONIBACTERIUM ACNES PROMOTES INFLAMMATION VIA TLRS

P. acnes is an anaerobic gram-positive, rod-shaped bacterium. It is a commensal organism that resides on most human skin (including non-acne-prone skin) and survives on fatty acids found in the sebum produced by sebaceous glands. It is unique in that its cell wall and outer envelope produce phosphatidyl inositol, which typically is produced only in eukaryotes. In addition, the peptidoglycan of the cell wall of *P. acnes* contains a cross-linkage region of peptide chains with L, L-diaminopimelic acid and D-alanine in which two glycine residues combine with amino and carboxyl groups. These features are notable as they may contribute to the recognition of *P. acnes* as a pathogen by human immune cells. In response to *P. acnes*, innate immune cells produce proinflammatory cytokines, including TNF-α and IL-1β (44). The chemotactic factor IL-8 is also induced by *P. acnes* (45,46). These soluble molecules play an important role in attracting neutrophils and monocytes/macrophages to the pilosebaceous follicles in acne lesions, which are then activated to further produce other inflammatory mediators.

The importance of *P. acnes* as an etiological factor of acne has long been known, and early studies demonstrated greater numbers of *P. acnes* in affected skin versus matched controls (47). Studies also showed that its injection into the skin promoted vigorous inflammatory responses (48). In a seminal paper, Vowels et al. found that the presence of a soluble factor of *P. acnes* induced proinflammatory cytokine production in monocytes, including TNF-α and IL-1β. Moreover, activation of inflammation was dependent on CD14, a known PRR for lipid-containing ligands, such as lipopolysaccharide (4).

Although the role of *P. acnes* as an etiological factor in inflammation associated with acne had been established, the exact mechanism of its action was described only recently. It is now known that *P. acnes* is recognized by TLRs and activates the innate immune system. Kim et al. demonstrated that transfection of TLR2 into a nonresponsive cell line was sufficient for NF-κB activation in response to *P. acnes* (16,17). Further, they demonstrated that *P. acnes* induces IL-12 and IL-8 production by human monocytes via activation of TLR2. They also demonstrated that TLR2 expression was found in macrophages in biopsied acne lesions, particularly in the perifollicular regions, and the quantity of TLR2-positive cells detected increased with the increasing age of the lesion. Following these findings, Jugeau et al. demonstrated that TLR2 and TLR4 expression are upregulated in acne lesions of patients with facial acne and that TLR2 and TLR4 expression increased within hours of incubating human keratinocytes with bacterial fractions (49). Although the exact *P. acnes* TLR2 ligand is unknown, it is postulated that *P. acnes* peptidoglycan on the cell wall serves as the PAMP for TLR2. Taken together, it seems that *P. acnes* contributes to the pathogenesis of acne by inducing inflammation through the activation of TLR2 and the subsequent release of cytokines, which regulate the local immune response.

PROPIONIBACTERIUM ACNES INDUCES MMP PRODUCTION

In addition to cytokines and chemokines, MMPs are also mediators of immunity and inflammation, tissue destruction, and scar formation. MMPs play a role in several inflammatory conditions, including rheumatoid arthritis and arterial inflammation, and possibly also in infectious diseases such as Lyme disease and tuberculosis. MMP-1, MMP-3, and MMP-9 have been found in acne lesions (10), and recent studies have shown that MMPs can participate in the innate immune response and induce inflammation. Jalian et al. showed that *P. acnes* upregulates MMP-1 and MMP-9 (18), and Choi et al. showed that *P. acnes* upregulates MMP-2 (19). The activation of MMP-1 and MMP-9 appears to occur through the transcription factor activator protein-1 (AP-1) (50), and recently the activation of MMP-1, MMP-9, and AP-1 has been shown to be found in acne lesions (51). Interestingly, Jalian et al. also demonstrated that all-*trans* retinoic acid (ATRA) inhibited *P. acnes*–induced upregulation of MMPs while downregulating tissue inhibitor of metalloproteinase (TIMP), suggesting that ATRA shifts a tissue-degrading phenotype to a tissue-preserving phenotype (18). This may explain the clinical findings that ATRA and other retinoids improve acne scarring. Furthermore, such studies suggest that ATRA may be useful for adjuvant therapy to prevent and treat acne scar formation.

PROPIONIBACTERIUM ACNES INDUCES ANTIMICROBIAL PEPTIDE PRODUCTION AND ANTIMICROBIAL RESPONSE

The innate immune system must rapidly recognize microbial pathogens and trigger direct host antimicrobial response to limit the infection, yet the activation of the innate immune system also results in inflammation and tissue injury that characterize the clinical manifestations of human disease. This "double-edged sword" of innate immunity is clearly evident in acne vulgaris in which innate immune cells mount an antimicrobial response to *P. acnes*, but they also induce an inflammatory response mediated by release of cytokines, chemokines, and

MMPs that contribute to clinical disease. The previous sections focused on the production of cytokines, chemokines, and MMPs. Here we discuss briefly the antimicrobial response in acne.

Antimicrobial peptides produced in the skin play a critical role in the elimination of the invading microorganisms. Important antimicrobial peptides in skin include human β-defensins 1 and 2 (HBD1 and HBD2). HBD2 is an important host defense molecule due to its ability to kill microorganisms and to recruit and activate macrophages and DCs (22). Antimicrobial peptide HBD2 is induced by proinflammatory cytokines such as IL-1β and TNFα and bacterial components (21). Chronnell et al. found that HBD2 expression is upregulated in acne lesions (22). Additionally, it has been shown that two different strains of *P. acnes* can induce HBD-2 in cultured keratinocytes and that *P. acnes* induces elevation of HBD2 and IL-8 via TLR2- and TLR4-mediated mechanisms (20). Furthermore, HBD2 has shown to have direct antimicrobial activity against *P. acnes* in synergy with cathelicidin (52).

Cathelicidin (LL-37) is another important antimicrobial peptide that is upregulated by *P. acnes* extracts in sebocytes, keratinocytes, and monocytes (53). It has also been demonstrated that cathelicidin and granulysin, another antimicrobial peptide, can kill *P. acnes* (52,53). Moreover, cathelicidin, HBD2, and psoriasin (another antimicrobial peptide found in acne lesions) provide synergistic action against *P. acnes* and other gram-positive organisms and recruit inflammatory mediators (20,21,53,54). Therefore, it is likely that antimicrobial peptides contribute to control local bacterial growth, but at the same time induce inflammatory responses in acne.

P. acnes has also been shown to directly induce the differentiation of cells involved in the phagocytosis of microbes, specifically the differentiation of monocytes to specific macrophages that express CD209. These CD209 macrophages are efficient phagocytic cells able to induce intracellular killing of pathogens. A study by Liu et al. demonstrated that CD209+ macrophages are able to phagocytose *P. acnes* and kill them intracellularly (56). While the mechanism of this killing was not demonstrated, the authors suggest that antimicrobial peptides such as HBD2 or LL-37 may play a role. Interestingly, the authors also demonstrated that ATRA alone induces the differentiation of human monocytes into CD209+ macrophages, suggesting an indirect antimicrobial property of ATRA. Studies in this and previous sections show that *P. acnes* activate two differential host innate immune responses—induction of inflammation that contributes to disease pathogenesis and induction of antimicrobial response by the host that contributes to control the growth of *P. acnes*. Future therapy should target and balance these two distinct innate immune responses found in acne.

SEBACEOUS GLAND LIPIDS INFLUENCE IMMUNE RESPONSES

Previously, the sebaceous glands were presumed to provide only a lubricating function for the skin and hair with its sole function of producing lipids. However, recent findings have shown that sebocytes as innate immune cells are capable of pattern recognition and mounting an immune response. A study by Nagy et al. demonstrated that *P. acnes* induce the expression of HBD2 and proinflammatory cytokines TNF-α and IL-1α and chemokine CXCL8 in a human sebocyte cell line (20,21). Nelson et al. have also shown that 13-*cis* retinoic acid can induce apoptosis of human sebocytes via a neutrophil gelatinase-associated lipocalin (NGAL) dependent mechanism, which may help to explain how this therapeutic works to treat severe acne (57). Therefore, similar to other innate immune cells, sebocytes recognize pathogens and are capable of inducing both inflammation and antimicrobial responses. Understanding the biology of sebocytes in the setting of both inflammation and antimicrobial responses may provide clues to the development of other therapeutics for acne.

Sebum production by the sebaceous gland is a well-established cause of acne. Sebum is a lipid-rich fluid that is a nutrient source for *P. acnes* and consists of cholesterol, fatty acids, fatty alcohols, di- and triglycerides, wax esters, sterol esters, and squalene (58). While other mammals have sebaceous glands, human sebum is specific and uniquely contains wax esters and squalene. Furthermore, humans are the only mammals to suffer from acne. The sebaceous gland is capable of synthesizing cholesterol de novo, under the influence of various steroidogenic genes that are regulated in a tissue-specific fashion, and converting this precursor to various cholesterol derivatives (6). Important lipids in acne pathogenesis include squalene (59), arachidonic acid, linoleic acid, palmitic acid, and sapneic acid, as these lipids have been shown to influence inflammation in acne (24).

In addition to antimicrobial peptides, there is also evidence to suggest that lipids could function as antimicrobial agents, for example, sapienic acid was found to be effective against *S. aureus* (55).

Sebaceous gland lipids have been found to exert direct inflammatory effects. Oxidized squalene can stimulate hyperproliferative behavior of keratinocytes and induce an initial upregulation of IL-6 production lipoxygenases activity, such as 5-lipoxygenase (5-LOX) (24,60). 5-LOX can subsequently metabolize arachidonic acid to leukotriene B4 (LTB4), which induces recruitment and activation of neutrophils, monocytes, and eosinophils. 5-LOX also stimulates the production of several proinflammatory cytokines and mediators that augment tissue inflammation. 5-LOX production is enhanced in the sebaceous glands of acne patients (60), and its in vivo inhibition reduces the production of proinflammatory sebaceous fatty acids as well as the number of inflammatory acne lesions (61,62). In addition, it has been shown that arachidonic acid and linoleic acid stimulate IL-6 and IL-8 synthesis and enhance the synthesis of sebaceous lipids (60) and that ceramides, another family of lipid molecules, contribute to neutrophil degranulation and increase integrin expression on leukocytes, which increases leukocyte recruitment to the area of inflammation. These studies suggest that lipids produced in the sebaceous gland, act in a direct, tissue-specific fashion to promote innate immune responses that contribute to acne pathogenesis.

In addition to directly promoting acne, sebum lipids have also been shown to promote downstream inflammatory pathways. These downstream effects include activation of nuclear receptors, which then regulate genes involved in inflammation and the innate immune system. Peroxisome proliferator–activated receptors (PPARs) are a class of nuclear receptors that are able to regulate transcription of DNA. It has been suggested that these nuclear receptors are regulated by fatty acid derivatives and can control inflammatory response genes. An example of this is the finding that LTB4, converted by 5-LOX from arachidonic acid, binds and activates PPARα, which can inhibit the expression of proinflammatory genes that regulate the production of cytokines, MMPs, and acute-phase proteins (63). In addition, a different prostaglandin (15d-PGJ2) has been reported to be an endogenous activator of PPARγ, which augments lipogenesis (64). Lastly, it has also been suggested that nuclear receptors activated by sebum lipids can activate T-cell signaling pathways and regulate further lipid production through AP-1 and NF-κB signals (65). More research is needed to further understand the downstream effects of sebum lipids on the innate immune system.

Taken together, these results support the view that sebum lipids induce inflammation and activate the innate immune system via direct and downstream effects. Furthermore, sebum lipids exert both pro- and anti-inflammatory effects, and the interplay between these in various skin sites and types could contribute to differences in acne expression.

CONCLUSION

The accepted pathogenic factors of acne have traditionally included complex interactions between sebum production by the sebaceous gland, *P. acnes* follicular colonization, alteration in the keratinization process, and hormone regulation. In this chapter, we discussed acne pathogenesis related to innate immunity. The skin is an efficient immune organ that uses the innate immune response to protect the host. On the other hand, the same mechanism that leads to antimicrobial responses can lead to the release of inflammatory mediators contributing to disease. While the precise mechanisms of these interactions are not fully understood, with the advent of cellular culture studies and advanced immunology techniques, it has been increasingly demonstrated that acne is a disease of innate immunity and that previously known pathogenic factors likely interact with various immune mechanisms to promote acne pathogenesis. While it has classically been thought that alterations in keratinization lead to inflammatory events, it is now believed that inflammatory events through IL-1 precede hyperkeratinization. Similarly, the role of *P. acnes* has been further elucidated to demonstrate that *P. acnes* activation of innate immune cells including keratinocytes, monocytes/macrophages, and sebocytes leads to inflammation, including the expression of cytokines, chemokines, and MMPs. In addition, it has been demonstrated that the sebaceous gland participates in the immune response and that sebum lipids exert both direct inflammatory effects and indirect regulation of downstream inflammatory pathways. It is becoming clear that acne is an inflammatory and immune-related disease and future acne therapies should target these pathways.

REFERENCES

1. Thiboutot D, Gollnick H, Bettoli V, et al. New insights into the management of acne: an update from the Global Alliance to Improve Outcomes in Acne group. J Am Acad Dermatol 2009; 60:S1–S50.
2. Oberemok SS, Shalita AR. Acne vulgaris, I: pathogenesis and diagnosis. Cutis 2002; 70:101–105.
3. Plewig G, Fulton JE, Kligman AM. Cellular dynamics of comedo formation in acne vulgaris. Arch Dermatol Forsch 1971; 242:12–29.
4. Vowels BR, Yang S, Leyden JJ. Induction of proinflammatory cytokines by a soluble factor of Propionibacterium acnes: implications for chronic inflammatory acne. Infect Immun 1995; 63:3158–3165.
5. Thiboutot D. Hormones and acne: pathophysiology, clinical evaluation, and therapies. Semin Cutan Med Surg 2001; 20:144–153.
6. Thiboutot D, Jabara S, McAllister JM, et al. Human skin is a steroidogenic tissue: steroidogenic enzymes and cofactors are expressed in epidermis, normal sebocytes, and an immortalized sebocyte cell line (SEB-1). J Invest Dermatol 2003; 120:905–914.
7. Thiboutot D. Acne: hormonal concepts and therapy. Clin Dermatol 2004; 22:419–428.
8. Thiboutot D. Regulation of human sebaceous glands. J Invest Dermatol 2004; 123:1–12.

9. Guy R, Green MR, Kealey T. Modeling acne in vitro. J Invest Dermatol 1996; 106:176–182.

10. Trivedi NR, Gilliland KL, Zhao W, et al. Gene array expression profiling in acne lesions reveals marked upregulation of genes involved in inflammation and matrix remodeling. J Invest Dermatol 2006; 126:1071–1079.

11. Gollnick H, Cunliffe W, Berson D, et al. Management of acne: a report from a Global Alliance to Improve Outcomes in Acne. J Am Acad Dermatol 2003; 49:S1–S37.

12. Thiboutot D, Chen W. Update and future of hormonal therapy in acne. Dermatology 2003; 206:57–67.

13. Downing DT, Stewart ME, Wertz PW, et al. Essential fatty acids and acne. J Am Acad Dermatol 1986; 14:221–225.

14. Jeremy AH, Holland DB, Roberts SG, et al. Inflammatory events are involved in acne lesion initiation. J Invest Dermatol 2003; 121:20–27.

15. Ingham E, Eady EA, Goodwin CE, et al. Pro-inflammatory levels of interleukin-1 alpha-like bioactivity are present in the majority of open comedones in acne vulgaris. J Invest Dermatol 1992; 98:895–901.

16. Kim J, Ochoa MT, Krutzik SR, et al. Activation of toll-like receptor 2 in acne triggers inflammatory cytokine responses. J Immunol 2002; 169:1535–1541.

17. Kim J. Review of the innate immune response in acne vulgaris: activation of Toll-like receptor 2 in acne triggers inflammatory cytokine responses. Dermatology 2005; 211:193–198.

18. Jalian HR, Liu PT, Kanchanapoomi M, et al. All-trans retinoic acid shifts Propionibacterium acnes-induced matrix degradation expression profile toward matrix preservation in human monocytes. J Invest Dermatol 2008; 128:2777–2782.

19. Choi JY, Piao MS, Lee JB, et al. Propionibacterium acnes stimulates pro-matrix metalloproteinase-2 expression through tumor necrosis factor-alpha in human dermal fibroblasts. J Invest Dermatol 2008; 128:846–854.

20. Nagy I, Pivarcsi A, Koreck A, et al. Distinct strains of Propionibacterium acnes induce selective human beta-defensin-2 and interleukin-8 expression in human keratinocytes through toll-like receptors. J Invest Dermatol 2005; 124:931–938.

21. Nagy I, Pivarcsi A, Kis K, et al. Propionibacterium acnes and lipopolysaccharide induce the expression of antimicrobial peptides and proinflammatory cytokines/chemokines in human sebocytes. Microbes Infect 2006; 8:2195–2205.

22. Chronnell CM, Ghali LR, Ali RS, et al. Human beta defensin-1 and -2 expression in human pilosebaceous units: upregulation in acne vulgaris lesions. J Invest Dermatol 2001; 117:1120–1125.

23. Zouboulis CC, Baron JM, Bohm M, et al. Frontiers in sebaceous gland biology and pathology. Exp Dermatol 2008; 17:542–551.

24. Ottaviani M, Alestas T, Flori E, et al. Peroxidated squalene induces the production of inflammatory mediators in HaCaT keratinocytes: a possible role in acne vulgaris. J Invest Dermatol 2006; 126:2430–2437.

25. Modlin Robert L, Kim J, Maurer D, et al. Innate and adaptive immunity in the skin. In: Wolff K, Goldsmith L, Katz S, et al., eds. Fitzpatrick's Dermatology in General Medicine. 7th ed. New York: McGraw-Hill, 2008.

26. Williams IR, Rich BE, Kupper TS. Cytokines. In: Wolff K, Goldsmith L, Katz S, et al., eds. Fitzpatrick's Dermatology in General Medicine. 7th ed. New York: McGraw-Hill, 2008.

27. Chu D. Development and structure of skin. In: Wolff K, Goldsmith L, Katz S, et al., eds. Fitzpatrick's Dermatology in General Medicine. 7th ed. New York: McGraw-Hill, 2008.

28. McInturff JE, Kim J. The role of toll-like receptors in the pathophysiology of acne. Semin Cutan Med Surg 2005; 24:73–78.

29. McInturff JE, Modlin RL, Kim J. The role of toll-like receptors in the pathogenesis and treatment of dermatological disease. J Invest Dermatol 2005; 125:1–8.

30. Yoshimura A, Lien E, Ingalls RR, et al. Cutting edge: recognition of gram-positive bacterial cell wall components by the innate immune system occurs via Toll-like receptor 2. J Immunol 1999; 163:1–5.

31. Poltorak A, Smirnova I, He X, et al. Genetic and physical mapping of the Lps locus: identification of the toll-4 receptor as a candidate gene in the critical region. Blood Cells Mol Dis 1998; 24:340–355.

32. Poltorak A, He X, Smirnova I, et al. Defective LPS signaling in C3H/HeJ and C57BL/10ScCr mice: mutations in Tlr4 gene. Science 1998; 282:2085–2088.

33. Hayashi F, Smith KD, Ozinsky A, et al. The innate immune response to bacterial flagellin is mediated by Toll-like receptor 5. Nature 2001; 410:1099–1103.

34. Hemmi H, Takeuchi O, Kawai T, et al. A Toll-like receptor recognizes bacterial DNA. Nature 2000; 408:740–745.

35. Alexopoulou L, Holt AC, Medzhitov R, et al. Recognition of double-stranded RNA and activation of NF-kappaB by Toll-like receptor 3. Nature 2001; 413:732–738.

36. Brightbill HD, Libraty DH, Krutzik SR, et al. Host defense mechanisms triggered by microbial lipoproteins through toll-like receptors. Science 1999; 285:732–736.

37. Ozinsky A, Underhill DM, Fontenot JD, et al. The repertoire for pattern recognition of pathogens by the innate immune system is defined by cooperation between toll-like receptors. Proc Natl Acad Sci U S A 2000; 97:13766–13771.

38. Sakamoto FH, Lopes JD, Anderson RR. Photodynamic therapy for acne vulgaris: a critical review from basics to clinical practice: part I. Acne vulgaris: when and why consider photodynamic therapy? J Am Acad Dermatol 2010; 63:183–193.

39. Harper JC, Thiboutot DM. Pathogenesis of acne: recent research advances. Adv Dermatol 2003; 19:1–10.

40. Perisho K, Wertz PW, Madison KC, et al. Fatty acids of acylceramides from comedones and from the skin surface of acne patients and control subjects. J Invest Dermatol 1988; 90:350–353.

41. Elias PM, Brown BE, Ziboh VA. The permeability barrier in essential fatty acid deficiency: evidence for a direct role for linoleic acid in barrier function. J Invest Dermatol 1980; 74:230–233.

42. Latkowski JM, Freedberg IM, Blumenberg M. Keratinocyte growth factor and keratin gene regulation. J Dermatol Sci 1995; 9:36–44.

43. Freedberg IM, Tomic-Canic M, Komine M, et al. Keratins and the keratinocyte activation cycle. J Invest Dermatol 2001; 116:633–640.

44. Kuwahara K, Kitazawa T, Kitagaki H, et al. Nadifloxacin, an antiacne quinolone antimicrobial, inhibits the production of proinflammatory cytokines by human peripheral blood mononuclear cells and normal human keratinocytes. J Dermatol Sci 2005; 38:47–55.

45. Yamanaka K, Tanaka M, Tsutsui H, et al. Skin-specific caspase-1-transgenic mice show cutaneous apoptosis and pre-endotoxin shock condition with a high serum level of IL-18. J Immunol 2000; 165:997–1003.

46. Tsutsui H, Yoshimoto Y, Hayashi N, et al. Induction of allergic inflammation by interleukin-18 in experimental animal models. Immunol Rev 2004; 202:115–138.

47. Miura Y, Ishige I, Soejima N, et al. Quantitative PCR of Propionibacterium acnes DNA in samples aspirated from sebaceous follicles on the normal skin of subjects with or without acne. J Med Dent Sci 2010; 57:65–74.

48. Strauss JS, Kligman AM. Pathologic patterns of the sebaceous gland. J Invest Dermatol 1958; 30:51–61.

49. Jugeau S, Tenaud I, Knol AC, et al. Induction of toll-like receptors by Propionibacterium acnes. Br J Dermatol 2005; 153:1105–1113.

50. Birkedal-Hansen H, Moore WG, Bodden MK, et al. Matrix metalloproteinases: a review. Crit Rev Oral Biol Med 1993; 4:197–250.

51. Kang S, Cho S, Chung JH, et al. Inflammation and extracellular matrix degradation mediated by activated transcription factors nuclear factor-kappaB and activator protein-1 in inflammatory acne lesions in vivo. Am J Pathol 2005; 166:1691–1699.

52. Hong I, Lee MH, Na TY, et al. LXRalpha enhances lipid synthesis in SZ95 sebocytes. J Invest Dermatol 2008; 128:1266–1272.

53. Lee DY, Yamasaki K, Rudsil J, et al. Sebocytes express functional cathelicidin antimicrobial peptides and can act to kill Propionibacterium acnes. J Invest Dermatol 2008; 128:1863–1866.

54. Ganceviciene R, Fimmel S, Glass E, et al. Psoriasin and follicular hyperkeratinization in acne comedones. Dermatology 2006; 213:270–272.

55. Drake DR, Brogden KA, Dawson DV, et al. Thematic review series: skin lipids. Antimicrobial lipids at the skin surface. J Lipid Res 2008; 49:4–11.

56. Liu PT, Phan J, Tang D, et al. CD209(+) macrophages mediate host defense against Propionibacterium acnes. J Immunol 2008; 180:4919–4923.

57. Nelson AM, Zhao W, Gilliland KL, et al. Neutrophil gelatinase-associated lipocalin mediates 13-cis retinoic acid-induced apoptosis of human sebaceous gland cells. J Clin Invest 2008; 118:1468–1478.

58. Kligman AM, Wheatley VR, Mills OH. Comedogenicity of human sebum. Arch Dermatol 1970; 102:267–275.

59. Motoyoshi K. Enhanced comedo formation in rabbit ear skin by squalene and oleic acid peroxides. Br J Dermatol 1983; 109:191–198.

60. Alestas T, Ganceviciene R, Fimmel S, et al. Enzymes involved in the biosynthesis of leukotriene B4 and prostaglandin E2 are active in sebaceous glands. J Mol Med 2006; 84:75–87.

61. Zouboulis CC. Acne and sebaceous gland function. Clin Dermatol 2004; 22:360–366.

62. Zouboulis CC. Propionibacterium acnes and sebaceous lipogenesis: a love-hate relationship? J Invest Dermatol 2009; 129:2093–2096.

63. Delerive P, Fruchart JC, Staels B. Peroxisome proliferator-activated receptors in inflammation control. J Endocrinol 2001; 169:453–459.
64. Trivedi NR, Cong Z, Nelson AM, et al. Peroxisome proliferator-activated receptors increase human sebum production. J Invest Dermatol 2006; 126:2002–2009.
65. Weindl G, Schafer-Korting M, Schaller M, et al. Peroxisome proliferator-activated receptors and their ligands: entry into the post-glucocorticoid era of skin treatment? Drugs 2005; 65:1919–1934.

1.4

Comedogenesis

Carol Heughebaert and Alan R. Shalita

INTRODUCTION

Despite extensive research over the past century, the pathogenesis of acne vulgaris remains unclear. In particular, the sequences of events that are involved in comedogenesis have yet to be elucidated. Comedogenesis is one of the four primary etiological factors of acne; the others are increased sebum production and secretion, follicular duct colonization with *Propionibacterium acnes* (*P. acnes*), and the inflammatory response. These four factors should not be seen as distinct phases, but rather as closely interrelated mechanisms that ultimately lead to the clinical disease acne vulgaris.

That comedones are essential lesions in acne was first suggested in 1960 (1). It is widely accepted that their pathogenesis is multifactorial, attributable to follicular hyperkeratinization, increased sebum production, increased androgen activity, alteration of sebum lipid quality, dysregulation of cutaneous steroido-genesis, neuropeptide production, inflammation, and follicular hypercolonization by the *P. acnes* bacteria (2,3).

This chapter focuses on the current etiologic aspects of comedogenesis, the factors controlling comedo formation and the various comedo subtypes.

COMEDONES: AN OVERVIEW

Acne vulgaris begins with the formation of microcomedones, subclinical lesions characterized by follicular epithelial hyperproliferation. These lesions can further evolve into inflammatory lesions or noninflammatory comedones, of which there are two types, open and closed. Clinically invisible, microcomedones are lesions present in regions of apparently healthy skin in a patient with acne (4).

They can only be observed via surface biopsy, a technique that employs cyanoacrylate glue to remove the follicular contents from the skin surface. These can then be microscopically examined (5). Histologic examination of microcomedones reveals dilated pilosebaceous ducts containing excessive keratinocytes and modified sebum, with a prominent granular layer in the ductal epithelium (4).

Under normal circumstances, keratinocytes are loosely arranged in normal pilosebaceous follicles. The flow of sebum transports them to the surface of the skin upon desquamation, maintaining a balance between new and desquamated keratinocytes. However, in comedones, this balance is disturbed, leading to keratinocyte accumulation in the pilosebaceous duct.

Hyperproliferation of basal keratinocytes, which line the wall of the infrainfundibulum, plays a central role in this accumulation (6,7). As more keratinous material accumulates, the follicular wall continues to distend and become thinner. Concurrently, sebaceous glands begin to atrophy and are replaced by undifferentiated epithelial cells. The thin walled, fully developed comedone contains very few, if any, sebaceous cells. The open comedo contains keratinous material arranged in a concentric lamellar fashion. The closed comedone contains less compact keratinous material and has a narrow follicular orifice.

The distal section of the pilosebaceous follicle, which is located above the junction of the sebaceous canal, is called the infundibulum. The infundibulum is composed of two parts: the deep infrainfundibulum (lower four-fifths) and the distal acroinfundibulum (upper fifth). The keratinocytes of the infrainfundibulum differentiate in a different manner than the epidermal keratinocytes and often have a subtle granular layer. Electronmicroscopically, the pattern of hyperkeratinization demonstrates retention hyperkeratosis with increased number and size of keratohyaline granules, accumulation of lipid droplets, and folding of the retained squames on themselves as a result of pressure effects (8). At the ultrastructural level, the follicular keratinocytes present in comedones display increased numbers of desmosomes and tonofilaments (9).

The mechanism of follicular hyperkeratinization is still unclear, and it is thought that several factors are responsible. These include changes in sebum lipid composition, abnormal responses to androgens, local cytokine production, and later, the presence and effects of *P. acnes*, each of which will be described below.

FOLLICULAR HYPERKERATINIZATION

Keratinocyte hyperproliferation and retention have been demonstrated by labeling comedones with ^{3}H-thymidine, a marker for cell proliferation (6). Immunohistochemical confirmation has been provided using a monoclonal antibody to Ki-67, another cellular marker for proliferation, which labels increased numbers of ductal keratinocytes (10). Further evidence of this ductal hyperproliferation was the increased expression of keratin K6, K16, and K17, the keratin markers of hyperproliferation in the wall of microcomedones and comedones (11).

In addition, clinically normal follicles in acne-prone skin have also been shown to overexpress Ki-67 and K16, which suggests that topical therapy should be applied not only to lesions but also to the surrounding healthy-looking skin as well (12). Further studies have provided evidence that the expression of keratin markers is upregulated by inflammatory cytokines, such as interleukin-1 (IL-1) and IFN-α, and growth factors, including TGF-α and EGF. This provides evidence for the involvement of inflammatory responses in the very early stage of acne lesion development (13–15).

Comedogenesis might also be due to reduced desquamation caused by increased cohesion between ductal keratinocytes, or a combination of keratinocyte hyperproliferation and reduced desquamation (6). Hydrolytic enzymes, produced by lamellar granules, are required for desquamation. When decreased lamellar granules were discovered in the follicle wall of comedones, it was assumed that lower levels of hydrolytic enzymes were available for desquamation (8). *P. acnes* biofilm production is believed to be another cause of increased cohesiveness of keratinocytes (16).

In summary, when more keratinocytes are produced or less keratinocytes are separated, they accumulate in the pilosebaceous duct, creating a bottleneck phenomenon and resulting in the formation of a nonvisible lesion, the microcomedone.

THE ROLE OF INFLAMMATION IN COMEDOGENESIS

Inflammation had generally been considered a secondary event in acne pathogenesis until it was demonstrated that inflammatory events in fact occur in the earliest stage of acne lesion development (17). Inflammatory markers can be detected even before hyperproliferation and abnormal differentiation of keratinocytes. The role of IL-1α in cutaneous inflammation and keratinocyte proliferation has since been closely studied. IL-1α is present in the perifollicular epidermis of uninvolved skin in acne patients before hyperproliferation or abnormal differentiation of the follicular epithelium takes place (17). IL-1α has been reported to induce in vitro and in vivo hyperkeratinization in the follicular infundibulum (18). IL-1α is comedogenic in pilosebaceous units (PSUs) that have been isolated in vitro (18,19). Addition of IL-1α to an isolated pilosebaceous infundibulum in vitro results in comedo-like hypercornification. An IL-1α antagonist can inhibit this reaction (19). When released into the dermis, IL-1α initiates an inflammatory response. Further, enough IL-1α has been shown to be present in a comedo for this to occur (20). The observed inflammatory response around uninvolved follicles consists of an infiltrate of CD4⁺ lymphocytes and macrophages (17).

It has been hypothesized that the cytokines produced in the follicle might be responsible for activating local endothelial cells, causing the upregulation of inflammatory vascular markers in the vasculature around the pilosebaceous follicles of the uninvolved skin (17). Further, it was suggested that the entire process is initiated by an increase in IL-1α activity. However, a matter of controversy exists about which factors might be responsible for the increased IL-1α expression and release (17).

THE ROLE OF SEBUM LIPID COMPOSITION ABNORMALITIES IN COMEDOGENESIS

Sebum, produced by sebaceous glands, is a complex mixture of triglycerides, wax esters, squalene, and, to a lesser extent, cholesterol and phospholipids. Abnormalities in its content are considered among the main factors implicated in acne pathogenesis, playing a role in both comedogenesis and the development of inflammatory reactions that lead to clinical acne lesions. Sebum production and secretion is a necessary condition for acne vulgaris, although hypersecretion is not sufficient to initiate lesion development. However, sebum in acne patients is both quantitatively and qualitatively different from that of the skin of normal individuals. The accumulation of comedogenic sebum components also plays a role.

In the late 1960s, studies with a rabbit ear model showed that sebaceous lipid abnormalities could all trigger hypercornification. These abnormalities include increased fatty acid, squalene, and squalene oxide, and decreased linoleic acid (21–23). Although it is unclear whether animal models accurately reflect the human sebaceous follicles, substances that are comedogenic in this model are capable of inducing comedones in the human model (5).

In the 1970s, comedogenesis was thought to be triggered by the presence of excessive follicular free fatty acids (24), the production of which is metabolized by bacterial lipases, predominantly from *P. acnes* and *Staphylococcus epidermidis* (25). Although this idea was later discounted, both topical and oral antibiotics have been shown to reduce comedones (26). Whether this reduction is due to the antibacterial effects of the antibiotics or the direct inhibition of lipase production is unclear. Regardless, it has since been discovered that the sebum lipid abnormalities that play a role in comedogenesis are more complex than a simple increase in amount.

One such abnormality is lipid polarity. Skin surface lipids in acne patients, as well as lipids in open and closed comedones, have an increased polar lipid content as compared with the skin surface lipids obtained from controls. These polar lipids appear to be derived mainly from the oxidation of squalene, a sebum-specific lipid, to squalene peroxide. Excessive accumulation of these peroxides may promote inflammatory changes in comedones, and their accumulation in comedones may lead to an increase in IL-1α expression via NF-κB and exacerbate comedogenesis by triggering follicular keratinization (27).

A link between a low sebum level of linoleic acid, an essential fatty acid, and comedogenesis was suggested in 1986 (23). Diminished linoleic acid content in intrafollicular sphingolipids may be involved in follicular hyperkeratosis, a crucial event in comedogenesis. Hyperkeratosis could possibly lead to a diminished epidermal barrier function, increased transepidermal water loss, and a scaly dermatosis. This can later predispose the follicular wall to increased permeability to proinflammatory substances (28). Further evidence of the importance of linoleic acid is provided by the fact that topically applied linoleic acid reduces the size of microcomedones (29). The concentration of linoleic acid in the sebum of acne patients increases after treatment with either oral iso-tretinoin or cyproterone acetate (30), although studies have found that this effect relates to the higher sebum secretion rate in acne patients rather than a direct effect on linoleic acid. It has been suggested that the linoleic acid level in human sebum depends on both the quantity of linoleic acid present in each sebaceous cell at the start of its differentiation and the extent to which this initial linoleic acid content is diluted by the sebum synthesized by each sebaceous cell (22). There is an inverse relationship between linoleic acid levels in sebum and the sebum secretion rate as endogenous lipid synthesis may dilute this essential fatty acid (23).

More recent studies have focused on the saturation pattern of fatty acids in acne. These have revealed differences in the ratio of saturated to unsaturated fatty acids in the skin surface triglycerides between acne patients and controls (31). In particular, an increased ratio of unsaturated to saturated fatty acids seems to be associated with increased sebogenesis.

THE ROLE OF ANDROGENS IN COMEDOGENESIS

Androgens influence various cutaneous functions, including sebaceous gland growth and differentiation, hair growth, epidermal barrier function, and wound healing. They play a central role in the stimulation of sebum production and keratinocyte proliferation (32,33).

Prohormone androgens, primarily produced in the gonads and adrenal glands, are converted in the skin to the more potent testosterone and dihy-drotestosterone (DHT). Type 1 5α-reductase, which is located within both the infrainfundibulum part of the duct and the sebaceous gland, catalyzes the cutaneous conversion of testosterone to the more potent DHT (34). The androgens then initiate changes in the sebaceous glands and pilosebaceous canals, both of which express androgen receptors. Androgens affect sebocytes and infundibular keratinocytes in a complex manner, having an effect on differentiation and proliferation of sebocytes, lipogenesis, and comedogenesis.

The role of androgens in the pathogenesis of acne has long been recognized. The principal link between androgens and acne is sebum, as the sebaceous glands are highly androgen sensitive. A significant proportion of patients with acne have systemic androgen abnormalities. Women experiencing excessive androgen states, as in polycystic ovary syndrome, suffer from acne (35). Skin in acne patients displays a higher androgen receptor density and higher 5α-reductase activity than nonacne skin (34,36). Systemic or topical administration of androgens (testosterone and DHT) or anabolic steroids increases the size and function of sebaceous glands (32). The close timing between the onset of microcomedonal acne during the prepubertal period and the adrenarchal rise in serum levels of DHEAS has been well documented (37,38). On the other hand, men who have been castrated before puberty, or individuals without functional androgen receptors, such as patients with androgen-insensitivity syndrome, neither produce sebum nor develop acne (39). Diet can also influence comedogenesis (40). In particular, dairy milk contains testosterone precursors (41) that, after conversion to DHT via testosterone, stimulate the PSU. The comedogenicity of milk is thought to be due to both testosterone precursors and 5α-reduced molecules (42,43). The consumption of milk might also exert a comedogenic effect via the IGF-1 pathway via the stimulation of androgen synthesis (44).

The role of androgens in follicular hyperkeratinization, and thus the possibility that local androgens might directly contribute to comedo formation, has been investigated in an in vitro study of cultured keratinocytes from the epidermis and the follicular infrainfundibulum. This study demonstrated a higher activity of type 1 5α-reductase in the infrainfundibular region, the region which is affected by hypercornification, as compared to epidermal keratinocytes, from subjects both with and without acne. Patients with acne have a slightly higher level of this enzyme compared to patients without acne, indicating increased capacity for producing androgens (33). The role of androgens in comedo formation, and whether the increase in enzyme level is a consequence of acne or its cause, remains to be determined. However, it is known that androgenic stimulation leads to excessive ductal and infundibular hyperkeratinization. This effect is potentiated by synergistic growth factors, neuropeptides and IL-1α, and hyperproliferation and hypercornification of the follicular wall could be blocked by the addition of IL-1 receptor antagonist (19).

Regarding the hormonal response, increased DHT may act on infundibular keratinocytes leading to abnormal hyperkeratinization (45). It remains to be determined whether higher activity of the type 1 5α-reductase detected in the follicular infrainfundibulum is associated with the abnormal differentiation of keratinocytes (45).

Further evidence for the comedogenic effects of androgens is the observation that anti-androgens reduce comedones. Oral contraceptives containing cyproterone acetate, such as Diane® and Dianette®, have a direct effect on comedogenesis (30).

THE ROLE OF CYTOKINES IN COMEDOGENESIS

There is increasing evidence that immune phenomena underlie both comedogenesis and the formation of inflammatory acne lesions (12,19,20,46,47). Cytokines, some of the most potent and diverse of the body's inflammatory mediators, have become the focus of study as possible comedogenic substances. Of particular interest is IL-1α, which has been found to be present in the inflammatory cytokine content of comedones (48). IL-1α seems to be produced by ductal keratinocytes in comedones (49) and, as previously mentioned, plays a role in the androgenic stimulation in comedogenesis. Indeed, elevated levels have been detected in most open comedones of acne vulgaris (20).

Direct evidence for involvement of IL-1α in comedogenesis has been demonstrated. The addition of IL-1α to an in vitro medium of normal PSUs leads to hyperproliferation and abnormal differentiation in isolated pilosebaceous follicles. Thus, IL-1α leads to comedonal features in the absence of other mediators. The addition of an IL-1α receptor antagonist to experimental acne systems inhibits the growth of comedones, confirming that this is indeed an IL-1α-specific response (12,19,47).

Because IL-1α influences hypercornification of the infundibulum in vitro, it might be responsible for creating the keratinous mass as well as the inflammatory response by inducing the production of vascular endothelial growth factor in dermal papilla cells and follicular keratinocytes of the PSU (50). Indeed, comedones have been found to contain enough IL-1α activity to initiate inflammation when released into the dermis. Further, it has been postulated that this cytokine causes the scaling seen in many inflammatory skin diseases (12,18,19,46,47). Aldana et al. reported increased IL-1α immunoreactivity in the follicle wall of PSUs of uninvolved skin and comedones (48,51). Recent evidence suggests that inflammatory events not only occur post hyperproliferation but are also involved in the early stages of acne lesion initiation, before the development of microcomedonal features (17). However, it is currently not clear what factors are responsible for the increased expression and release of IL-1α.

THE ROLE OF *PROPIONIBACTERIUM ACNES*

P. acnes is a gram-positive bacterium whose close association with acne vulgaris has long been recognized (52). Initially thought to be the primary causative factor of acne lesions, *P. acnes* is now regarded as one of several interconnected factors in the pathophysiology of acne vulgaris. The role that *P. acnes* plays in comedogenesis has not yet been entirely elucidated. However, studies have shown that *P. acnes* is frequently present in high concentrations in microcomedones (53); and that it plays a part in the induction of cytokines, integrins, and inflammation; and that the biofilm produced by the bacteria might have a role in follicular hyperkeratinization. *P. acnes* is not only important in the development of inflammatory acne lesions but also in the formation of the microcomedo. However, the presence of microorganisms is not a strict prerequisite for comedo formation (54). Further, *P. acnes* belongs to the resident cutaneous flora. It is possible, however, that *P. acnes* may play a role in comedogenesis by secreting lipase that hydrolyzes the triglycerides of sebum into free fatty acids and glycerol. Free fatty acids are likely to be comedogenic.

Cytokines

Cytokines are present in normal sebaceous glands (55), but under pathological conditions, the amount of cytokines released increases significantly. *P. acnes*, by acting on TLR-2, has been shown to be able to induce cytokines in the pilosebaceous unit (56,57). IL-6 and IL-8 are thus produced by follicular keratinocytes and IL-8 and IL-12 by macrophages. Barely detectable in the sebaceous glands of healthy skin, IL-6 concentrations are slightly higher in the uninvolved skin of acne patients and significantly higher in the acne-involved skin of the same patients (58). IL-1α has been implicated in the hypercornification of the infundibulum, which plays a central role in comedogenesis (19).

Inflammation

The importance of the bacteria in the induction and maintenance of the inflammatory phase of acne is well recognized. In contrast to what was initially thought, it is now generally accepted that inflammation is not only the result of comedone rupture but is also involved in initiating comedogenesis. This is achieved via the elaboration of IL-1α, whose expression and production is induced by *P. acnes*. An innate immune response to *P. acnes* also induces inflammation.

Integrin and Filaggrin

In vitro studies have confirmed that *P. acnes* is able to modulate the differentiation and proliferation of keratinocytes, by inducing the expression of integrin and filaggrin (filament-aggregating protein) derived from *P. acnes* (59,60), and thus playing a role in the formation of comedones. Biopsies of acne lesions that the keratinocyte differentiation alterations are associated with altered integrin expression (17). Integrins, which are cell adhesion proteins, play an important role in the modulation of keratinocyte proliferation and differentiation. In 1998, it was suggested that integrins might play a role in the initial events of acne lesion formation, as abnormal α2 and α3 integrin expression was observed around comedones and uninvolved follicles of acne patients, whereas the basal membrane was still intact (61). This disorder of integrin expression appears to coincide with the inflammatory events, suggesting that it precedes hyperproliferation, although whether it is responsible for it remains to be seen. Abnormal infundibular keratinization has been associated with a disorder in terminal differentiation of infundibular keratinocytes, which is related to increased filaggrin expression (62). Acneic skin has been shown to carry large amounts of filaggrin in the intermediate layers of the sebaceous duct and infundibulum, suggesting a premature terminal differentiation process in these particular areas of the PSU. Additionally, electron microscopy images have shown an increase in the number of keratohyaline granules in acne skin (62).

Biofilm

P. acnes biofilms appear to play a role in comedogenesis (16). A biofilm is an aggregation of microorganisms encased within a polysaccharide lining secreted by the microorganisms upon adherence to a surface. This lining allows for intermicrobial coherence as well as adherence to the surface. It has been recently discovered that *P. acnes* resides within a biofilm in the follicles, allowing the bacteria to adhere to the interior follicular surface. A *P. acnes* biofilm that penetrates into the sebum may act like an adhesive, leading to the increased sebum stickiness and thus corneocyte cohesiveness seen in the keratin plug in microcomedones. The recent decoding of the genome of *P. acnes* further supports the existence of a *P. acnes* biofilm (63,64). Further, the presence of a biofilm greatly increases bacterial resistance to antibiotic therapy.

THE DIFFERENT COMEDONAL SUBTYPES

Comedones can be categorized into several different subtypes, based on several factors including morphology, size, and chronology of appearance. In most patients, the various subtypes of comedones coexist. However, it is occasionally important to differentiate the different types to prescribe the appropriate treatment.

Microcomedones

Microcomedones represent the first subclinical acne lesions. These precursor lesions, which are clinically invisible, and only evident histologically, can be found in uninvolved skin of acne-prone individuals (4). Despite their subclinical nature, they require special therapeutic attention, because they represent the initial lesions that can eventually change into both noninflammatory and inflammatory acne lesions. Further, the number of microcomedones increases in correlation with worsening of acne severity (7).

As previously discussed, the factors that induce microcomedones include aberrant proliferation and differentiation of the follicular epithelium, excessive sebum production, and inflammatory events. Microcomedones can be sampled and studied by using cyanoacrylate follicular biopsies to sample material from the upper portion of the follicular duct (29).

Open and Closed Comedones

Open and closed comedones are the primary characteristics of noninflammatory acne. They are easily recognizable, follicle-based lesions that develop from microcomedones. Comedones may be open, as with blackheads, or closed, as with whiteheads, depending on the size of the follicular opening (65). Closed comedones are typically small, white-, or skin-colored papules and are usually found in higher numbers than open comedones. These lesions frequently go unrecognized. Bright light and stretching of the skin are sometimes necessary for visualization (66). Open comedones are then recognizable as papules with a dark central plug. Melanin deposition and lipid oxidation give the material in the follicle the typical black color (66).

Sand Paper Comedones

Sand paper comedones are confluent closed comedones frequently found on the forehead, which give the skin a rough, "sandpaper-like" feel (67). These dreaded comedones can be very difficult to treat, being frequently resistant to topical retinoid therapy and antibiotic treatment. Treatment with oral isotretinoin is often necessary for resistant cases.

Submarine Comedones

As with closed comedones, stretching of the skin may be necessary to see these lesions. Despite their large size, up to 1 cm in diameter, they are located deeper in the skin, away from the surface. They are probably best treated with cautery under local anesthesia.

Macrocomedones

Macrocomedones refer to closed or more commonly open comedones that are larger than 1 mm. The treatment of these cosmetically unflattering lesions may be very challenging. They are known for their potentially poor response to, or to slow down the effect of, oral isotretinoin (68). Macrocomedones can produce devastating acne flares, particularly if patients are inappropriately prescribed oral isotretinoin (69). Different treatment options have been proposed such as cautery therapy, specific extraction techniques, and photodynamic therapy (70,71).

Drug-Induced Comedones

Corticosteroids, androgens, and anabolic steroids are known potential triggers for comedonal drug-induced acne (67).

Chloracne

Chloracne is caused by exposure to halogenated aromatic compounds via cutaneous, pulmonary, or gastrointestinal exposure. This type of acne is primarily characterized by numerous persistent comedones that are frequently abnormally large. These large comedones can become confluent and form plaques. The lesion location is also typical: lesions in pre- and postauricular lesions and in the axillae or male genital region are well recognized. Systemic effects may persist years after exposure to the chloracne-producing agent.

Nevoid Comedones

Nevus comedonicus, first described by Kofmann in 1895, is a rare developmental abnormality of the PSU that presents as plaque of confluent comedones. The nevus comedonicus syndrome is characterized by a combination of nevus comedonicus with ipsilateral ocular, skeletal, or central nervous system abnormalities (72). Its treatment is challenging and numerous therapies have been reported, including surgical excision, dermabrasion, manual extraction, topical retinoids, oral isotretinoin, and laser treatments (73).

Conglobate Comedones

Acne conglobata is an uncommon, often therapy-resistant nodulocystic condition usually seen in males. This disorder typically begins in adulthood and is characterized by papules, pustules, nodules, abscesses, draining sinus tracts, and characteristically grouped polypored comedones involving the posterior neck and trunk (74).

REFERENCES

1. Strauss JS, Kligman AM. The pathologic dynamics of acne vulgaris. Br J Dermatol 1960; F50082:779–790.
2. Zouboulis CC. Acne and sebaceous gland function. Clin Dermatol 2004; 22: 360–366.
3. Georgel P, Crozat K, Lauth X, et al. A toll-like receptor 2-responsive lipid effector pathway protects mammals against skin infections with Gram-positive bacteria. Infect Immun 2005; 73:4512–4521.
4. Norris JF, Cunliffe WJ. A histological and immunocytochemical study of early acne lesions. Br J Dermatol 1988; 118:651–659.
5. Mills OH, Kligman AM. Human model for assessing comedogenic substances. Arch Dermatol 1982; 118:903–905.
6. Plewig G, Fulton JE, Kligman AM. Cellular dynamics of comedo formation in acne vulgaris. Arch Dermatol Forsch 1971; 242:12–29.
7. Holmes RL, Williams M, Cunliffe WJ. Pilosebaceous duct obstruction and acne. Br J Dermatol 1972; 87:327–332.
8. Knutson DD. Ultrastructural observations in acne vulgaris: the normal sebaceous follicle and acne lesions. J Invest Dermatol 1974; 62:288–307.
9. Toyoda M, Morohashi M. Pathogenesis of acne. Med Electron Microsc 2001; 34(1):29–40.
10. Knaggs HE, Holland DB, Morris C, et al. Quantification of cellular proliferation in acne using the monoclonal antibody Ki-67. J Soc Invest Dermatol 1994; 102:89–92.
11. Hughes BR, Morris C, Cunliffe WJ, et al. Keratin expression in pilosebaceous epithelia in truncal skin of acne patients. Br J Dermatol 1996; 134(2):247–256.
12. Cunliffe WJ, Holland DB, Clark SM, et al. Comedogenesis: some new aetiological, clinical and therapeutic strategies. Br J Dermatol 2000; 142(6):1084–1091.
13. Jiang CK, Magnaldo T, Ohtsuki M, et al. Epidermal growth factor and transforming growth factor α specifically induce the activation and hyperproliferation associated keratins 6 and 16. Proc Natl Acad Sci U S A 1993; 90:6786–6790.
14. Blumenberg M, Komine M, Rao L, et al. Blueprint to footprint to toeprint to culprit: regulation of K6 keratin gene promoter by extracellular signals and nuclear transcription factors. J Invest Dermatol 1998; 110:495.
15. Jiang CK, Flanagan S, Ohtsuki M, et al. Disease activated transcription factor: allergic reactions in human skin cause nuclear translocation of STAT-91 and induce synthesis of keratin 17. Mol Cell Biol 1994; 14:4759–4769.
16. Burkhart CG, Burkhart CN. Expanding the microcomedone theory and acne therapeutics: Propionibacterium acnes biofilm produces biological glue that holds corneocytes that form plug. J Am Acad Dermatol 2007; 57(4):722–724.

17. Jeremy AH, Holland DB, Roberts SG, et al. Inflammatory events are involved in acne lesion initiation. J Invest Dermatol 2003; 121:20–27.
18. Guy R, Kealey T. The effects of inflammatory cytokines on the isolated human sebaceous infundibulum. J Invest Dermatol 1998; 110(4):410–415.
19. Guy R, Green MR, Kealey T. Modeling acne in vitro. J Invest Dermatol 1996; 106:176–182.
20. Ingham E, Eady EA, Goodwin CE, et al. Pro-inflammatory levels of interleukin-1 alpha-like bioactivity are present in the majority of open comedones in acne vulgaris. J Invest Dermatol 1992; 98:895–901.
21. Kligman AM, Katz AC. Pathogenesis of acne vulgaris: I. Comedogenic properties of human sebum in external ear canal of the rabbit. Arch Dermatol 1968; 98:53–57.
22. Motoyoshi K. Enhanced comedo formation in rabbit ear skin by squalene and oleic acid peroxides. Br J Dermatol 1983; 109:191–198.
23. Downing DT, Stewart ME, Wertz PW, et al. Essential fatty acids and acne. J Am Acad Dermatol 1986; 14:221–225.
24. Shalita AR. Genesis of free fatty acids. J Invest Dermatol 1974; 62(3):332–335.
25. Cunliffe WJ, Gollnick H (BOEK). Acne: Diagnosis and Management. London: Martin Dunitz Ltd 2001; 15.
26. Voss JG. Acne vulgaris and free fatty acids. Arch Dermatol 1974; 109(6):894–898.
27. Tochio T, Tanaka H, Nakata S, et al. Accumulation of lipid peroxide in the content of comedones may be involved in the progression of comedogenesis and inflammatory changes in comedones. J Cosmet Dermatol 2009; 8(2):152–158.
28. Ziboh VA, Chapkin RS. Biologic significance of polyunsaturated fatty acids in the skin. Arch Dermatol 1987; 123:1688–1690.
29. Letawe C, Boone M, Pierard GE. Digital image analysis of the effect of topically applied linoleic acid on acne microcomedones. Clin Exp Dermatol 1998; 23:56–58.
30. Stewart ME, Greenwood R, Cunliffe WJ, et al. Effect of cyproterone acetate-ethinyl estradiol treatment on the proportions of linoleic and sebaleic acids in various skin surface lipid classes. Arch Dermatol Res 1986; 278(6):481–485.
31. Smith RN, Braue A, Varigos GA, et al. The effect of a low glycemic load diet on acne vulgaris and the fatty acid composition of skin surface triglycerides. J Dermatol Sci 2008; 50(1):41–52.
32. Pochi PE, Strauss JS. Sebaceous gland response in man to the administration of testosterone, delta-4-androstendione and dehydroisoandrosterone. J Invest Dermatol 1969; 52:32–36.
33. Thiboutot D, Knaggs H, Gilliland K, et al. Activity of 5-alpha-reductase and 17-betahydroxysteroid dehydrogenase in the infrainfundibulum of subjects with and without acne vulgaris. Dermatology 1998; 196:38–42.
34. Thiboutot D, Harris G, Iles V, et al. Activity of the type 1 5 alpha-reductase exhibits regional differences in isolated sebaceous glands and whole skin. J Invest Dermatol 1995; 105(2):209–214.
35. Maluki AH. The frequency of polycystic ovary syndrome in females with resistant acne vulgaris. J Cosmet Dermatol 2010; 9(2):142–148.
36. Schmidt JB, Spona J, Huber J. Androgen receptor in hirsutism and acne. Gynecol Obstet Invest 1986; 22(4):206–211.

37. Stewart ME, Downing DT, Cook JS, et al. Sebaceous gland activity and serum dehydroepiandrosterone sulfate levels in boys and girls. Arch Dermatol 1992; 128(10):1345–1348.

38. Lucky AW, Biro FM, Huster GA, et al. Acne vulgaris in premenarchal girls. An early sign of puberty associated with rising levels of dehydroepiandrosterone. Arch Dermatol 1994; 130(3):308–314.

39. Imperato-McGinley J, Gautier T, Cai LQ, et al. The androgen control of sebum production: studies of subjects with dihydrotestosterone deficiency and complete androgen insensitivity. J Clin Endocrinol Metab 1993; 76:524–528.

40. Bowe WP, Joshi SS, Shalita RR. Diet and acne. J Am Acad Dermatol 2010; 63(1):124–141.

41. Darling JA, Laing AH, Harkness RA. A survey of the steroids in cows' milk. J Endocrinol 1974; 62:291–297.

42. Adebamowo CA, Spiegelman D, Danby FW, et al. High school dietary dairy intake and teenage acne. J Am Acad Dermatol 2005; 52:207–214.

43. Hartmann S, Lacorn M, Steinhart H. Natural occurrence of steroid hormones in food. Food Chem 1998; 62:7–20.

44. Adebamowo CA, Spiegelman D, Berkey CS, et al. Milk consumption and acne in teenaged boys. J Am Acad Dermatol 2008; 58:787–93.

45. Thiboutot DM, Knaggs H, Gilliland K, et al. Activity of type 1 5 alpha-reductase is greater in the follicular infrainfundibulum compared with the epidermis. Br J Dermatol 1997; 136:166–171.

46. Eady EA, Cove JH. Is acne an infection of blocked pilosebaceous follicles? Implications for antimicrobial treatment. Am J Clin Dermatol 2000; 1:201–209.

47. Guy R, Kealey T. Modeling the infundibulum in acne. Dermatology 1998; 196:32–37.

48. Webster GF. Inflammation in acne vulgaris. J Am Acad Dermatol 1995; 33: 247–253.

49. Eady EA, Ingham E, Walters CE, et al. Modulation of comedonal levels of interleukin-1 in acne patients treated with tetracyclines. J Invest Dermatol 1993; 101:86–91.

50. Kealey T, Guy R. Modeling the infundibulum in acne. J Invest Dermatol 1997; 108:376.

51. Aldana OL, Holland DB, Cunliffe WJ. A role for interleukin-1α in comedogenesis (abstr). J Invest Dermatol 1998; 110:558.

52. Unna P. The Histopathology of Disease of the Skin. New York: Macmillan and Co., 1896.

53. Leyden JJ, McGinley KJ, Vowels B. Propionibacterium acnes colonization in acne and nonacne. Dermatology 1998; 196:55–58.

54. Leeming JP, Holland KT, Cunliffe WJ. The pathological and exological significance of microorganisms colonizing acne vulgaris comedones. J Med Microbiol 1985; 20(1):11–16.

55. Clarke SB, Nelson AM, George RE, et al. Pharmacologic modulation of sebaceous gland activity: mechanisms and clinical applications. Dermatol Clin 2007; 25: 137–146.

56. Kim J, Ochoa MT, Krutzik SR, et al. Activation of toll-like receptor 2 in acne triggers inflammatory cytokine responses. J Immunol 2002; 169:1535–1541.

57. Nagy I, Pivarcsi A, Koreck A, et al. Distinct strains of Propionibacterium acnes induce selective human beta-defensin-2 and interleukin-8 expression in human keratinocytes through toll-like receptors. J Invest Dermatol 2005; 124:931–938.

58. Alestas T, Ganceviciene R, Fimmel S, et al. Enzymes involved in the biosynthesis of leukotriene B4 and prostaglandin E2 are active in sebaceous glands. J Mol Med 2006; 84:75–87.

59. Jugeau S, Tenaud I, Knol AC, et al. Induction of toll-like receptors by Propionibacterium acnes. Br J Dermatol 2005; 153:1105–1113.

60. Jarrousse V, Castex-Rizzi N, Khammari A, et al. Modulation of integrins and filaggrin expression by Propionibacterium acnes extracts on keratinocytes. Arch Dermatol Res 2007; 299:441–447.

61. Holland DB, Aldana OL, Cunliffe WJ. Abnormal integrin expression in acne. J Invest Dermatol 1998; 110:559.

62. Kurokawa I, Mayer-da-Silva, Gollnick H, et al. Monoclonal antibody labeling for cytokeratins and filaggrin in the human pilosebaceous unit of normal, seborrhoeic and acne skin. J Invest Dermatol 1988; 91:566–571.

63. Bruggeman H, Henne A, Hoster F. The complete genome sequence of Propionibacterium acnes, a commensal of human skin. Science 2004; 205:671–673.

64. Burkhart CN, Burkhart CG. Genome sequence of Propionibacterium acnes reveals immunologic and surface-associated genes confirming existence of the acne biofilm. Int J Dermatol 2006; 45:872.

65. Shalita AR. Clinical aspects of acne. Dermatology 1998; 196(1):93–94.

66. Zaenglein AL, Thiboutot DM. Dermatology. In Bolognia JL, et al. (eds.). 2nd ed., Elsevier 2008.

67. Cunliffe WJ, Holland DB, Jeremy A. Comedone formation: etiology, clinical presentation, and treatment. Clin Dermatol 2004; 22(5):367–374.

68. Plewig G, Kligman AM. Induction of acne by topical steroids. Arch Dermatol Forsch 1973; 247(1):29–52.

69. Bottomley WW, Cunliffe WJ. Severe flares of acne following isotretinoin: large closed comedones (macrocomedones) are a risk factor. Acta Derm Venereol 1993; 73(1):74.

70. Kaya TI, Tursen U, Kokturk A, et al. An effective extraction technique for the treatment of closed macrocomedones. Dermatol Surg 2003; 29(7):741–744.

71. Fabbrocini G, Cacciapuoti S, De Vita V, et al. The effect of aminolevulinic acid photodynamic therapy on microcomedones and macrocomedones. Dermatology 2009; 219(4):322–328; [Epub October 23, 2009].

72. Happle R. The group of epidermal nevus syndromes. Part I. Well defined phenotypes. J Am Acad Dermatol 2010; 63(1):1–22.

73. Givan J, Hurley MY, Glaser DA. Nevus comedonicus: a novel approach to treatment. Dermatol Surg 2010; 36(5):721–725.

74. Shirakawa M, Uramoto K, Harada FA. Treatment of acne conglobata with infliximab. J Am Acad Dermatol 2006; 55(2):344–346.

1.5

Scarring

Thy Thy Do, Manisha Patel, and Sewon Kang

INTRODUCTION

A scar is defined as "fibrous tissue that replaces normal tissue destroyed by injury or disease" (1). In acne vulgaris, scarring is the end result of abnormal wound healing from damage to the pilosebaceous unit and surrounding tissue. Clinically, it may present as increased (hypertrophic or keloidal) or more commonly as loss (atrophy) of tissue.

Few studies have examined the incidence of acne scarring, with Goulden et al. reporting an 11% frequency of acne scars in men and 14% in women (2), while Layton et al. observed some degree of facial scarring in up to 95% of both men and women, but a higher incidence of scarring on the trunk was seen in men, as were hypertrophic and keloidal scars in these sites (3). Not surprisingly, there was a significant correlation between the severity of acne and degree of scarring in both sexes at all sites. Scars are often cosmetically unacceptable to patients, and they add to the significant psychosocial distress that is observed in patients with acne vulgaris (4). Concern for scar formation is one of the main motivating factors in patients seeking treatment for acne.

As in all wounded tissues, acne scars are the end result of various phases of healing that includes inflammation, formation of granulation and fibrous tissues, neovascularization, wound contracture, and tissue remodeling (5). However, the exact mechanism that initiates and leads to scarring in acne is not fully understood and is likely multifactorial in nature.

PATHOGENESIS

Several key factors are involved in acne pathogenesis including follicular hyperkeratinization, obstruction of sebaceous follicles, stimulation of sebaceous gland secretion by androgens, and colonization by the gram-positive bacteria *Propionibacterium acnes* (6). How inflammatory lesions develop is unclear, but the resulting inflammation is believed to play a key role in subsequent scarring. Similar to wound healing, acne scarring is a consequence of the complex interplay between the type of inflammatory response, dermal matrix remodeling, repetitive injury, and resulting imperfect repair (7).

A Study of Acne Scars

Although it is generally accepted that acne scars result from inflammatory lesions, few studies have vigorously examined their evolution. A recent photographic tracking study of facial acne scars over a 12-week period demonstrated that the most common type of scar in patients with mild to moderate acne is ice pick (69%), followed by boxcar (29%) and rolling scars (2%) (8). At week 12, a total of 104 scars were identified in 22 subjects. When all the atrophic scars were tracked to week 0, 53 were clinically normal skin, 30 were established scars, and 21 were acne lesions (7 papules, 6 erythematous macules, 4 pustules, and 4 closed comedones). No open comedones at baseline corresponded to atrophic scars. Papules, closed comedones, and erythematous macules at baseline were mostly associated with ice pick, followed by boxcar, and then rolling scars. Interestingly, all pustular lesions present at week 0 corresponded with only boxcar scars at week 12. These results confirm that inflammatory acne lesions often lead to atrophic scarring. Furthermore, it suggests that 12 weeks is long enough to develop and establish atrophic scars.

Interestingly, this study also suggests that some scarring may arise from initially noninflammatory lesions. Jeremy et al. demonstrated that inflammatory events are involved in acne lesion initiation (9). Biopsy specimens of clinically normal pilosebaceous follicles from acne patients showed vascular endothelial cell activation, an increased number of macrophages, and upregulation of the proinflammatory cytokine interleukin (IL)-1. Furthermore, biopsies of clinically noninflamed facial comedones showed significant upregulation of inflammatory mediators including human β-defensin 2, IL-8, matrix metalloproteinase (MMP)-1, MMP-9, and MMP-13 (10). Taken together, aggressive treatment of inflammatory and noninflammatory acne is likely warranted to minimize acne scarring.

Stages of Wound Healing

Although normal wound healing is not an exact mirror to acne scar formation, it provides an important framework to better understand the mechanism of scarring. The three phases that define wound healing are inflammatory, proliferative, and remodeling (11).

1. The inflammatory phase is composed of cellular and vascular responses. Inflammatory cells such as neutrophils and monocytes are induced to migrate to the wound by chemotactic factors and inflammatory mediators, which also serve to upregulate adhesion molecules that mediate cell-cell binding. Other mediators such as histamine, complements, and growth factors contribute to the inflammatory phase resulting in vasodilation, fibroblast proliferation, and mast cell activation. The increased fluid leakage into the extravascular space and blockade of lymphatic drainage give rise to the signs of inflammation—rubor (redness), tumor (swelling), and calor (heat). However, macrophages are considered the most important regulatory cell in the inflammatory reaction and allow for induction of angiogenesis and formation of granulation tissue. The acute inflammatory reaction usually lasts 24 to 48 hours but can persist up to two weeks or longer in some patients.

2. The proliferative phase is characterized by cellular responses that involve angiogenesis and fibroplasia three to five days after wounding. Angiogenesis refers to new vessel formation (revascularization) that provides oxygen and nutrients to the wound. Hypoxia in wounds can stimulate the profibrotic cytokine transforming growth factor (TGF)-β and collagen synthesis and therefore promote increased fibrosis (12). Fibroplasia is the reinforcement of injured tissue with new granulation tissue, consisting of new vessels and fibroblasts that produce matrix materials including elastin, proteoglycans, and collagen (predominantly type III), during early wounding.

3. The remodeling phase is a dynamic process of deposition and changes in the extracellular matrix. Importantly, it heralds the change from type III collagen that is made in the early phase of healing to type I collagen that normally makes up 80% of the collagen found in preinjured dermis. Enzymatic activities of collagenases facilitate this transition, and the stimulus for this conversion between collagen types may be the mechanical strain on the wound (13). Therefore, more scar tissue is necessary in areas of the body that are on mobile extremities, which may also explain why hypertrophic and keloidal scars in acne have a greater predilection for the shoulders than, for example, the face.

Inflammatory Cascade in Acne Scarring

In addition to the changes described above, an inflammatory cascade involving activated protein (AP)-1, nuclear factor (NF)-κB signaling, and MMPs have been shown to have a crucial role in acne scarring (7). MMPs are a family of zinc-dependent endopeptidases that are capable of degrading extracellular matrix proteins including collagen. In inflammatory acne lesions, there is increased gene transcription of AP-1 regulated MMPs (Fig. 1.5.1) (7).

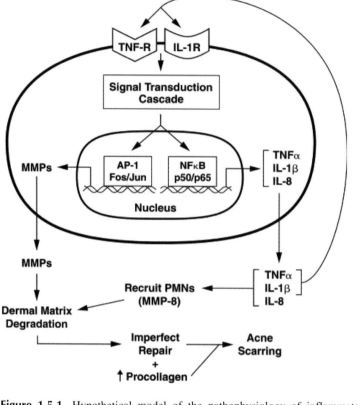

Figure 1.5.1 Hypothetical model of the pathophysiology of inflammatory acne and dermal damage. In inflammatory acne lesions, NF-κB signaling is activated. As a consequence, NF-κB-driven inflammatory cytokine genes (e.g., TNF-α and IL-1β) are induced. These primary cytokines will propagate the inflammatory response by acting on endothelial cells to elaborate adhesion molecules (e.g., ICAM-1) to facilitate recruitment of inflammatory cells into the skin. TNF-α and IL-1β will also stimulate the production of secondary cytokines, such as IL-8, which can aid in chemotaxis of inflammatory cells. By working through their cell surface receptors, TNF-α and IL-1β not only amplify the NF-κB signaling cascade but also activate MAP kinases to stimulate AP-1-mediated gene transcription. As a consequence of AP-1 activation (c-Jun induction), AP-1-driven MMPs are elaborated by resident skin cells. Along with MMP-8 and neutrophil elastase brought in by PMNs, they degrade the surrounding dermal matrix. This is followed by matrix synthesis and repair, which is imperfect. Most of the imperfections would leave clinically undetectable deficits in the organization or composition, or both of the extracellular matrix. However, when they occur to a significant extent throughout time, accompanied by sustained procollagen synthesis, acne scarring becomes clinically visible. *Abbreviations*: NF-κB, nuclear factor-κB; TNF, tumor necrosis factor; IL, interleukin; MAP, mitogen-activated protein; AP-1, activated protein-1. *Source*: From Ref. 7.

1. *NF-κB* is a transcription factor important in the upregulation of many proinflammatory cytokine genes, including tumor necrosis factor (TNF)-α and IL-1β that propagate the inflammatory response by acting on endothelial cells to increase the expression of adhesion molecules and thus facilitate recruitment of inflammatory cells into the skin. TNF-α and IL-1β also stimulate the production of secondary cytokines such as IL-8 by keratinocytes, which increases the influx of inflammatory cells such as neutrophils. Although TNF-α and IL-1β primarily signal through the NF-κB signaling pathway, they also activate the AP-1 pathway through mitogen-activated protein (MAP) kinases.

2. *AP-1* is a critical regulator of several MMPs including MMP-1 (collagenase-I), MMP-3 (stromelysin-I), and MMP-9 (92-kD gelatinase or collagenase-4), all of which are overexpressed in inflammatory acne lesions (7). MMP-1 is critical in the degradation of mature type 1 collagen, which is the predominant collagen in the dermis. Upon initial cleavage of collagen by collagenases (MMP-1, MMP-8, MMP-13), resulting gelatin is further degraded by other MMPs such as gelatinase and stromeolysin.

Matrix Synthesis and Repair in Acne Scarring

As part of wound healing, matrix degradation is followed by matrix synthesis and repair, with increased expression of procollagens I and III, which are increased in inflammatory acne lesions. Concomitant increase in TGF-β1 level suggests participation of this profibrotic cytokine (7). These sequences of events would leave imperfections in the organization, composition, or both of the extracellular matrix that may not be clinically detectable. That may explain why some and not all inflammatory lesions progress to scarring. However, with significant magnitude in their changes (matrix degradation and procollagen synthesis), clinically visible acne scars are expected to result. When acne lesions are physically manipulated by patients, this process is aggravated. Therefore, an aberration in the dynamic interactions between the various components of wound healing that govern the direction of repair can lead to clinical expression of acne scars (excessive hypertrophic scars at one end and loss of substance in atrophic scars at the other end of the spectrum) (14).

FACTORS INFLUENCING SCAR FORMATION

Genetics are important in determining individual susceptibility to acne. In a study of 204 patients over the age of 25 with facial acne that persisted from adolescence, the risk of adult acne occurring in a relative was significantly higher than that for the relative of an unaffected individual (15). Although similar studies examining the familial risk of scarring are lacking, genetics are likely to play a role as not all patients with inflammatory acne will scar and patients often report that their parents also have severe scarring from acne in their youths.

Data suggest that the likelihood of scarring is associated with the type of inflammatory response. Holland et al. observed that in inflammatory lesions from patients who have less scarring, there is a brisk inflammatory cellular infiltrate composed of T-helper lymphocytes, macrophages, and Langerhans cells, with accompanying angiogenesis that quickly resolves compared with patients who are prone to scarring, where the inflammation and angiogenesis start slowly but is maintained over a longer period. It is speculated that the prolonged inflammatory response in patients prone to scarring is a delayed-type hypersensitivity reaction to persistent antigenic stimulus that they were initially unable to eliminate (16). As there is no tool to predict who will develop this delayed-type reaction, treating early inflammation is the best approach in preventing acne scarring.

CLASSIFICATION OF ACNE SCARS

Acne scars are broadly divided into either increased tissue formation (hypertrophic or keloidal) or, more commonly, loss of tissue (atrophic). They can have associated color changes including erythema with or without associated telangiectasias and hyper and/or hypopigmentation. Hypertrophic/keloidal scars can be symptomatic with pruritus or pain (6).

Hypertrophic/Keloidal Scars

Hypertrophic and keloidal scars are associated with excess collagen formation and decreased collagenase activity. Hypertrophic scars are usually pink, raised, and firm lesions that remain within the borders of the original site of injury. In contrast, keloids form as reddish-purple papules and nodules that proliferate beyond the borders of the original wound. Histologically, hypertrophic scars and keloids both exhibit excess collagen in whorled masses with varying numbers of fibroblastic cells. In addition, keloids demonstrate characteristic hyalinized hypocellular zones of fibrous tissue in contrast to more cellular nodules in hypertrophic scars (17). Acne-associated hypertrophic and keloidal scars are often found on the upper trunk, more commonly seen in men and in people with darker-pigmented skin (18).

Atrophic Scars

Different types of atrophic scars have been defined according to the degree and depth of scarring, a reflection of the extent of inflammation, which is usually below the epidermis, at the infrainfundibular region of the pilosebaceous unit. The widely used atrophic scar categories as proposed by Jacob et al. are "ice pick," "rolling," and "boxcar" (19). Ice pick scars are narrow (<2 mm), sharply delineated, and tapered at the base in the dermis or subcutaneous tissue forming a "V" shape. It is usually too deep for treatment with conventional skin resurfacing. Rolling scars occur from subdermal tethering, creating a shallow broad scar that is usually 4 to 5 mm wide, and successful treatment depends on correcting the subdermal component. Boxcar scars are broad and can be shallow or deep with sharp vertical edges that do not taper at the base like ice pick scars. However, although the precise categorization helps facilitate choosing the type of therapy, acne scars are sometimes mixed and not easily classifiable (Fig. 1.5.2). To help standardize grading of acne scar severity, a few systems have been proposed including the ECCA scale (échelle d'évaluation Clinique des cicatrices d'acné) designed for clinical use. The authors reported good interobserver reliability for the scale, which is based on qualitative assessment of six scar types (using their own classification of atrophic scars) and a quantitative score for each scar type identified (determined semiquantitatively by a four-point scale from no scar to many scars >20) multiplied by a weighting factor (keloid scars have the highest weight) to produce the final score of severity (20). Goodman and Baron also developed a quantitative global scarring grading system, which assigns points based on the type and number of scars, with fewer points given for macular and mild atrophic scars (21). These grading systems help standardize discussions on acne scars in clinical practice and research.

TREATMENT

Treatment of acne scars depends on several factors including the individual patient, types of scars present, and costs involved. There are numerous available options with varying efficacy including medical (e.g., corticosteroids, silicone, retinoids), surgical (e.g., primary elliptical excision, punch excision, punch elevation, subcision, skin grafting, debulking), procedural (cryotherapy, chemical peels, microdermabrasion), and emerging new technologies including lasers (e.g., ablative, nonablative, and light) and tissue augmentation (e.g., dermal fillers) (22). The optimal therapy depends on the scar type. For example, intralesional corticosteroids is usually the first line of treatment for hypertrophic and keloid scars. Punch excision is best for ice pick scars with deep bases and narrow (<3 mm) deep boxcar scars. Wide (>3 mm), deep boxcar scars can be treated with either punch excision or punch elevation, while shallow boxcar scars are best treated with laser resurfacing. Dermal fillers can be used for rolling scars; however, the benefit is temporary, and therefore, subcision may be preferred (19).

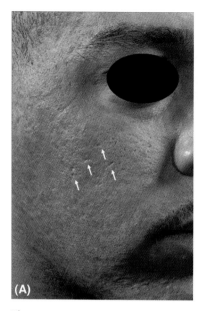 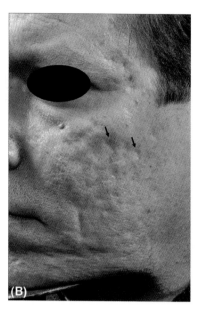

Figure 1.5.2 (**A**) Multiple acne scars on the cheeks and chin, likely a result of previous significant inflammatory acne with no active areas of inflammation. The predominant scar type is ice pick (*white arrows*), characterized by small (usually <2 mm), sharply delineated scars that are tapered at the base forming a "V" shape. (**B**) This patient's acne scars are predominantly the rolling type (*black arrows*). They are usually broad (4–5 mm) and shallow with sloping edges. (**C**) Patients can have a combination of different types of atrophic scars, including ice pick (*white arrow*), rolling (*black arrow*), and boxcar (*black arrowhead*). The latter are broad and can be shallow or deep with sharp vertical edges, forming a "U" shape, and they do not taper at the base like ice pick scars. Often patients have atrophic scars that do not neatly fit into any category. (**D**) Although patients often demonstrate different types of atrophic scarring, many often have a predominant subtype. A recent study demonstrated that ice pick scars (*white arrow*) are the most common type, followed by boxcar (*arrowhead*) and rolling (*black arrow*). (**E**) Acne scarring is often the unwanted complication of inflammatory acne, as demonstrated in this patient who already has several atrophic scars including ice pick (*white arrow*) and boxcar (*black arrowhead*), in addition to inflammatory papules and pustules. (**F**) This patient has prominent ice pick (*white arrow*) and rolling scars (*black arrow*) on the cheeks, in addition to several closed comedones. Comedones are considered precursors to inflammatory acne lesions and can sometimes result in scarring. (**G**) Atrophic acne scars can be erythematous, hyper-, or hypopigmented as demonstrated in this patient who has a number of hypopigmented rolling scars (*white arrowhead*). *Source*: All photographs courtesy of the University of Michigan, Program for Clinical Research in Dermatology.

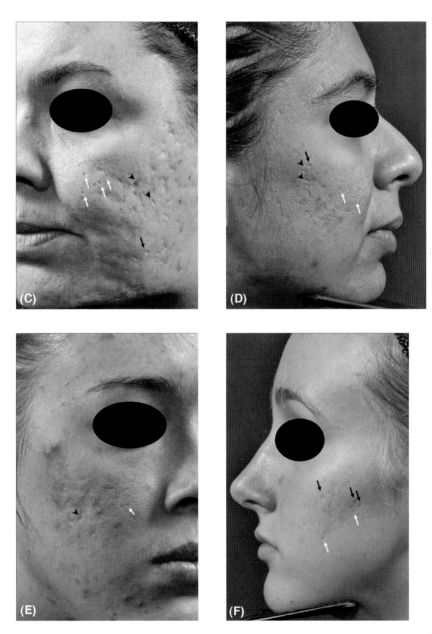

(*Continued*)

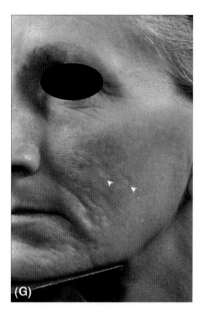

Figure 1.5.2 (*Continued*)

However, prevention is always preferred. Retinoids have been shown to reduce inflammation in acne through inhibition of migration of leukocytes in the skin (23). In addition, isotretinoin reduces the expression of MMP-9 and MMP-13 in the sebum of acne patients (24). Therefore, these agents may reduce the risk of subsequent scar formation by shifting the balance of MMPs and tissue inhibitors toward normal (6).

CONCLUSION

Scarring is an untoward result in patients with mild to severe acne vulgaris. It is a consequence of the complex interplay between inflammation, repetitive injury, and wound healing, which can be compounded by host and environmental factors. Further elucidation into the complexity of acne scar development is needed to help prevent this outcome as effective scar therapies remain limited.

REFERENCES

1. Scar. The American Heritage Stedman's Medical Dictionary. Houghton Mifflin Company. Available at: http://dictionary.reference.com/browse/scar. Accessed September 4, 2010.

2. Goulden V, Stables GI, Cunliffe WJ. Prevalence of facial acne in adults. J Am Acad Dermatol 1999; 41(4):577–580.

3. Layton AM, Henderson CA, Cunliffe WJ. A clinical evaluation of acne scarring and its incidence. Clin Exp Dermatol 1994; 19(4):303–308.

4. Koo J. The psychosocial impact of acne: patients' perceptions. J Am Acad Dermatol 1995; 32(5 pt 3):S26–S30.

5. Goodman GJ. Post-acne scarring: a short review of its pathophysiology. Australas J Dermatol 2001; 42(2):84–90.

6. Thiboutot D, Gollnick H, Bettoli V, et al. New insights into the management of acne: an update from the Global Alliance to Improve Outcomes in Acne group. J Am Acad Dermatol 2009; 60(5 suppl):S1–S50.

7. Kang S, Cho S, Chung JH, et al. Inflammation and extracellular matrix degradation mediated by activated transcription factors nuclear factor-kappa and activator protein-1 in inflammatory acne lesions in vivo. Am J Pathol 2005; 166(6):1691–1699.

8. Patel MJ, Antony A, Do TT, et al. Atrophic acne scars may arise from both inflammatory and non-inflammatory acne lesions. J Investig Dermatol 2010; 130 (suppl 1s):S58.

9. Jeremy AH, Holland DB, Roberts SG, et al. Inflammatory events are involved in acne lesion initiation. J Invest Dermatol 2003; 121(1):20–27.

10. Lee W, Do TT, Wang F, et al. Upregulation of pro-inflammatory markers in open and closed comedones in acne vulgaris. J Investig Dermatol 2009; 129(suppl 1s): S58.

11. Li J, Chen J, Krasner R. Pathophysiology of acute wound healing. Clin Dermatol 2007; 25(1):9–18.

12. Falanga V, Martin TA, Takagi H, et al. Low oxygen tension increases mRNA levels of alpha 1 (I) procollagen in human dermal fibroblasts. J Cell Physiol 1993; 157(2):408–412.

13. Wang Z, Fong KD, Pham TT, et al. Increased transcriptional response to mechanical strain in keloid fibroblasts due to increased focal adhesion complex formation. J Cell Physiol 2006; 206(2):510–517.

14. Tuan TL, Nichter LS. The molecular basis of keloid and hypertrophic scar formation. Mol Med Today 1998; 4(1):19–24.

15. Goulden V, McGeown CH, Cunliffe WJ. The familial risk of adult acne: a comparison between first-degree relatives of affected and unaffected individuals. Br J Dermatol 1999; 141(2):297–300.

16. Holland DB, Jeremy AH, Roberts SG, et al. Inflammation in acne scarring: a comparison of the responses in lesions from patients prone and not prone to scar. Br J Dermatol 2004; 150(1):72–81.

17. Beer TW, Lam MH, Heenan PJ. Tumors of fibrous tissue involving the skin. In: Elder DE, Elenitsas R, Johnson BL Jr., et al., eds. Lever's Histopathology of the Skin. 10th ed. Philadelphia: Lippincott Williams & Wilkins, 2009.

18. Child FJ, Fuller LC, Higgins EM, et al. A study of the spectrum of skin disease occurring in a black population in south-east London. Br J Dermatol 1999; 141(3):512–517.

19. Jacob CI, Dover JS, Kaminer MS. Acne scarring: a classification system and review of treatment options. J Am Acad Dermatol 2001; 45(1):109–117.
20. Dréno B, Khammari A, Orain N, et al. ECCA grading scale: an original validated acne scar grading scale for clinical practice in dermatology. Dermatology 2007; 214(1):46–51.
21. Goodman GJ, Baron JA. Postacne scarring–a quantitative global scarring grading system. J Cosmet Dermatol 2006; 5(1):48–52.
22. Rivera AE. Acne scarring: a review and current treatment modalities. J Am Acad Dermatol 2008; 59(4):659–676.
23. Zouboulis CC. Isotretinoin revisited: pluripotent effects on human sebaceous gland cells. J Invest Dermatol 2006; 126(10):2154–2156.
24. Papakonstantinou E, Aletras AJ, Glass E, et al. Matrix metalloproteinases of epithelial origin in facial sebum of patients with acne and their regulation by isotretinoin. J Invest Dermatol 2005; 125(4):673–684.

2.1

Enhancing the success of acne therapy

Alan R. Shalita

Current concepts of acne therapy date to the mid-20th century with the introduction of broad-spectrum antibiotics, notably the tetracyclines, and estrogen, in the form of oral contraceptives. This was followed by enhanced topical therapy with the introduction of benzoyl peroxide in the 1950s, topical tretinoin in the early 1970s, and, a short time later, by topical antibiotics. Topical acne therapy was augmented further by improved formulations for all available agents, and the introduction of adapalene and tazarotene in the mid-1990s. Estrogen therapy for acne was enhanced by combination with antiandrogens, cyproterone in other countries, and drospirenone, a spironolactone derivative, in the United States. The introduction of oral isotretinoin in 1982 was a monumental step forward, revolutionizing the treatment of severe, refractory acne. More recently, combinations of benzoyl peroxide with antibiotics or retinoids and retinoids with antibiotics have simplified compliance with treatment programs. All of these will be covered in this section.

The issue of compliance, however, remains a principle concern in all forms of acne treatment. Acne can have devastating physical as well as emotional effects, and thus it is critical that the patient be made aware of the nature of the disease process and what is to be expected from the treatment regimen prescribed. Failure to take the time to do this is a "key to the highway" of therapeutic failure in many patients. There are, of course, other factors that can affect compliance with acne treatment. The reluctant child with the dominant parent often leads to a lack of adherence to the prescribed treatment and provides a source of increased friction between parents and children, particularly in teenage acne. Some young, teenage boys are not yet concerned about their acne, yet their parents insist on dragging them to the dermatologist. The physician needs to deftly "connect" with both the patient and parent, explaining in an understandable manner how acne can continue to worsen the potential benefits of "staying on top of it" with treatment, and the importance of working the use of their medication into their daily routine. Overprescribing is another common reason for poor compliance. I have seen many patients who have been prescribed topical medication morning and evening with oral antibiotics and then sold cleansers, moisturizers and/or heating instruments, cleansing brushes, etc. It is much better to begin simply, albeit with a regimen tailored to the severity of acne, and add medication as necessary, all the time explaining the treatment program, the anticipated time course of response, and gaining the trust of the patient with sincere "eye-to-eye" contact. Above all, anticipate and explain the common side effects, and arrange the treatment to minimize unwanted effects in the beginning to allow the patient to gradually accommodate. Finally, it is useful to use examples the patient can relate to, in order to explain proper use of medication. For example, we usually tell our patients to apply an amount of medication equivalent to a small green pea for each cheek and spread it out evenly. For oral isotretinoin, we not only tell the patient that it is a fat-soluble vitamin, best absorbed with food, but also use the illustration of a cheeseburger with a milkshake, for illustration purposes and not as a recommended "diet for life." Ultimately, success occurs not only with their consistency but also with yours.

2.2

The relationship between acne and diet

Whitney P. Bowe, Maria C. Kessides, and Alan R. Shalita

INTRODUCTION

After the publication of a few landmark studies in the 1960s concluding that there is no relationship between diet and acne, the dogmatic teaching among dermatologists was as such for the next several decades. Interestingly, during this time of skepticism, the perception of a relationship between diet and acne persisted among patients across the world (1–3) and even among young medical school graduates (4). In the last 5 to 10 years, several compelling studies have introduced some intriguing new evidence supporting the link between diet and acne. Here we present the most up-to-date and strongest evidence regarding a relationship between acne and the intake of carbohydrates, dairy, ω-3 fatty acids, antioxidants, zinc, vitamin A, and iodine.

CARBOHYDRATES AND ACNE

The strongest evidence favoring a relationship between diet and acne lies in a correlation between acne severity and carbohydrate intake. It has been observed through a survey-based study that acne severity may be related to intake of foods high in sugar (5), but the research in this area has broadened to quantify carbohydrate intake in general. Most of the studies in the area of carbohydrate intake utilize the glycemic index (GI) as a tool for quantifying serum glucose and insulin levels for various foods and then relating these measurements to clinical outcome. For instance, some of the most interesting evidence on glycemic index and its correlation with acne severity comes from studies on acne among peoples of non-Western societies where they consume very little highly refined foods with high glycemic indices. A cross-sectional study conducted in 2002 by Cordain et al. among peoples in Papua New Guinea and Paraguay found no acne among a total of 1300 subjects (6), although environmental influence and genetic pool were not taken into account (7,8).

Developed in 1981, the glycemic index is a numerical unit assigned to a given food that reflects the rate at which its consumption increases serum glucose and insulin (9). Similarly, the glycemic load was developed in 1997 to quantify total increase in serum glucose and insulin after multiplying glycemic index by carbohydrate content and serving size (10,11). In short, foods of a low glycemic index tend to be raw vegetables and multigrains, whereas those with higher glycemic index are comprised of more refined carbohydrates such as white spaghetti, cereal, chips, cookies, or foods made with white flour (12). While there is a perpetual challenge of isolating diet as a single variable among many with potential influences on acne, there is a common conclusion among these aforementioned studies that those foods with the highest glycemic index are associated with greater acne severity.

To date, the mechanism for this correlation is still theoretical. One notion holds that acne pathogenesis is the downstream effect of hyperinsulinemia and its upregulation and stimulation of various endocrinological pathways that include androgens, insulin-like growth factor 1 (IGF-1), insulin-like growth factor binding protein 3 (IGFBP-3), and retinoid signaling cascades (13). Growth hormone (GH) is released by the anterior pituitary gland and stimulates GH receptors in the liver to form and release IGF-1, which then mediates the effects of GH (14). IGF-1 also serves as a surrogate marker for GH, which is potentially involved in acne pathogenesis (15). IGFBP-3 binds to both IFG-1 and IFG-2 and stabilizes it for transport in the serum, but then frees IFG at its receptors so that it may be biologically active (16). Thus, levels of IGFBP-3 are negatively correlated with levels of biologically active IGF-1. All of these pathways may influence various factors in acne pathogenesis such as sebum production, overgrowth of follicular epithelium, and abnormal keratinization (13).

The best clinical illustration of hyperinsulinemia and its concomitant endrocrinologic pathways that affect acne is in adult women with polycystic ovarian syndrome (PCOS). This condition is marked by hyperinsulinemia, insulin resistance, hyperandrogenemia, and resulting hyperandrogenism characterized by hirsutism and acne (17). When the hyperinsulinemia is targeted for therapy, symptoms improve, illustrating that hyperandrogenism and hyperinsulinemia may be linked. For instance, it has been shown that these patients have improvements in symptoms when treated with medications to improve insulin sensitivity such as metformin, tobutamide, pioglitazone, and acarbose (18,19). Furthermore, when they consume a diet comprised of foods with a low glycemic index, their androgen levels normalize (20).

Elevated IGF-1 levels and testosterones such as dehydroepiandrosterone sulfate (DHEAS) and dihydrotestosterone (DHT) have been reported to be correlated with acne lesion count, and IGF-1 may influence testosterone production and vice versa (21). In one study, adult women with acne were found to have elevated IGF-1 levels, and IGF-1, in addition to DHEAS and DHT, correlated with comedonal and inflammatory lesion count. However, men with acne did not have significantly higher levels of IGF-1 when compared with their controls, nor did the levels correlate with acne count (21). A study in which postmenopausal women were administered DHEA found that IGF-1 levels rose in addition to testosterone (22), and IGF-1 has been shown to promote expression of steroidogenic enzymes that create precursors to both DHEAS and androgens (23).

Nonetheless, GH may influence acne severity independently of androgen levels. A study from 1995 on postadolescent eumenorrheic women with acne found that in comparison with their age- and sex-matched controls, they possessed higher IGF-1 levels. However, higher IGF-1 levels did not necessarily correlate with higher androgens (free and total testosterone, DHEA-S) or acne severity (15). A subsequent study also among postadolescent eumenorrheic women with acne attempted to correlate androgen levels with both basal insulin levels and insulin measured after an oral glucose tolerance test (OGTT). The OGTT involves administering 75 grams of oral glucose and then measuring serum insulin levels two hours thereafter. When compared with their age- and sex-matched controls, the women with acne had higher levels of DHEA-S, DHT, and serum free testosterone, but comparable levels of basal insulin. However, the subjects with acne showed evidence of insulin resistance after administration of the OGTT in that they demonstrated significantly higher levels of summed insulin. Also at the two-hour mark, androgen levels were drawn in both the acne patients and their controls, and neither total nor free testosterone was shown to have changed significantly with administration of the OGTT (24). Thus, while adult women with acne and higher levels of androgens show evidence of postprandial hyperinsulinemia, it does not appear to have a direct or at least immediate effect on androgen levels.

A series of two cohort studies by Smith et al. on males with acne showed evidence that foods with a low glycemic load may decrease androgen bioavailability and improve insulin resistance, but the role of weight loss as it relates to these outcomes is unclear. When 23 young males with acne adhered to a diet with a low glycemic load, they experienced reductions in weight and BMI, decreased free androgen index, increased IGFBP-1, and improved insulin sensitivity. Nonetheless, whether weight reduction or low glycemic load improved these parameters is unclear, as adjustment for BMI resulted in a loss of significance in the association of low glycemic load and both lesion count and insulin resistance (25,26). A subsequent prospective cohort study randomized males with acne to diets of low and high glycemic indices, and designed their food intake to avoid weight changes. The results indicated that in comparison with the subjects who consumed a diet with a low glycemic load, those consuming a high glycemic load showed evidence of higher androgen ability, and the subjects who consumed a low glycemic load had evidence of increases in IGF-1-binding proteins and, therefore, decreased IGF-1 bioavailability (27). While neither of these studies are generalizable to women and are limited by small sample size, their results question whether glycemic load or its frequent result in weight reduction is responsible for the changes in serum free androgens, insulin sensitivity, or IGF-1 bioavailability.

Several of the aforementioned studies conducted on acne severity as it relates to glycemic load and glycemic index are limited by small sample size, failure to control for weight changes that may affect serum insulin levels, and inability to generalize results to women or nonadolescent males. Nonetheless, the results across all studies are consistent in suggesting that low glycemic loads may improve acne severity, and more carefully designed studies should certainly be conducted to validate these preliminary findings.

DAIRY

Many of the studies conducted to investigate the connection between dairy and acne relied on self-reported questionnaires regarding dairy intake, and yet the conclusions remained consistent. For instance, two retrospective studies separated by over 50 years assessed the acne severity in their subjects as it related to self-reported dairy intake (28,29). Both studies concluded that not only dairy intake was related to acne severity but also the type of milk most frequently implicated was skim milk (28,29). Two prospective studies in 2006 and 2008 upheld these previous findings (30,31). In two cohorts of adult women (29,31) and boys (30), a positive correlation remained between skim milk and acne severity.

The aforementioned studies published from 2005 onward demonstrate an association between milk and acne in three separate populations. Nonetheless, they were limited by their reliance on subjects' self-reports rather than objective measures as well as their observational design that falls short of the gold standard randomized controlled clinical trial (29–31). Lastly, the associations that were detected were all weak by epidemiological standards in that the odds ratios of associations were consistently close to one.

The comedogenicity of milk draws on its tendency to increase IGF-1 levels, and its containing testosterone prescursors such as androstenedione and DHEA-S (32). These precursors are reduced by 5α-reductase to form DHT, which directly stimulates sebum production at hair follicles. At the same time, DHT may be formed directly from 5α-reduced testosterones such as 5α-androstanedione and 5α-pregnanedione, both of which are found in milk (32,33). Thus, endogenous testosterone precursors, in addition to 5α-reduced testosterones, ingested with milk are channeled toward the same hormonal pathway to form DHT, which stimulates sebum production and hyperkeratinization of the pilosebaceous unit.

FATTY ACIDS

The effects of glycemic load may extend beyond hormonal pathways to include an effect on sebum composition, which was recently shown to be related to acne severity (34). That is, adolescent males who consumed a low glycemic load diet produced sebum with a higher ratio of skin surface fatty acids (SFAs) to monounsaturated fatty acids (MUFAs), and they also had fewer acne lesions. Also, increased sebum production or the stimulation of sebum production was associated with a higher proportion of MUFAs, suggesting that desaturase enzyme in sebaceous lipogenesis may play a key role in sebum production, modification, and then acne development.

Moreover, the role of polyunsaturated fatty acids and specifically the relative ratio of ω-6 to ω-3 fatty acids may have direct effects on the inflammatory pathway involved in acne development (35,36). Whereas fat intake in a typical Western diet is mainly comprised of ω-6 fatty acids, the fat intake of non-Western or hunter-gather societies is mainly comprised of ω-3 fatty acids with a higher intake of fish, wild game, and vegetables (37). In fact, the current ratio of ω-6 to ω-3 fatty acids intake in North America is 20:1, which is stark contrast to the 2:1 ratio recommendation by lipid panel experts (38). Although a previous study by Cordain et al. attributed lower acne prevalence among non-Western societies to their intake of foods with lower glycemic load (6), it has been postulated that the intake of a higher ratio of ω-3 to ω-6 fatty acids among these non-Western societies could be another factor in decreasing acne prevalence through both hormonal and anti-inflammatory effects (37). First, ω-3 polyunsaturated fatty acids (PUFAs) have been associated with lower IGF-1 levels (39). Second, ω-3 PUFAs may suppress cytokine production (36) in that they inhibit the formation of leukotriene B4 (LTB4), which is linked with inflammatory acne (40). Proinflammatory eicosanoids such as prostaglandin E2 (PGE2) and LTB4 are derived from ω-6 fatty acids such as arachidonic acid (AA) (41). Omega-6 fatty acids found in fish such as eicosapentaenoic acid (EPA) and docosahexaenoic acid (DHA) may act as competitive inhibitors of AA conversion into PGE2 or LTB4.

However, one study has suggested that the relative concentration of ω-3 fatty acids in the body may also be affected by estrogen, thereby suggesting a new mechanism of birth control pills and their effects on acne. Women have been found to have higher levels of DHA, and consumption of birth control pills increases DHA, while administration of testosterone decreases it; at the same time, administration of estradiols to male to female transsexual subjects resulted in an increase in DHA. Thus, it is possible that estradiols in birth control pills exert their positive effect on improving acne by increasing the ratio of ω-3 fatty acids in the body (42).

Nonetheless, very few studies among humans have been conducted to establish the role of fatty acid consumption and acne. An epidemiologic study conducted in 1961 associated the consumption of large amounts of fish, a potent source of ω-3 fatty acids, with fewer acne lesions (43), while a limited case series from 2008 attributed consumption of an ω-3 dietary supplement with fewer inflammatory acne lesions and improved well-being (44). Further clinical studies must be conducted to verify the findings in the basic science literature.

ANTIOXIDANTS

Oxidative stress and the production of reactive oxygen species (ROS) by neutrophils may contribute to acne severity (45). There is evidence that acne patients have lower levels of certain antioxidants and therefore may be less capable of removing ROS, suggesting a potential role for antioxidant supplementation (46,47). Cross-sectional studies have found that levels of endogenous antioxidants such as glucose-6-phosphate dehydrogenase and catalase (46) as well as vitamins A and E (48) are lower in acne patients. Furthermore, compared with their controls, acne patients have demonstrated higher than normal levels of malondialdehyde (MDA), which is a marker of lipid peroxidation and oxidative damage (46,47). Both selenium and selenium-dependant glutathione peroxidase activities are lower in acne patients compared with their controls (49), and yet the data from one study supporting a benefit of selenium supplementation lacked a control (50).

Basic science experiments continue to elaborate on the role of ROS and antioxidants in acne, paving the way for further human-based experimentation. For instance, epigallocatechin-3-gallate (EGCG), an antioxidant found in green tea, has been linked to lower sebum production when applied to male hamster foreskin (51). A flavonoid with antioxidant properties known as nobiletin, found in the juice of *Citrus depressa,* was applied to hamster auricles and shown to decrease lipogenesis and cell proliferation in sebaceous glands, while facilitating the excretion of sebum from mature sebocytes (52). The flower *Impatiens balsamina*, which is used in Eastern medicine, possesses the flavonoids kaempferol and quercetin, both of which have demonstrated bactericidal activity against *Propionibacterium acnes.* The well-known phytoalexin resveratrol that is found in red grape skin, red wine, peanuts, mulberries, spruce, and eucalyptus has been shown in vitro to also be bactericidal against *P. acnes* (53).

The conclusions regarding the role of antioxidants in acne improvement are primarily presumptive and based on evidence of higher ROS in these patients. Nonetheless, the evidence from the basic science literature suggests that administration of exogenous antioxidants may improve acne severity, such that clinical trials are needed to confirm this theory.

VITAMIN A

As mentioned previously, levels of vitamin A, an antioxidant, have been shown to be lower in acne patients (48). Humans consume vitamin A in one of two forms: *preformed vitamin A*, which is from animal sources and absorbed by the gut in the form of retinol, and *provitamin A carotenoid*, which is from colorful fruits and vegetables. Retinol is one of the most active forms of vitamin A and is easily absorbed in the gut. Once absorbed, it is made into retinal and retinoic acids, which are two other active forms of vitamin A. Preformed vitamin A is most prevalent in liver, whole milk, and fortified food products. In contrast, provitamin A carotenoid is from fruits and vegetables, and must be converted into retinol once absorbed during ingestion. Of the 563 identified carotenoids, fewer than 10% can be converted into vitamin A by the body, with β-carotene being the most easily absorbed (54). In general, vitamin A deficiency is rare in the United States and is really only seen in the developing world along with extreme malnourishment. Nonetheless, it may be seen in conjunction with strict dietary restrictions, alcoholism, zinc deficiency (zinc is needed to make retinol-binding protein), and conditions predisposing patients to low fat absorption such as celiac disease and Crohn's disease (54).

The Institute of Medicine recommends about 900 μg/day and 700 μg/day of vitamin A daily for men and women, respectively, over 19 years of age (55). However, dermatologists have traditionally been reluctant to give oral supplementation for fear of inducing hypervitaminosis A, which may cause birth defects, hepatotoxicity, reduced bone mineral density, and central nervous system abnormalities such as pseudotumor cerebri (55,56). The upper limit of tolerable daily intake of vitamin A for otherwise healthy individuals is 3000 μg/day, which should not induce toxicity (55).

The role of high doses of vitamin A in treating refractory and severe acne is well known since isotretinoin was first approved by the FDA in 1982 (57). Isotretinoin is a synthetic retinoid, which is a compound that is chemically similar to vitamin A (54). In 1981, Kligman et al. first reported that with doses as high as 300,000 IU in women and 400,000 to 500,000 IU in men, severe acne and other disorders of the pilosebaceous unit could be treated effectively. This study had followed subjects for up to four months and concluded that the fears of hypervitaminosis were, for the most part, exaggerated. They reported that the most common side effects of these high doses of medications were xerosis and cheilitis (58).

ZINC AND IODINE

Zinc is an essential element for proper skin development and function (59), has a bacteriostatic effect against *P. acnes,* and may decrease production of TNF-α, a proinflammatory cytokine (60). Up until the 1980s, zinc sulfate was the only form of the element available for supplementation, after which it become available as zinc gluconate, a more tolerable form for ingestion. Acne patients have been found to have lower levels of zinc (61,62), and randomized double-blind clinical trials comparing zinc with placebo (63–68) have shown that patients with severe acne improve with zinc supplementation. However, patients with mild or moderate inflammatory acne may not benefit when compared with placebo (69), and zinc may be most beneficial for inflammatory and not comedonal lesions (70). Most of these previous studies on zinc were comprised of small sample sizes, lacked controlling for dietary intake, and administered high doses of both zinc gluconate (200 mg) and zinc sulfate (400 or 600 mg), which were associated with gastrointestinal side effects such as nausea, vomiting, and diarrhea (64,65,68,70). Nonetheless, a few randomized and controlled clinical trials have shown that zinc supplementation is as effective as or less so than oral tetracyclines (71,72). The studies on acne and zinc supplementation have utilized doses of zinc with high side effect profiles while failing to show any benefit over oral antibiotics. Nonetheless, since the aforementioned experiments comparing zinc with placebo seem to show a benefit with zinc supplementation, further studies are warranted, especially in light of increasing resistance of *P. acnes* to many traditionally used oral antibiotics.

Iodine consumption in the form of iodine-rich foods such as kelp or systemic medications containing iodine may create a monomorphic eruption of pustules (73,74). Studies that have claimed an association with certain foods containing iodine and acne severity have been confounded by the other contents of these foods. For instance, a study from 1961 concluded that adolescents consuming high amounts of seafood, which is very high in iodine, also have decreased severity of acne (43), and yet it is impossible to attribute these results to iodine alone when seafood also contains high amounts of ω-3 fatty acids. Similarly, that milk consumption may be associated with acne severity as found in previous experiments (28–31) could be determined by the iodine content of milk (75), which may vary depending on the location of the milk farm, the season, the use of fortified animal feed, and the use of iodophor sanitizing solutions (76).

CONCLUSION

It has long been posited that diet has no impact on acne, but recent clinical trials have suggested that a relationship does indeed exist. While the clinical evidence is compelling, much of what we can attribute to diet as a factor in acne severity draws from inferences based on our expanding knowledge of hormonal and endocrinologic pathways.

The association between glycemic load and acne is especially convincing. Further studies should include a thorough analysis of women with PCOS, as it is these patients who would likely most benefit from dietary intervention, given their metabolic abnormalities. Indeed, further clinical trials among a wider patient base could better define recommendations for modifying carbohydrate intake, but until then, it is appropriate for dermatologists to recommend a lower glycemic load diet among patients with acne.

Although the link between dairy and acne is less convincing than that between a high glycemic load diet and acne, both deserve consideration during any dietary counseling efforts. The exact mechanism by which dairy may impact acne, whether it is via a hormonal pathway or upregulated IGF-1, remains to be further clarified. If physicians choose to counsel their patients that dairy consumption may indeed exacerbate their acne, it is reasonable to simultaneously advise patients to supplement their diets with vitamin D and calcium, the levels of which may suffer with a decrease in dairy intake.

The role of ω-3 fatty acids, antioxidants, zinc, vitamin A, and iodine in acne vulgaris remains to be elucidated. Given the level of evidence available, the authors currently advise their patients to supplement their diets on the basis of personal preferences and experiences, remaining vigilant for signs of intolerance or toxicity.

In light of the last decade of research investigating the relationship between diet and acne, it is no longer dermatological dogma to state that any association between diet and acne is mere myth. If a particular patient notes an association between a certain dietary factor and acne severity, it is best to support that patient's dietary supplementation or restriction and to encourage the patient to keep a food diary to test his or her hypothesis.

REFERENCES

1. Tallab TM. Beliefs, perceptions and psychological impact of acne vulgaris among patients in the Assir region of Saudi Arabia. West Afr J Med 2004; 23(1):85–87.
2. Al-Hoqail IA. Knowledge, beliefs and perception of youth toward acne vulgaris. Saudi Med J 2003; 24(7):765–768.
3. Tan JK, Vasey K, Fung KY. Beliefs and perceptions of patients with acne. J Am Acad Dermatol 2001; 44(3):439–445.

4. Green J, Sinclair RD. Perceptions of acne vulgaris in final year medical student written examination answers. Australas J Dermatol 2001; 42(2):98–101.
5. Ghodsi SZ, Orawa H, Zouboulis CC. Prevalence, severity, and severity risk factors of acne in high school pupils: a community-based study. J Invest Dermatol 2009; 129(9):2136–2141.
6. Cordain L, Lindeberg S, Hurtado M, et al. Acne vulgaris: a disease of Western civilization. Arch Dermatol 2002; 138(12):1584–1590.
7. Thiboutot DM, Strauss JS. Diet and acne revisited. Arch Dermatol 2002; 138(12):1591–1592.
8. Bershad S. The unwelcome return of the acne diet. Arch Dermatol 2003; 139(7):940–941.
9. Attia N, Tamborlane WV, Heptulla R, et al. The metabolic syndrome and insulin-like growth factor I regulation in adolescent obesity. J Clin Endocrinol Metab 1998; 83(5):1467–1471.
10. Liu S, Willett WC. Dietary glycemic load and atherothrombotic risk. Curr Atheroscler Rep 2002; 4(6):454–461.
11. Brand-Miller JC, Thomas M, Swan V, et al. Physiological validation of the concept of glycemic load in lean young adults. J Nutr 2003; 133(9):2728–2732.
12. Foster-Powell K, Holt SH, Brand-Miller JC. International table of glycemic index and glycemic load values. Am J Clin Nutr 2002; 76(1):5–56.
13. Cordain L, Eades MR, Eades MD. Hyperinsulinemic diseases of civilization: more than just syndrome X. Comp Biochem Physiol A Mol Integr Physiol 2003; 136(1):95–112.
14. Melnik BC, Schmitz G. Role of insulin, insulin-like growth factor-1, hyperglycaemic food and milk consumption in the pathogenesis of acne vulgaris. Exp Dermatol 2009; 18(10):833–841.
15. Aizawa H, Niimura M. Elevated serum insulin-like growth factor-1 (IGF-1) levels in women with postadolescent acne. J Dermatol 1995; 22(4):249–252.
16. National Institutes of Health. IGFBP3 insulin-like growth factor binding protein 3, 2010. Available at: http://www.ncbi.nlm.nih.gov/sites/entrez?Db=gene&Cmd=ShowDetailView&TermToSearch=3486. Accessed December 17, 2010.
17. Marsh K, Brand-Miller J. The optimal diet for women with polycystic ovary syndrome? Br J Nutr 2005; 94(2):154–165.
18. De Leo V, Musacchio MC, Morgante G, et al. Metformin treatment is effective in obese teenage girls with PCOS. Hum Reprod 2006; 21(9):2252–2256.
19. Ciotta L, Calogero AE, Farina M, et al. Clinical, endocrine and metabolic effects of acarbose, an alpha-glucosidase inhibitor, in PCOS patients with increased insulin response and normal glucose tolerance. Hum Reprod 2001; 16(10):2066–2072.
20. Mavropoulos JC, Yancy WS, Hepburn J, et al. The effects of a low-carbohydrate, ketogenic diet on the polycystic ovary syndrome: a pilot study. Nutr Metab (Lond) 2005; 2:35.
21. Cappel M, Mauger D, Thiboutot D. Correlation between serum levels of insulin-like growth factor 1, dehydroepiandrosterone sulfate, and dihydrotestosterone and acne lesion counts in adult women. Arch Dermatol 2005; 141(3):333–338.
22. Genazzani AD, Stomati M, Strucchi C, et al. Oral dehydroepiandrosterone supplementation modulates spontaneous and growth hormone-releasing hormone-induced

growth hormone and insulin-like growth factor-1 secretion in early and late post-menopausal women. Fertil Steril 2001; 76(2):241–248.

23. Pham-Huu-Trung MT, Villette JM, Bogyo A, et al. Effects of insulin-like growth factor I (IGF-I) on enzymatic activity in human adrenocortical cells. Interactions with ACTH. J Steroid Biochem Mol Biol 1991; 39(6):903–909.

24. Aizawa H, Niimura M. Mild insulin resistance during oral glucose tolerance test (OGTT) in women with acne. J Dermatol 1996; 23(8):526–529.

25. Smith RN, Mann NJ, Braue A, et al. A low-glycemic-load diet improves symptoms in acne vulgaris patients: a randomized controlled trial. Am J Clin Nutr 2007; 86 (1):107–115.

26. Smith RN, Mann NJ, Braue A, et al. The effect of a high-protein, low glycemic-load diet versus a conventional, high glycemic-load diet on biochemical parameters associated with acne vulgaris: a randomized, investigator-masked, controlled trial. J Am Acad Dermatol 2007; 57(2):247–256.

27. Smith R, Mann N, Makelainen H, et al. A pilot study to determine the short-term effects of a low glycemic load diet on hormonal markers of acne: a nonrandomized, parallel, controlled feeding trial. Mol Nutr Food Res 2008; 52(6):718–726.

28. Robinson HM. The acne problem. South Med J 1949; 42(12):1050–1060, illustration.

29. Adebamowo CA, Spiegelman D, Danby FW, et al. High school dietary dairy intake and teenage acne. J Am Acad Dermatol 2005; 52(2):207–214.

30. Adebamowo CA, Spiegelman D, Berkey CS, et al. Milk consumption and acne in teenaged boys. J Am Acad Dermatol 2008; 58(5):787–793.

31. Adebamowo CA, Spiegelman D, Berkey CS, et al. Milk consumption and acne in adolescent girls. Dermatol Online J 2006; 12(4):1.

32. Darling JA, Laing AH, Harkness RA. A survey of the steroids in cows' milk. J Endocrinol 1974; 62(2):291–297.

33. Danby FW. Diet and acne. Clin Dermatol 2008; 26(1):93–96.

34. Smith RN, Braue A, Varigos GA, et al. The effect of a low glycemic load diet on acne vulgaris and the fatty acid composition of skin surface triglycerides. J Dermatol Sci 2008; 50(1):41–52.

35. Simopoulos AP. Omega-3 fatty acids in inflammation and autoimmune diseases. J Am Coll Nutr 2002; 21(6):495–505.

36. Cordain L. Implications for the role of diet in acne. Semin Cutan Med Surg 2005; 24(2):84–91.

37. Logan AC. Omega-3 fatty acids and acne. Arch Dermatol 2003; 139(7):941–942; author reply 942–943.

38. Simopoulos AP, Leaf A, Salem N Jr. Workshop on the Essentiality of and Recommended Dietary Intakes for Omega-6 and Omega-3 Fatty Acids. J Am Coll Nutr 1999; 18(5):487–489.

39. Bhathena SJ, Berlin E, Judd JT, et al. Effects of omega 3 fatty acids and vitamin E on hormones involved in carbohydrate and lipid metabolism in men. Am J Clin Nutr 1991; 54(4):684–688.

40. Zouboulis CC, Nestoris S, Adler YD, et al. A new concept for acne therapy: a pilot study with zileuton, an oral 5-lipoxygenase inhibitor. Arch Dermatol 2003; 139(5):668–670.

41. James MJ, Gibson RA, Cleland LG. Dietary polyunsaturated fatty acids and inflammatory mediator production. Am J Clin Nutr 2000; 71(1 suppl):343S–348S.

42. Giltay EJ, Gooren LJ, Toorians AW, et al. Docosahexaenoic acid concentrations are higher in women than in men because of estrogenic effects. Am J Clin Nutr 2004; 80(5):1167–1174.
43. Hitch JM, Greenburg BG. Adolescent acne and dietary iodine. Arch Dermatol 1961; 84:898–911.
44. Rubin MG, Kim K, Logan AC. Acne vulgaris, mental health and omega-3 fatty acids: a report of cases. Lipids Health Dis 2008; 7:36.
45. Briganti S, Picardo M. Antioxidant activity, lipid peroxidation and skin diseases. What's new. J Eur Acad Dermatol Venereol 2003; 17(6):663–669.
46. Arican O, Kurutas EB, Sasmaz S. Oxidative stress in patients with acne vulgaris. Mediators Inflamm 2005; 2005(6):380–384.
47. Abdel Fattah NS, Shaheen MA, Ebrahim AA, et al. Tissue and blood superoxide dismutase activities and malondialdehyde levels in different clinical severities of acne vulgaris. Br J Dermatol 2008; 159(5):1086–1091.
48. El-Akawi Z, Abdel-Latif N, Abdul-Razzak K. Does the plasma level of vitamins A and E affect acne condition? Clin Exp Dermatol 2006; 31(3):430–434.
49. Michaelsson G. Decreased concentration of selenium in whole blood and plasma in acne vulgaris. Acta Derm Venereol 1990; 70(1):92.
50. Michaelsson G, Edqvist LE. Erythrocyte glutathione peroxidase activity in acne vulgaris and the effect of selenium and vitamin E treatment. Acta Derm Venereol 1984; 64(1):9–14.
51. Liao S. The medicinal action of androgens and green tea epigallocatechin gallate. Hong Kong Med J 2001; 7(4):369–374.
52. Sato T, Takahashi A, Kojima M, et al. A citrus polymethoxy flavonoid, nobiletin inhibits sebum production and sebocyte proliferation, and augments sebum excretion in hamsters. J Invest Dermatol 2007; 127(12):2740–2748.
53. Docherty JJ, McEwen HA, Sweet TJ, et al. Resveratrol inhibition of *Propionibacterium acnes*. J Antimicrob Chemother 2007; 59(6):1182–1184.
54. National Institutes of Health Office of Dietary Supplements. Dietary supplement fact sheet: vitamin A and carotenoids, 2006. Available at: http://ods.od.nih.gov/factsheets/vitamina/. Accessed December 17, 2010.
55. Institute of Medicine. Dietary Reference Intakes for Vitamin A, Vitamin K, Arsenic, Boron, Chromium, Copper, Iodine, Iron, Manganese, Molybdenum, Nickel, Silicon, Vanadium, and Zinc, 2001. Available at: http://www.nap.edu/openbook.php?record_id=10026&page=1. Accessed December 17, 2010.
56. Wall M. Idiopathic intracranial hypertension. Neurol Clin 2010; 28(3):593–617.
57. Concerns Regarding Accutane (isotretinoin). Subcommittee on Oversight and Investigations House Committee on Energy and Commerce, December 11, 2002. Washington, D.C., FDA, 2002.
58. Kligman AM, Mills OH Jr., Leyden JJ, et al. Oral vitamin A in acne vulgaris. Preliminary report. Int J Dermatol 1981; 20(4):278–285.
59. Prasad AS. Zinc deficiency. BMJ 2003; 326(7386):409–410.
60. Bowe WP, Shalita AR. Effective over-the-counter acne treatments. Semin Cutan Med Surg 2008; 27(3):170–176.

61. Amer M, Bahgat MR, Tosson Z, et al. Serum zinc in acne vulgaris. Int J Dermatol 1982; 21(8):481–484.
62. Michaelsson G, Vahlquist A, Juhlin L. Serum zinc and retinol-binding protein in acne. Br J Dermatol 1977; 96(3):283–286.
63. Dreno B, Amblard P, Agache P, et al. Low doses of zinc gluconate for inflammatory acne. Acta Derm Venereol 1989; 69(6):541–543.
64. Goransson K, Liden S, Odsell L. Oral zinc in acne vulgaris: a clinical and methodological study. Acta Derm Venereol 1978; 58(5):443–448.
65. Hillstrom L, Pettersson L, Hellbe L, et al. Comparison of oral treatment with zinc sulphate and placebo in acne vulgaris. Br J Dermatol 1977; 97(6):681–684.
66. Liden S, Goransson K, Odsell L. Clinical evaluation in acne. Acta Derm Venereol Suppl (Stockh) 1980; (suppl 89):47–52.
67. Michaelsson G, Juhlin L, Vahlquist A. Effects of oral zinc and vitamin A in acne. Arch Dermatol 1977; 113(1):31–36.
68. Verma KC, Saini AS, Dhamija SK. Oral zinc sulphate therapy in acne vulgaris: a double-blind trial. Acta Derm Venereol 1980; 60(4):337–340.
69. Orris L, Shalita AR, Sibulkin D, et al. Oral zinc therapy of acne. Absorption and clinical effect. Arch Dermatol 1978; 114(7):1018–1020.
70. Weimar VM, Puhl SC, Smith WH, et al. Zinc sulfate in acne vulgaris. Arch Dermatol 1978; 114(12):1776–1778.
71. Cunliffe WJ. Unacceptable side-effects of oral zinc sulphate in the treatment of acne vulgaris. Br J Dermatol 1979; 101(3):363.
72. Michaelsson G, Juhlin L, Ljunghall K. A double-blind study of the effect of zinc and oxytetracycline in acne vulgaris. Br J Dermatol 1977; 97(5):561–566.
73. Harrell BL, Rudolph AH. Letter: kelp diet: a cause of acneiform eruption. Arch Dermatol 1976; 112(4):560.
74. Jackson R. Nonbacterial pus-forming diseases of the skin. Can Med Assoc J 1974; 111(8):801, 804–806.
75. Arbesman H. Dairy and acne—the iodine connection. J Am Acad Dermatol 2005; 53 (6):1102.
76. Pennington JAT. Iodine Concentrations in U.S. Milk: variation due to time, season and region. J Dairy Sci 1990; 73:3421.

Overview of treatment principles for skin of color

Marcelyn K. Coley, Diane S. Berson, and Valerie D. Callender

INTRODUCTION

Treating acne in patients of color requires special consideration of the unique differences within this heterogeneous patient population. While pathogenesis, clinical presentation, and treatment are similar among all patients regardless of color, two important complications occur more frequently in ethnic skin—postinflammatory hyperpigmentation (PIH) and scarring (1). Acne and its consequences may have a significant psychosocial impact, reducing quality of life (2). In fact, PIH and scarring are oftentimes the motivating factors for patients to seek medical attention in people of color (3).

    Skin of color is traditionally classified as Fitzpatrick skin phototypes IV through VI and encompasses a spectrum of pigmented skin (4). People of color make up the majority of the world's population (5) and are projected to represent half of the population in the United States by 2050 (6). This further highlights the importance of understanding management of acne in this patient population.

EPIDEMIOLOGY

Acne vulgaris is the most common dermatological condition among patients of color just as it is in the general population (7–12). It affects 40 to 50 million people nationwide (13). Most data regarding prevalence of acne in patients of color come from survey studies. In 1983, Halder et al. conducted a survey (of predominantly black and white private practices in Washington, D.C.) reporting that acne was the most common dermatologic diagnosis in both black (27.7%) and white (29.5%) patients. In 2007, Alexis et al. found similar results at the Skin of Color Center in New York City, with acne being the top diagnosis in both black (28.4%) and white (21.0%) patients seen. The incidence does not seem to differ in the Latino or Hispanic population (14). However, one study reported a higher prevalence of acne in Mexican-American indigent adolescents when compared with their white or African-American counterparts (15). Additionally, a survey of Arab Americans documented acne as the most common self-reported diagnosis (16). In Singapore, a large study of 74,589 Asian patients was conducted, and similarly, acne was among the most common diagnoses observed there (17). A 2010 study by Perkins et al. (1) examined acne prevalence and subtypes among 2,895 Caucasian, Asian, continental Indian, and African-American women and noted somewhat different findings, reporting that African-American and Hispanic women showed a higher prevalence of clinical acne when compared to groups with lighter skin types.

PATHOGENESIS

The development of acne in skin of color is thought to occur by the same mechanisms as in Caucasians. Pathogenesis is multifactorial, including abnormal keratinization, excess sebum production, and infection with *Propionibacterium acnes*. Pathogenesis is discussed in detail in Part 1.

Structure and Function

Structural and functional differences among darkly pigmented skin types have important clinical implications for diagnosis and treatment of acne. One significant difference in the skin of darker-pigmented individuals is that it contains an increased amount of melanin. Melanin is derived from melanocytes located in the basal cell layer of the epidermis. These dendritic cells produce pigment via membrane-bound granules, known as melanosomes, in which melanin synthesis takes place (18). There is no major difference in the number of melanocytes between ethnic groups, but in darker skin types, melanosomes are more numerous, larger, and singly dispersed when compared with fair skin types. In addition to higher melanin content, melanosomes undergo a slower rate of degradation in darker skin (18). The variation in number and distribution of melanosomes may help to explain the differences seen with pigment disturbances associated with acne in patients of color. An exaggerated response of melanocytes to cutaneous injury (i.e., ultraviolet (UV) irradiation, irritating topical medications, or inflammatory medical conditions) (19) has also been observed in darker skin and may play a part in the development of dyschromias. Labile melanocytes seem to demonstrate increased melanogenesis or greater melanin release in the setting of inflammation or trauma (20,21).

A thicker, compact dermis containing many fragments of collagen fibrils and glycoprotein has also been described in darker skin types (22). Fibroblasts are reportedly larger and more numerous than those found in white skin, suggesting heightened activity (or reactivity), which may influence keloid and hypertrophic scar formation—complications particularly common in individuals of African and Asian ancestry (22).

There is conflicting evidence on sebum production. Studies have shown no difference in sebum production between African-Americans and Caucasians (23,24), while others report that African-Americans have larger sebaceous glands, increased sebum secretion, and a greater pore count fraction (25). A positive correlation between darker pigmentation and the amount of skin surface lipids has been noted in Asian women (26). A recent study noted a negative correlation between pore size and skin lightness, that is, larger pores were associated with darker skin types. However, the authors did not find an association between pore size or pore count fraction and acne (1).

CLINICAL PRESENTATION

Acne typically manifests with characteristic lesions including comedones, papules, pustules, nodules, and/or cysts affecting primarily the face, chest, and upper back. The physical examination should not only document the location and type of lesion but also assess for discoloration (hypo- or hyperpigmentation) and acne scarring (keloidal, hypertrophic, or atrophic). Clinical features that are of particular importance in skin of color patients are PIH and scarring. Therefore, along with the classic lesions mentioned above, hyperpigmented macules or patches are often found at sites of previous acne eruption and may be present alongside active lesions (Fig. 2.3.1). Scars may take the form of atrophic (ice pick, boxcar, or rolling), hypertrophic, or keloidal scars (Fig. 2.3.2A, B) (27). It is common for dyschromia and scarring to remain after the acne lesions themselves have resolved and thus serve as a primary complaint for many patients of color affected by acne. One study reported a high incidence of PIH, where 47%, 53%, and 65% of Asian, Hispanic, and black patients, respectively, were found to have acne and acne-related hyperpigmented macules (28). Nodulocystic acne is reportedly less common in blacks as compared with Caucasian or Hispanic patients (29).

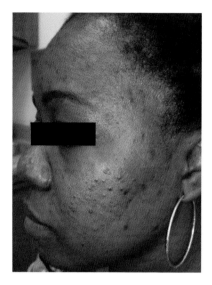

Figure 2.3.1 Acne with postinflammatory hyperpigmentation. African-American woman with multiple comedones, hyperpigmented papules and macules.

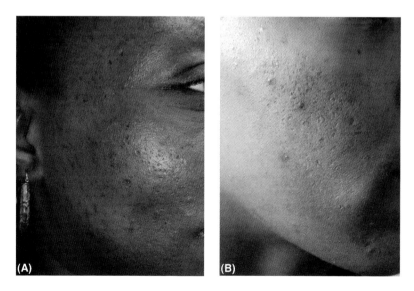

Figure 2.3.2 Acne with scarring and postinflammatory hyperpigmentation. (**A**) Pitted scars and hyperpigmented macules. (**B**) Boxcar-type scars with few inflammatory papules.

Cultural Practices and Considerations

Cultural practices must also be taken into account when evaluating patients. Some common practices known to exacerbate acne in patients of color include the use of occlusive products such as cocoa butter, hair pomades (*hair grease*), or steroid-containing fade creams used by some populations to lighten the complexion. Pomade acne is a type of acne generally limited to patients of African descent and are to lesser degree seen in Hispanic patients who use lubricating products on the hair (30,31). Several cases have also been reported in East Africa in response to the practice of treating the face of children with petroleum jelly up to twice daily (32). The lesions typically consist of closed or open comedones on the forehead along the anterior hairline in a patient giving the history of pomade and/or oils used in the hair. This may be worsened when hairstyles allow direct contact on the face (i.e., bangs). Pomade acne is less prevalent today than previous decades because of changes in hair care practices and the introduction of more sophisticated formulations of hair lubricants such as silicone-based products (33,34).

HISTOPATHOLOGY

Even acne lesions in clinically mild cases may prove to be very inflamed and hyperactive. Noninflammatory lesions (i.e., comedones) and seemingly uninvolved skin beyond the lesion have shown marked inflammation on histopathology in black patients (35). This may contribute to the high prevalence of PIH and scarring in ethnic patients.

TREATMENT

Although treatment of acne vulgaris is similar among all skin types, the potential for disfiguring PIH and scarring as a result of acne in darker skin types warrants early and aggressive treatment. Nonetheless, balance between effective treatment of acne and the risk of inducing potential adverse reactions secondary to irritating preparations must be considered. Inappropriate selection and overzealous use of treatments may lead to worsening inflammation and/or secondary irritant dermatitis with resultant dyspigmentation.

Topical Therapy

Retinoids

As in all acne patients, topical therapy is the first line in treatment of mild-to-moderate acne. Topical retinoids continue to be the leading choice in skin of color.

Retinoids are vitamin A derivatives, which have comedolytic effects as well as antikeratinization and anti-inflammatory properties. These agents also facilitate melanin dispersion and removal by increasing epidermal turnover (36), making topical retinoids particularly effective in the treatment of acne and associated PIH in pigmented skin (37–44). Adapalene, tazarotene, and tretinoin are frequently used and available in the United States. A common concern when using retinoids, however, is the potential risk of irritant dermatitis, which may lead to secondary PIH. To reduce this potential adverse effect, it is important to start treatment with lower doses and more tolerable formulations (i.e., creams vs. gels) (33). Microsphere formulations and aqueous-based gels are now available and tend to be well tolerated. Starting treatment with alternate-day dosing (three times weekly to every other night) and titrating up (once nightly) as tolerated is one approach commonly utilized.

Antimicrobials

Topical antimicrobials are often used in combination therapy in mild-to-moderate cases of inflammatory acne in skin of color patients. Macrolides and lincosamides, such as erythromycin and clindamycin, respectively, are effective in reducing *P. acnes* and inflammation. These antibiotic agents are often combined with topical benzoyl peroxide, an oxidizer of bacterial proteins, which reduces the development of bacterial resistance commonly seen when topical antibiotics are used as monotherapy. Available in concentrations ranging from 2.5% to 10% as lotions, creams, gels, masks, pads, foams, and cleansers, benzoyl peroxide is sometimes used as monotherapy. However, clinical studies have shown increased efficacy with combination therapy (45).

Like retinoids, benzoyl peroxide can be both drying and irritating, and therefore, it is important to minimize the risk of irritation by choosing lower concentrations and careful vehicle selection (33). In general, creams are better tolerated than gels, and aqueous gels better than alcohol-based gels. Patients should be informed that benzoyl peroxide can bleach hair and color fabrics.

Dapsone

Topical dapsone is one of the latest additions to the list of acne therapeutic agents. Approved for the treatment of acne, dapsone is classified as a sulfone. It carries anti-inflammatory and antimicrobial properties. Historically, systemic sulfones have shown positive effects on acne (46); however, systemic toxicities have limited its widespread use. A particularly problematic complication with use of systemic sulfones is dose-dependent hemolytic anemia in patients with glucose-6-phoshate dehydrogenase (G6PD) deficiency (47). G6PD deficiency commonly affects certain ethnic groups of African, Asian, Middle-Eastern, and Mediterranean ancestry, with an estimated prevalence in approximately 1 in 10 African-Americans in the United States (48,49). Studies have shown that topical dapsone 5% gel is both safe and effective for the treatment of acne (50,51). When compared with oral dapsone, topical dapsone was found to have systemic exposures of 100-fold or less, even when given along with trimethoprim/sulfamethoxazole (TMP/SMX) (52), which is known to increase systemic absorption of oral dapsone (53). Piette et al. conducted a study in which 64 ethnic patients with G6PD deficiency and acne vulgaris were treated with topical dapsone. The authors demonstrated no clinical or laboratory evidence of drug-induced hemolytic anemia in this group (54). Investigators noted a slight decrease in hemoglobin concentration of 0.32 g/dL from baseline to two weeks during dapsone gel treatment. This was not accompanied by changes in other laboratory parameters (i.e., reticulocytes, haptoglobin, bilirubin, and lactate dehydrogenase levels). There was no apparent decrease in hemoglobin at 12 weeks as treatment continued. Thus, topical dapsone 5% gel imposes no significant risk of hemolytic anemia in patients with G6PD deficiency and is safe in all patients (54). Use of benzoyl peroxide along with topical dapsone may cause a temporary yellow or orange discoloration of the skin (55).

Other Topical Agents

Azelaic Acid

Topical azelaic acid is a naturally occurring dicarboxylic acid derivative, which has been reported to successfully reduce both inflammatory and noninflammatory acne lesions as well as decrease hyperpigmentation via its inhibitory effect on tyrosine (56,57). It has activity against *P. acnes* and *Staphylococcus epidermidis* in vitro, and antiproliferative effects against hyperactive and abnormal melanocytes (57,58). The latter property is beneficial in acne-associated PIH. Azelaic acid is formulated as a 20% cream for acne, its efficacy profile has been reported to be similar to that of tretinoin 0.05% cream, BPO 5% gel, erythromycin 2% ointment, and clindamycin 1% gel (59). Its low irritation potential, however, makes it well tolerated and suited for patients of color, especially those with sensitive skin (e.g., atopic dermatitis). The typical dose is azelaic acid 20% cream applied twice daily. More recently, azelaic 15% gel, indicated for rosacea, is increasingly used for acne vulgaris with good results (60,61).

Systemic Agents

Antimicrobials

Systemic agents are generally reserved for moderate-to-severe inflammatory acne and are often used in conjunction with topical therapy. Oral antibiotics are used in skin of color patients as in the general population. Commonly used oral antibiotics include the tetracyclines (e.g., tetracycline, doxycycline, minocycline) and the macrolides (e.g., erythromycin). Systemic antibiotics target *P. acnes* and reduce inflammation, improving acne and subsequently reducing the risk of PIH and scarring. Clinical studies have shown success when combining oral antibiotics with topical agents. Examples include minocycline along with tazarotene (62), or doxycycline plus adapalene (63).

Retinoids

The treatment of choice for severe or nodulocystic acne is oral isotretinoin (13-*cis*-retinoic acid). Although nodulocystic acne is reportedly less common in blacks as compared with Caucasian or Hispanic patients, some experts have proposed use of systemic retinoids in mild-to-moderate acne in skin of color as a way to avoid disfiguring PIH and acne scarring (33). When considering this systemic agent, the safety profile must be considered along with a careful examination of the risks and benefits. Of note, retinoids may cause adverse effects including teratogenicity, psychiatric disorders, hepatic toxicity, elevation in lipid profile, and mucocutaneous side effects. Therefore, careful patient selection and close monitoring are required.

Hormonal Therapy

Hormonal therapy for acne may be very effective in women even when androgen levels are normal. Several antiandrogenic therapies have been used to treat acne, including oral contraceptives (64) androgen receptor antagonists (e.g., spironolactone, flutamide, cyproterone acetate), finasteride, and corticosteroids. Thus, oral contraceptives, like norgestimate/ethinyl estradiol, Ortho Tri-Cyclen Lo[®] (Ortho-McNeil-Janssen Pharmaceuticals, Inc., New Jersey, U.S.), have been viable options in appropriately selected women who concurrently desire family-planning alternatives. It is important to consider that oral contraceptives may cause several side effects and can sometimes trigger the development of melasma (65), patchy hyperpigmentation predominantly on the face, which is especially common in patients of color.

Adjunctive Treatments

Intralesional Corticosteroids

Intralesional corticosteroids are often used as an adjunct for acutely inflamed nodules and cysts and offer a rapid response with marked improvement, generally within 48 to 72 hours (66). Preparations of triamcinolone 10 mg/mL diluted with sterile water or lidocaine to concentrations of 2.5 to 5.0 mg/mL are commonly used (67,68). Concentrations as low as 0.63 mg/mL have also been reported to be effective in the treatment of nodulocystic acne (66). If keloidal or hypertrophic scarring is present, individual lesions may be injected with 10 to 20 mg/mL triamcinolone to flatten the lesions. This is generally repeated at two- to four-week intervals (33).

Rare complications of intralesional corticosteroid therapy include development of atrophy, telangiectasias, and hypopigmentation. The latter tends to be more visible in darkly pigmented individuals. Lower concentrations and wider intervals of treatment help to circumvent these potential effects. Suppression of the hypothalamic-pituitary-adrenal axis has been reported with repeated injections or higher total doses (69,70).

Chemical Peels

Chemical peels are effective and safe in skin of color when limited to superficial peeling agents such as salicylic acid and glycolic acid (71,72). These agents induce epidermolysis and comedolysis (73,74). Salicylic acid and glycolic acid are often found in over-the-counter acne treatments in low concentrations. At higher concentrations, as chemical peels, they may aid in effective improvement of primary and secondary acne lesions, including PIH, as well as facilitates absorption of other topical agents (72). As a general rule, deeper peels are not used in darker skin types as the risk of complications is significantly greater. A series of peels with salicylic acid (20–30%) or glycolic acid (30–70%) performed at four-week intervals are usually performed for acne vulgaris. Concomitant use of topical retinoids may actually deepen the depth of the peel. For this reason, topical retinoids should be held for at least one week prior to treatment and may be resumed five to seven days after the peel. Some clinicians have suggested resuming all topical acne medications as soon as the skin 'feels' normal to the patient. Potential complications include scarring, hyperpigmentation, or hypopigmentation. Because of the risk of post-peel hyperpigmentation, pretreatment with hydroquinone 4% cream for one to two weeks before has been suggested as a way to minimize this risk in skin types IV to VI (71,72). Spot testing with the selected chemical peeling agent prior to full treatment is advisable in skin of color.

Microdermabrasion

Indications for microdermabrasion are similar to that of chemical peels and include acne, acne scarring, and hyperpigmentation. It is a noninvasive procedure that can be safely performed in all skin types (75), although acute skin inflammation, such as pustular acne, is a relative contraindication (76). Efficacy was noted in one study with 25 patients with grade II or III acne (77).

Fade Creams/Lightening Agents

Treatment of PIH is often incorporated into the acne treatment regimen and is best initiated after the acne itself is under control. Commonly used lightening agents include hydroquinone, azelaic acid, and kojic acid. Hydroquinone inhibits the action of tyrosinase, inhibiting melanin synthesis. Spot treatment with hydroquinone 4% cream twice daily following the application of acne medications is recommended. Care must be taken to avoid inadvertent application to surrounding normal skin as a halo effect, with a noticeable hypopigmented ring surrounding the lesion may occur on the adjacent skin. This is generally transient. Cotton-swab application may help to minimize this effect.

Azelaic acid has activity against tyrosinase in addition to mild anti-inflammatory and comedolytic effects (57,60) and has also been effective in the treatment of melasma (78).

Sun protection is an important measure in treating skin of color patients with acne and PIH as UV exposure may exacerbate PIH. Sun protection factor (SPF) 15 or greater with both UVA and UVB protection and sun avoidance has been suggested as a necessary adjunct (79).

Laser Devices

Given the considerable risk for dyschromia and keloids, ablative resurfacing in darker skin types is generally not recommended. As many as 66% to 100% of patients with Fitzpatrick skin types IV to VI will develop some degree of hyperpigmentation, in contrast to up to 40% in skin types I to III (80). Ablative devices cause full thickness injury and include the carbon dioxide (CO_2) and erbium:yttrium-aluminum-garnet (Er:YAG) lasers. Nonablative resurfacing is theoretically safer in darker skin types and is associated with less side effects and downtime. Few studies have examined the efficacy and safety of nonablative laser modalities in skin types IV to VI. A recent study by Mahmoud and colleagues (81) found significant improvement in facial acne scars in patients skin types IV to VI after five sessions with the fractionated erbium 1550-nm laser at monthly intervals. No difference was found between those treated with 10-mJ versus 40-mJ fluences at a constant treatment density. Other devices have reportedly shown some effect in pigmented skin, including the nonablative 1450-nm diode (82).

Common side effects include pain and hyperpigmentation. These effects seem to be more severe with increasing skin phototype type (greatest in skin type VI) (81). Other commonly used nonablative laser systems include the 1064-nm Q-switched Nd:YAG laser (83,84), 1320-nm Nd:YAG laser (85,86),1450-nm diode laser (86), and 1540-nm Er:Glass laser (87). It is important that no oral isotretinoin be used at least one year prior because there is a reportedly higher risk of abnormal postoperative healing and scarring (80).

Dermal Fillers

The concept of using injectable agents such as collagen, hyaluronic acid, and silicone to fill atrophic scarring has long been established (88–90). Of late, dermal fillers have gained popularity among various ethnic groups. Few studies have looked specifically at darker skin types however. Poly-L-lactic acid (PLLA) (91) has been reported to be effective and safe for treatment of macular atrophic scars. For some darker-skinned patients, injection site dyschromia may occur but generally resolves spontaneously within several weeks. No reports of keloid formation or hypertrophic scars post injection have been found.

A combination of procedures generally produces the best results. One case report noted satisfactory results in one Hispanic patient and one African-American patient where several procedures were performed including chemical peeling, punch grafting, subcision, dermal grafting, and dermabrasion (92).

Patient Education

Patient education is paramount to ensuring patient compliance with any treatment regimen. In patients of color, it is important to understand and be sensitive to differences in cultural practices and to educate patients as to potential exacerbating factors such as those mentioned above. Questioning patients regarding their daily routine (i.e., cleansers, scrubs, astringents, and other over-the-counter topicals) is a great place to start. Gentle cleansers are best when prescribing any treatment regimen. Setting realistic expectations is essential. For example, informing patients of the risks of various medications, giving instructions in case they experience an adverse effect, or explaining that dark spots may take months to fade will aid in the patient's compliance, outcome, and overall satisfaction.

REFERENCES

1. Perkins A, Cheng C, Hillebrand G, et al. Comparison of the epidemiology of acne vulgaris among Caucasian, Asian, Continental Indian and African American women. J Eur Acad Dermatol Venereol 2010.
2. Yazici K, Baz K, Yazici AE, et al. Disease-specific quality of life is associated with anxiety and depression in patients with acne. J Eur Acad Dermatol Venereol 2004; 18(4):435–439.
3. Taylor SC. Cosmetic problems in skin of color. Skin Pharmacol Appl Skin Physiol 1999; 12(3):139–143.
4. Fitzpatrick TB. The validity and practicality of sun-reactive skin types I through VI. Arch Dermatol 1988; 124(6):869–871.
5. Shah SK, Alexis AF. Defining skin of color. In: Alam M, Bhatia AC, Kundu RV, et al. eds. Cosmetic Dermatology for Skin of Color. New York: McGraw Hill, 2009:1–11.
6. Projections of the population by sex, race, and Hispanic origin for the United States: 2010 to 2050 [database on the Internet]. U.S. Census Bureau. 2008 [cited April 1, 2009]. Available at: http://www.census.gov/population/www/projections/files/nation/summary/np2008-t4.xls.

7. Alexis AF, Sergay AB, Taylor SC. Common dermatologic disorders in skin of color: a comparative practice survey. Cutis 2007; 80(5):387–394.
8. Arsouze A, Fitoussi C, Cabotin PP, et al. Presenting skin disorders in black Afro-Caribbean patients: a multicentre study conducted in the Paris region. Ann Dermatol Venereol 2008; 135(3):177–182.
9. Child F, Fuller L, Higgins E, et al. A study of the spectrum of skin disease occurring in a black population in south-east London. Br J Dermatol 1999; 141 (3):512–517.
10. Dunwell P, Rose A. Study of the skin disease spectrum occurring in an Afro-Caribbean population. Int J Dermatol 2003; 42(4):287–289.
11. Halder RM, Grimes PE, McLaurin CI, et al. Incidence of common dermatoses in a predominantly black dermatologic practice. Cutis 1983; 32(4):388, 390.
12. Taylor SC. Epidemiology of skin diseases in people of color. Cutis 2003; 71(4): 271–275.
13. White GM. Recent findings in the epidemiologic evidence, classification, and sub-types of acne vulgaris. J Am Acad Dermatol 1998; 39(2 pt 3):S34–S37.
14. Sanchez MR. Cutaneous diseases in Latinos. Dermatol Clin 2003; 21(4):689–697.
15. Fitzpatrick SB, Fujii C, Shragg GP, et al. Do health care needs of indigent Mexican-American, black, and white adolescents differ? J Adolesc Health Care 1990; 11(2):128–132.
16. El-Essawi D, Musial JL, Hammad A, et al. A survey of skin disease and skin-related issues in Arab Americans. J Am Acad Dermatol 2007; 56(6):933–938.
17. Chua-Ty G, Goh CL, Koh SL. Pattern of skin diseases at the National Skin Centre (Singapore) from 1989-1990. Int J Dermatol 1992; 31(8):555–559.
18. Bolognia JL, Pawelek JM. Biology of hypopigmentation. J Am Acad Dermatol 1988; 19(2 pt 1):217–255.
19. Andersen KE, Maibach HI. Black and white human skin differences. J Am Acad Dermatol 1979; 1(3):276–282.
20. Grimes PE. Pigmentary disorders in blacks. Dermatologic Clinics 1988; 6(2):271.
21. Taylor SC. Skin of color: biology, structure, function, and implications for derma-tologic disease. J Am Acad Dermatol 2002 Feb; 46 (2 suppl Understanding):S41–62.
22. Yosipovitch G, Theng CTS. Asian skin: its architecture, function and differences from Caucasian skin. Cosmet Toil 2002; 117(9):104–110.
23. Grimes PE, Edison B, Green B, et al. Evaluation of inherent differences between African American and white skin surface properties using subjective and objective measures. Cutis 2004; 73(6):392–396.
24. Pochi PE, Strauss JS. Sebaceous gland activity in black skin. Dermatol Clin 1988; 6(3):349–351.
25. Rawlings AV. Ethnic skin types: are there differences in skin structure and function? Int J Cosmet Sci 2006; 28(2):79–93.
26. Abe T, Arai S, Mimura K, et al. Studies of physiological factors affecting skin susceptibility to ultraviolet light irradiation and irritants. J Dermatol 1983; 10(6):531–537.
27. Jacob CI, Dover JS, Kaminer MS. Acne scarring: a classification system and review of treatment options. J Am Acad Dermatol 2001; 45(1):109–117.

28. Taylor SC, Cook-Bolden F, Rahman Z, et al. Acne vulgaris in skin of color. J Am Acad Dermatol 2002; 46(2 Suppl Understanding):S98–S106.
29. Wilkins JW Jr., Voorhees JJ. Prevalence of nodulocystic acne in white and Negro males. Arch Dermatol 1970; 102(6):631–634.
30. Halder RM, Nootheti PK, Richards GM. Dermatological disorders and cultural practices: understanding practices that cause skin conditions in non-Caucasian populations. Skin Aging 2002; 10(8):46–50.
31. Ravanfar P, Dinulos JG. Cultural practices affecting the skin of children. Curr Opin Pediatr 2010; 22(4):423–431.
32. Verhagen AR. Pomade acne in black skin. Arch Dermatol 1974; 110(3):465.
33. Callender VD. Acne in ethnic skin: special considerations for therapy. Dermatol Ther 2004; 17(2):184–195.
34. Halder RM, Brooks HL, Caballero JC. Common dermatological diseases in pigmented skins. In: Halder RM, ed. Dermatology and Dermatological Therapy of Pigmented Skins. Boca Raton: Taylor & Francis, 2006:17–39.
35. Halder RM. A clinicopathological study of acne vulgaris in black females. J Invest Dermatol 1996; 106:888 (abstr).
36. Ortonne JP, Passeron T. Melanin pigmentary disorders: treatment update. Dermatol Clin 2005; 23(2):209–226.
37. Czernielewski J, Poncet M, Mizzi F. Efficacy and cutaneous safety of adapalene in black patients versus white patients with acne vulgaris. Cutis 2002; 70(4):243–248.
38. Grimes P, Callender V. Tazarotene cream for postinflammatory hyperpigmentation and acne vulgaris in darker skin: a double-blind, randomized, vehicle-controlled study. Cutis 2006; 77(1):45–50.
39. Halder RM. The role of retinoids in the management of cutaneous conditions in blacks. J Am Acad Dermatol 1998; 39(2 pt 3):S98–S103.
40. Jacyk WK. Adapalene in the treatment of African patients. J Eur Acad Dermatol Venereol 2001; 15(suppl 3):37–42.
41. Tanghetti E, Dhawan S, Green L, et al. Randomized comparison of the safety and efficacy of tazarotene 0.1% cream and adapalene 0.3% gel in the treatment of patients with at least moderate facial acne vulgaris. J Drugs Dermatol 2010; 9 (5):549–558.
42. Thiboutot D, Arsonnaud S, Soto P. Efficacy and tolerability of adapalene 0.3% gel compared to tazarotene 0.1% gel in the treatment of acne vulgaris. J Drugs Dermatol 2008; 7(6 suppl):s3–s10.
43. Zhu XJ, Tu P, Zhen J, et al. Adapalene gel 0.1%: effective and well tolerated in the topical treatment of acne vulgaris in Chinese patients. Cutis 2001; 68(4 suppl):55–59.
44. Bulengo-Ransby SM, Griffiths CE, Kimbrough-Green CK, et al. Topical tretinoin (retinoic acid) therapy for hyperpigmented lesions caused by inflammation of the skin in black patients. N Engl J Med 1993; 328(20):1438–1443.
45. Ko HC, Song M, Seo SH, et al. Prospective, open-label, comparative study of clindamycin 1%/benzoyl peroxide 5% gel with adapalene 0.1% gel in Asian acne patients: efficacy and tolerability. J Eur Acad Dermatol Venereol 2009; 23(3):245–250.

46. Barranco VP. Dapsone—other indications. Int J Dermatol 1982; 21(9):513–514.
47. Jollow DJ, Bradshaw TP, McMillan DC. Dapsone-induced hemolytic anemia. Drug Metab Rev 1995; 27(1–2):107–124.
48. Glucose-6-phosphate dehydrogenase deficiency. U.S. National Library of Medicine, 2010 [updated November 22, 2010; cited 2010 November 27, 2010]. Available at: http://ghr.nlm.nih.gov/condition/glucose-6-phosphate-dehydrogenase-deficiency.
49. Beutler E. G6PD deficiency. Blood 1994; 84(11):3613–3636.
50. Draelos ZD, Carter E, Maloney JM, et al. Two randomized studies demonstrate the efficacy and safety of dapsone gel, 5% for the treatment of acne vulgaris. J Am Acad Dermatol 2007; 56(3):439 e1–439 e10.
51. Lucky AW, Maloney JM, Roberts J, et al. Dapsone gel 5% for the treatment of acne vulgaris: safety and efficacy of long-term (1 year) treatment. J Drugs Dermatol 2007; 6(10):981–987.
52. Thiboutot DM, Willmer J, Sharata H, et al. Pharmacokinetics of dapsone gel, 5% for the treatment of acne vulgaris. Clin Pharmacokinet 2007; 46(8):697–712.
53. Lee BL, Medina I, Benowitz NL, et al. Dapsone, trimethoprim, and sulfamethoxazole plasma levels during treatment of Pneumocystis pneumonia in patients with the acquired immunodeficiency syndrome (AIDS). Evidence of drug interactions. Ann Intern Med 1989; 110(8):606–611.
54. Piette WW, Taylor S, Pariser D, et al. Hematologic safety of dapsone gel, 5%, for topical treatment of acne vulgaris. Arch Dermatol 2008; 144(12):1564–1570.
55. ACZONE® (dapsone) Gel 5% Prescribing Information. Irvine, CA 2008 March 2009.
56. Fitton A, Goa KL. Azelaic acid. A review of its pharmacological properties and therapeutic efficacy in acne and hyperpigmentary skin disorders. Drugs 1991; 41 (5):780–798.
57. Hsu S, Quan LT. Topical antibacterial agents. In: Wolverton SE, ed. Comprehensive Dermatologic Drug Therapy. Philadelphia: Saunders, 2001:472–496.
58. Woody JLCM. Antimicrobial drugs. In: Bolognia JL, Jorizzo JL, Rapini RP, et al. eds. Dermatology. 2nd ed. Spain: Mosby Elsevier, 2008.
59. Webster G. Combination azelaic acid therapy for acne vulgaris. J Am Acad Dermatol 2000; 43(2 pt 3):S47–S50.
60. Gollnick HP, Graupe K, Zaumseil RP. Azelaic acid 15% gel in the treatment of acne vulgaris. Combined results of two double-blind clinical comparative studies. J Dtsch Dermatol Ges 2004; 2(10):841–847.
61. Thiboutot D. Versatility of azelaic acid 15% gel in treatment of inflammatory acne vulgaris. J Drugs Dermatol 2008; 7(1):13–16.
62. Leyden J, Thiboutot DM, Shalita AR, et al. Comparison of tazarotene and minocycline maintenance therapies in acne vulgaris: a multicenter, double-blind, randomized, parallel-group study. Arch Dermatol 2006; 142(5):605–612.
63. Thiboutot DM, Shalita AR, Yamauchi PS, et al. Combination therapy with adapalene gel 0.1% and doxycycline for severe acne vulgaris: a multicenter, investigator-blind, randomized, controlled study. Skinmed 2005; 4(3):138–146.
64. Redmond GP, Olson WH, Lippman JS, et al. Norgestimate and ethinyl estradiol in the treatment of acne vulgaris: a randomized, placebo-controlled trial. Obstet Gynecol 1997; 89(4):615–622.

65. Halder RM, Brooks HL, Callender VD. Acne in ethnic skin. Dermatol Clin 2003; 21(4):609–615, vii.

66. Levine RM, Rasmussen JE. Intralesional corticosteroids in the treatment of nodulocystic acne. Arch Dermatol 1983; 119(6):480–481.

67. Khunger N. Standard guidelines of care for acne surgery. Indian J Dermatol Venereol Leprol 2008; 74(suppl):S28–S36.

68. Taub AF. Procedural treatments for acne vulgaris. Dermatol Surg 2007; 33(9): 1005–1026.

69. Jarratt MT, Spark RF, Arndt KA. The effects of intradermal steroids on the pituitary-adrenal axis and the skin. J Invest Dermatol 1974; 62(4):463–466.

70. Potter RA. Intralesional triamcinolone and adrenal suppression in acne vulgaris. J Invest Dermatol 1971; 57(6):364–370.

71. Grimes PE. The safety and efficacy of salicylic acid chemical peels in darker racial-ethnic groups. Dermatol Surg 1999; 25(1):18–22.

72. Roberts WE. Chemical peeling in ethnic/dark skin. Dermatol Ther 2004; 17(2): 196–205.

73. Lewis AB. Alpha-hydroxy acids. In: Wolverton SE, ed. Comprehensive Dermatologic Drug Therapy. Philadelphia: Saunders, 2001:659–670.

74. Hessel AB, Cruz-Ramon JC, Lin AN. Agents used for treatment of hyperkeratosis. In: Wolverton SE, ed. Comprehensive Dermatologic Drug Therapy. Philadelphia: Saunders, 2001:671–684.

75. Shim EK, Barnette D, Hughes K, et al. Microdermabrasion: a clinical and histopathologic study. Dermatol Surg 2001; 27(6):524–530.

76. Callender VD, Cherie MY. Cosmetic procedures in skin of color: chemical peels, microdermabrasion, hair transplantation, augmentation, and sclerotherapy. In: Kelly AP, Taylor SC, eds. Dermatology for Skin of Color. China: McGraw Hill, 2009:513–528.

77. Lloyd JR. The use of microdermabrasion for acne: a pilot study. Dermatol Surg 2001; 27(4):329–331.

78. Balina LM, Graupe K. The treatment of melasma. 20% azelaic acid versus 4% hydroquinone cream. Int J Dermatol 1991; 30(12):893–895.

79. Cayce KA, McMichael AJ, Feldman SR. Hyperpigmentation: an overview of the common afflictions. Dermatol Nurs 2004; 16(5):401–406, 13–16; quiz 17.

80. Chilukuri S, Bhatia AC. Nonablative dermal resurfacing in ethnic skin: laser and intense pulsed light. In: Alam M, Bhatia AC, Kundu RV, et al., eds. Cosmetic Dermatology for Skin of Color. McGraw Hill, 2009:51–57.

81. Mahmoud BH, Srivastava D, Janiga JJ, et al. Safety and efficacy of erbium-doped yttrium aluminum garnet fractionated laser for treatment of acne scars in type IV to VI skin. Dermatol Surg 2010; 36(5):602–609.

82. Chua SH, Ang P, Khoo LS, et al. Nonablative 1450-nm diode laser in the treatment of facial atrophic acne scars in type IV to V Asian skin: a prospective clinical study. Dermatol Surg 2004; 30(10):1287–1291.

83. Goldberg D, Metzler C. Skin resurfacing utilizing a low-fluence Nd:YAG laser. J Cosmet Laser Ther 1999; 1(1):23–27.

84. Goldberg DJ, Silapunt S. Histologic evaluation of a Q-switched Nd:YAG laser in the nonablative treatment of wrinkles. Dermatol Surg 2001; 27(8):744–746.

85. Goldberg DJ. Non-ablative subsurface remodeling: clinical and histologic evaluation of a 1320-nm Nd:YAG laser. J Cosmet Laser Ther 1999; 1(3):153–157.

86. Tanzi EL, Alster TS. Comparison of a 1450-nm diode laser and a 1320-nm Nd:YAG laser in the treatment of atrophic facial scars: a prospective clinical and histologic study. Dermatol Surg 2004; 30(2):152–157.

87. Lupton JR, Williams CM, Alster TS. Nonablative laser skin resurfacing using a 1540 nm erbium glass laser: a clinical and histologic analysis. Dermatol Surg 2002; 28(9):833–835.

88. Barnett JG, Barnett CR. Treatment of acne scars with liquid silicone injections: 30-year perspective. Dermatol Surg 2005; 31(11 pt 2):1542–1549.

89. Klein AW, Rish DC. Substances for soft tissue augmentation: collagen and silicone. J Dermatol Surg Oncol 1985; 11(3):337–339.

90. Langdon RC. Regarding dermabrasion for acne scars. Dermatol Surg 1999; 25 (11):919–920.

91. Sadove R. Injectable poly-L: -lactic acid: a novel sculpting agent for the treatment of dermal fat atrophy after severe acne. Aesthetic Plast Surg 2009; 33(1):113–116.

92. Swinehart JM. Case reports: surgical therapy of acne scars in pigmented skin. J Drugs Dermatol 2007; 6(1):74–77.

3.1

Topical retinoids

Andrea M. Hui and Alan R. Shalita

ACNE VULGARIS: PATHOPHYSIOLOGY

Acne vulgaris is a common dermatological complaint, accounting for over 30% of all visits to dermatologists. It is a multifactorial disease in which genetics and hormonal changes play a role in its development. The clinical lesions of acne develop from several steps, beginning with androgen stimulation of the sebaceous glands at or around puberty (1). This stimulates sebum production; the constituents of sebum are comedogenic and contribute to early changes of the follicle that lead to the microcomedo, the precursor lesion of acne vulgaris.

The microcomedo is a dense and cohesive corneal layer that accumulates along with sebum and occludes the follicle instead of naturally desquamating. Through resultant distention, the follicle may mature into open comedones of noninflammatory acne. This occluded, anaerobic, and lipid-rich environment supports the proliferation of the bacterium *Propionibacterium acnes* (*P. acnes*), a resident member of cutaneous flora. *P. acnes* was discovered to play a role in acne pathogenesis in the mid-1970s when treatment with tetracycline was associated with a decrease in *P. acnes* and free fatty acids in the surface lipid film.

P. acnes secretes chemotactic factors, attracting neutrophils to the occluded follicle. After phagocytosing *P. acnes*, hydrolytic enzymes are released by the neutrophils, activating complement and inflammation and breaks down the follicular wall. This leads to the characteristic inflammatory papules and pustules of acne vulgaris (2).

TOPICAL RETINOIDS

Topical retinoids play a major role in dermatology for the treatment of acne vulgaris. Retinoids are also used for the treatment of an array of dermatoses including acne and other acneiform disorders, photoaging, preneoplastic and neoplastic lesions, ichthyosiform disorders, psoriasiform disorders, keloids, and pigmentation disorders (3). These disorders all demonstrate an abnormal or dysfunctional epidermis.

Retinoids are a class of biologically active compounds that are structurally and functionally related to vitamin A (4). They have a wide range of biologic functions affecting cellular growth. Retinoids promote the proliferation of basal keratinocytes and prevent terminal stages of epithelial differentiation, instead directing keratinocytes to follow a normal or hyperproliferative state, and thus functions as an anti-keratinization agent (5,6). Reversal of abnormal keratinization by retinoids is due in part to the reduction of filaggrin expression and suppression of the proteolysis of keratins 1 and 14 (6). This contributes to the normalization of the epidermis.

The advantage of a topical retinoid over a systemic retinoid is its site specificity. This allows treatment of cutaneous lesions without inducing the various adverse effects of systemic retinoids. There are several topical retinoids available, and thus it is important for the clinician to understand their similarities and differences when choosing agents to manage their patients. The most widely used retinoids include topical tretinoin, adapalene, tazarotene, and oral and topical isotretinoin. Topical retinoids inhibit the formation of noninflammatory microcomedones and inflammatory acne lesions, as well as decrease the number of lesions (7). Recently, evidence has shown that inflammatory events can occur prior to microcomedo formation and that the development of plugs is influenced in part by the inflammation caused by *P.* acnes (8). Retinoids also exhibit direct anti-inflammatory activity (9).

Alterations of cellular growth, differentiation, and maintenance of epidermal tissue by retinoids are mediated by two classes of nuclear receptors: retinoic acid receptors (RARs) and retinoic X receptors (RXRs). RARs are divided into three subtypes: α, β, and γ. RAR-α is widely found in embryonic and adult tissues; RAR-β is found only in dermal fibroblasts; and RAR-γ is widely found in human epidermis and is thought to be the major receptor regulating the effects of retinoids on keratinocytes (10). Tretinoin, a first-generation retinoid, has shown nearly equal affinity for all three receptors, but it may have the highest affinity for the γ-receptor. Adapalene, a third-generation retinoid, has shown to bind strongly to RAR-β and -γ; RAR-γ is the prominent receptor found in epidermal and epithelial cells, allowing for topical retinoids to specifically affect comedonal proliferation.

The major adverse effect of topical retinoids is local irritation, including dry skin, discomfort, erythema, and scaling. Other elements contributing to irritation include quantity applied, site and frequency of application, irritation from washing, other medications, and skin type (11). With use of topical retinoids over time, skin irritation subsides. Additionally, several studies have demonstrated that topical tretinoin is neither photoallergic nor a photosensitizer. Furthermore, because of insignificant percutaneous absorption of tretinoin, long-term application of topical tretinoin has not been associated with the teratogenic effects shown with systemic use (12).

TRETINOIN

Topical tretinoin was the first FDA-approved topical retinoid and has remained a standard for acne therapy since the pioneer study of Kligman et al. in 1969 (13). In this study, Kligman et al. demonstrated that a 0.1% tretinoin solution most significantly reduced acne lesion counts in comparison with benzoyl peroxide, sulfur-resorcinol, and vehicle (13). Kligman et al. also noted spontaneous extrusion of comedonal material, which correlated with the histology of tretinoin-treated skin, including acanthosis, parakeratosis, and thinning and decreased cohesiveness of the stratum corneum (13). By its ability to thin the stratum corneum, topical tretinoin allows improved penetration and efficacy of topical antimicrobial agents such as benzoyl peroxide (14).

Tretinoin binds with equal affinity to all RAR subtypes. It is available as a cream (0.025%, 0.05%, 0.1%, and 0.4%), gel (0.01%, 0.025%, and 0.05%), microsphere gel (0.04% and 0.1%), liquid (0.025%, 0.05%, and 0.1%), lotion (0.1%), ointment (0.05%), compress (0.05%), and polymer cream (0.025%) (15). It is also available in Canada in combination with erythromycin and/or with a sunscreen. Many trials have demonstrated that tretinoin as a single agent significantly reduces both noninflammatory and inflammatory acne lesions, and global severity for periods of up to 12 weeks (16,17). A reduction in lesions may be noted after two to three weeks, but the greatest improvement is noted after three to four months. Common cutaneous adverse effects include desquamation, erythema, burning, and pruritus. Tretinoin binds and upregulates cellular retinoic acid–binding protein II (CRABP II), an intracellular binding protein found widely in the skin. The action that tretinoin exerts on CRABP II is a possible reason for the greater level of irritation caused by tretinoin compared with topical retinoids of later generations (18). Tretinoin is also highly unstable when exposed to oxygen and light. Improved tolerability has been achieved by a microsphere formulation, which gradually releases tretinoin over time (Retin-A Micro). This microsphere formulation also prevents degradation by oxidants such as benzoyl peroxide and ultraviolet light (19).

ISOTRETINOIN

Topical isotretinoin, the 13-*cis*-isomer of tretinoin, although not available in the United States, is widely available throughout most of the rest of the world and has an established record of safety and efficacy in the treatment of acne. It is available as a single agent topical formulation and, in some countries, combined with erythromycin.

TAZAROTENE

Tazarotene is a member of the third generation of receptor subtype–specific retinoids, which maintain efficacy while offering a reduced adverse effect profile. It regulates keratinocytes through the RAR-β and RAR-γ subtypes. It is available in a gel and cream formulation, containing either 0.05% or 0.1% of tazarotene. Both formulations were found to significantly reduce noninflammatory acne and lesion counts when compared with vehicle at 4 to 8 weeks; the 0.1% formulation continued to reduce inflammatory lesions at 12 weeks (20). In a trial comparing tazarotene 0.1% with tretinoin 0.1% microsponge gel, tazarotene was shown to be more efficacious than tretinoin in reducing noninflammatory lesion count (21). When adapalene was introduced, a trial comparing adapalene 0.1% gel with tazarotene 0.1% gel demonstrated that tazarotene was more effective in decreasing numbers inflammatory and noninflammatory lesions than adapalene (22). Additionally, topical tazarotene plus oral minocycline showed greater efficacy as a maintenance therapy for acne vulgaris, but did not show statistically significant reductions in lesion count when compared with tazarotene alone (23).

For the treatment of noninflammatory lesions, tazarotene has been shown to work best as monotherapy; several studies comparing the efficacy of tazarotene with standard acne therapy agents such as benzoyl peroxide gel, erythromycin/benzoyl peroxide cream, and clindamycin showed that monotherapy was superior to all combinations for the reduction of noninflammatory lesions (24). In combination, tazarotene plus clindamycin was superior for overall improvement. Additionally, a recent study demonstrated that tazarotene 0.1% cream appeared to be more effective and nearly as well tolerated as adapalene 0.3% gel in reducing lesion count and acne severity, and was more effective than adapalene 0.3% gel in reducing postinflammatory hyperpigmentation (25).

ADAPALENE

Adapalene is a member of the third generation of receptor subtype–specific retinoids, available in 0.1% and 0.3% gel, and 0.1% cream formulations. Adapalene shows the greatest affinity for the RAR-γ and RAR-β subtypes. Topical adapalene is a safe and effective retinoid for the treatment of acne vulgaris (26,27). Compared with tretinoin 0.025% gel, adapalene 0.1% gel showed similar efficacy in reducing inflammatory and noninflammatory lesions, and global severity in several randomized trials (28–32). In a trial comparing adapalene 0.1% gel with tazarotene 0.1% gel, daily tazarotene 0.1% was more effective than daily adapalene 0.1% gel in reducing inflammatory and non-inflammatory lesions (22). However, this study did not include the microsphere formulation of topical tretinoin. When combined with doxycycline, adapalene has been shown to be significantly more effective for the treatment of acne than doxycycline alone (33). Several studies demonstrated that a combination of adapalene 0.1% gel plus clindamycin 1% lotion twice daily was significantly more effective in reducing acne lesions and global severity compared with clindamycin 1% lotion twice daily plus gel vehicle (34).

Adapalene is well tolerated and shows a lower adverse effect profile when compared with other topical retinoids including tretinoin gel and cream at 0.01%, 0.025%, and 0.05%, tretinoin 0.1% and 0.04% microsphere gel, 0.5% and 0.1% tazarotene gel and benzoyl peroxide (35–39).

NEW DEVELOPMENTS

The current consensus for the treatment of both noninflammatory and inflammatory acne is the use of both topical retinoids and antimicrobial therapy to provide combination therapy, targeting the different pathophysiologies of acne. Recent in vitro studies have shown that the third-generation retinoid adapalene was significantly more stable than the first-generation retinoid treti-noin in the presence of light, clindamycin, and oxidizing agents such as benzoyl peroxide. The unstable, light-sensitive double bonds present in the chemical structure of tretinoin are absent and are replaced by the more stable naphthoic acid aromatic rings in adapalene (40). This is important because benzoyl per-oxide is often given concurrently with retinoids for its safe, effective anti-microbial activity against *P. acnes*. Additionally, adapalene has demonstrated targeted delivery to the microcomedo. Clinical trials comparing adapalene 0.3% with another third-generation retinoid tazarotene 0.1% have shown these to be therapeutically similar in efficacy for the reduction of inflammatory and non-inflammatory lesions, but adapalene was significantly better tolerated than tazarotene.

Topical retinoids have been shown to permit greater penetration and efficacy of topical antimicrobials because of their effect of thinning of the stratum corneum, as mentioned previously. This allows for a multitude of combination therapies to suppress the proliferation of *P. acnes* in micro-comedones to treat inflammatory lesions (41). Recently, a fixed-combination therapy containing topical adapalene 0.1% and benzoyl peroxide 2.5% has demonstrated significant efficacy in addressing comedones, *P. acnes*, and inflammatory lesions of acne vulgaris (42). Adapalene 0.1%/benzoyl peroxide 2.5% fixed-combination therapy offers an advantage over monotherapies, with significant differences in lesion counts observed as early as one week after initiating therapy (43). Adapalene 0.1%/benzoyl peroxide 2.5% fixed-combination therapy is safe and effective for up to 52 weeks of use (44).

Another recent fixed-combination therapy containing topical tretinoin 0.025% and clindamycin 1.2% has been shown in a large randomized control study to significantly reduce inflammatory, noninflammatory, and total acne lesions after 12 weeks of treatment (45). This combination therapy was significantly more effective than monotherapy or vehicle alone, and demonstrated excellent tolerability and safety after 52 weeks of use (45).

Topical retinoids have been a safe and efficacious treatment of acne vulgaris for decades. Recent advances in retinoid development have allowed for other treatment modalities to be administered in fixed-combination formulations, offering clinicians and their patients increased tolerability and efficacy.

REFERENCES

1. Leyden JJ, Shalita AR. Rational therapy for acne vulgaris: an update on topical treatment. J Am Acad Dermatol 1986; 15(4 pt 2):907–915.
2. Leyden JJ. The evolving role of Propionibacterium acnes in acne. Semin Cutan Med Surg 2001; 20(3):139–143.
3. Haas AA, Arndt KA. Selected therapeutic applications of topical tretinoin. J Am Acad Dermatol 1986; 15(4 pt 2):870–877.
4. Bollag W. The development of retinoids in experimental and clinical oncology and dermatology. J Am Acad Dermatol 1983; 9(5):797–805.
5. Eichner R. Epidermal effects of retinoids: in vitro studies. J Am Acad Dermatol 1986; 15(4 pt 2):789–797.
6. Eichner R, Kahn M, Capetola RJ, et al. Effects of topical retinoids on cytoskeletal proteins: implications for retinoid effects on epidermal differentiation. J Invest Dermatol 1992; 98(2):154–161.
7. Lavker RM, Leyden JJ, Thorne EG. An ultrastructural study of the effects of topical tretinoin on microcomedones. Clin Ther 1992; 14(6):773–780.
8. Thiboutot D, Gollnick H, Bettoli V, et al. Global Alliance to Improve Outcomes in Acne. New insights into the management of acne: an update from the Global Alliance to Improve Outcomes in Acne group (review). J Am Acad Dermatol 2009; 60(5 suppl):S1–S50.
9. Jones DA. The potential immunomodulatory effects of topical retinoids (review). Dermatol Online J 2005; 11(1):3.
10. Czernielewski J, Michel S, Bouclier M, et al. Adapalene biochemistry and the evolution of a new topical retinoid for treatment of acne (review). J Eur Acad Dermatol Venereol 2001; 15(suppl 3):5–12.
11. Papa CM. The cutaneous safety of topical tretinoin. Acta Derm Venereol Suppl (Stockh) 1975; 74:128–132.

12. Loureiro KD, Kao KK, Jones KL, et al. Minor malformations characteristic of the retinoic acid embryopathy and other birth outcomes in children of women exposed to topical tretinoin during early pregnancy. Am J Med Genet A 2005; 136(2):117–121.

13. Kligman AM, Fulton JE Jr., Plewig G. Topical vitamin A acid in acne vulgaris. Arch Dermatol 1969; 99(4):469–476.

14. Leyden JJ, Marples RR, Mills OH, et al. Tretinoin and antibiotic therapy in acne vulgaris. South Med J 1974; 67(1):20–25.

15. Thielitz A, Gollnick H. Topical retinoids in acne vulgaris: update on efficacy and safety. Am J Clin Dermatol 2008; 9(6):369–381.

16. Krautheim A, Gollnick HP. Acne: topical treatment (review). Clin Dermatol 2004; 22(5):398–407.

17. Webster GF. Topical tretinoin in acne therapy (review). J Am Acad Dermatol 1998; 39(2 pt 3):S38–S44.

18. Martin B, Meunier C, Montels D, et al. Chemical stability of adapalene and tretinoin when combined with benzoyl peroxide in presence and in absence of visible light and ultraviolet radiation. Br J Dermatol 1998; 139(suppl 52):8–11.

19. Nyirady J, Lucas C, Yusuf M, et al. The stability of tretinoin in tretinoin gel microsphere 0.1%. Cutis 2002; 70(5):295–298.

20. Shalita AR, Chalker DK, Griffith RF, et al. Tazarotene gel is safe and effective in the treatment of acne vulgaris: a multicenter, double-blind, vehicle-controlled study. Cutis 1999; 63(6):349–354.

21. Leyden JJ, Tanghetti EA, Miller B, et al. Once-daily tazarotene 0.1 % gel versus once-daily tretinoin 0.1 % microsponge gel for the treatment of facial acne vulgaris: a double-blind randomized trial. Cutis 2002; 69(2 suppl):12–19.

22. Webster GF, Guenther L, Poulin YP, et al. A multicenter, double-blind, randomized comparison study of the efficacy and tolerability of once-daily tazarotene 0.1% gel and adapalene 0.1% gel for the treatment of facial acne vulgaris. Cutis 2002; 69(2 suppl):4–11.

23. Leyden J, Thiboutot DM, Shalita AR, et al. Comparison of tazarotene and minocycline maintenance therapies in acne vulgaris: a multicenter, double-blind, randomized, parallel-group study. Arch Dermatol 2006; 142(5):605–612.

24. Draelos ZD, Tanghetti EA; Tazarotene Combination Leads to Efficacious Acne Results (CLEAR) Trial Study Group. Optimizing the use of tazarotene for the treatment of facial acne vulgaris through combination therapy. Cutis 2002; 69(2 suppl):20–29.

25. Tanghetti E, Dhawan S, Green L, et al. Randomized comparison of the safety and efficacy of tazarotene 0.1% cream and adapalene 0.3% gel in the treatment of patients with at least moderate facial acne vulgaris. J Drugs Dermatol 2010; 9 (5):549–558.

26. Pariser DM, Thiboutot DM, Clark SD, et al.; Adapalene Study Group. The efficacy and safety of adapalene gel 0.3% in the treatment of acne vulgaris: a randomized, multicenter, investigator-blinded, controlled comparison study versus adapalene gel 0.1% and vehicle. Cutis 2005; 76(2):145–151.

27. Thiboutot D, Pariser DM, Egan N, et al.; Adapalene Study Group. Adapalene gel 0.3% for the treatment of acne vulgaris: a multicenter, randomized, double-blind, controlled, phase III trial. J Am Acad Dermatol 2006; 54(2):242–250.

28. Tu P, Li GQ, Zhu XJ, et al. A comparison of adapalene gel 0.1% vs. tretinoin gel 0.025% in the treatment of acne vulgaris in China. J Eur Acad Dermatol Venereol 2001; 15(suppl 3):31–36.

29. Ellis CN, Millikan LE, Smith EB, et al. Comparison of adapalene 0.1% solution and tretinoin 0.025% gel in the topical treatment of acne vulgaris. Br J Dermatol 1998; 139(suppl 52):41–47.

30. Grosshans E, Marks R, Mascaro JM, et al. Evaluation of clinical efficacy and safety of adapalene 0.1% gel versus tretinoin 0.025% gel in the treatment of acne vulgaris, with particular reference to the onset of action and impact on quality of life. Br J Dermatol 1998; 139(suppl 52):26–33.

31. Cunliffe WJ, Caputo R, Dreno B, et al. Clinical efficacy and safety comparison of adapalene gel and tretinoin gel in the treatment of acne vulgaris: Europe and U.S. multicenter trials. J Am Acad Dermatol 1997; 36(6 pt 2):S126–S134.

32. Shalita A, Weiss JS, Chalker DK, et al. A comparison of the efficacy and safety of adapalene gel 0.1% and tretinoin gel 0.025% in the treatment of acne vulgaris: a multicenter trial. J Am Acad Dermatol 1996; 34(3):482–485.

33. Thiboutot DM, Shalita AR, Yamauchi PS, et al.; Differin Study Group. Combination therapy with adapalene gel 0.1% and doxycycline for severe acne vulgaris: a multicenter, investigator-blind, randomized, controlled study. Skinmed 2005; 4(3):138–146.

34. Wolf JE Jr., Kaplan D, Kraus SJ, et al. Efficacy and tolerability of combined topical treatment of acne vulgaris with adapalene and clindamycin: a multicenter, randomized, investigator-blinded study. J Am Acad Dermatol 2003; 49(3 suppl):S211–S217.

35. Queille-Roussel C, Poncet M, Mesaros S, et al. Comparison of the cumulative irritation potential of adapalene gel and cream with that of erythromycin/tretinoin solution and gel and erythromycin/isotretinoin gel. Clin Ther 2001; 23(2):205–212.

36. Galvin SA, Gilbert R, Baker M, et al. Comparative tolerance of adapalene 0.1% gel and six different tretinoin formulations. Br J Dermatol 1998; 139(suppl 52):34–40.

37. Caron D, Sorba V, Clucas A, et al. Skin tolerance of adapalene 0.1% gel in combination with other topical antiacne treatments. J Am Acad Dermatol 1997; 36(6 pt 2):S113–S115.

38. Toole JW, Lockhart L, Potrebka J, et al. Comparative irritancy study among retinoid creams and gels. J Cutan Med Surg 1999; 3(6):298–301.

39. Dosik JS, Homer K, Arsonnaud S. Cumulative irritation potential of adapalene 0.1% cream and gel compared with tazarotene cream 0.05% and 0.1%. Cutis 2005; 75(5):289–293.

40. Martin B, Meunier C, Montels D, et al. Chemical stability of adapalene and tretinoin when combined with benzoyl peroxide in presence and in absence of visible light and ultraviolet radiation. Br J Dermatol 1998; 139(suppl 52):8–11.

41. Jain GK, Ahmed FJ. Adapalene pretreatment increases follicular penetration of clindamycin: in vitro and in vivo studies. Indian J Dermatol Venereol Leprol 2007; 73(5):326–329.

42. Gold LS, Tan J, Cruz-Santana A, et al.; Adapalene-BPO Study Group. A North American study of adapalene-benzoyl peroxide combination gel in the treatment of acne. Cutis 2009; 84(2):110–116.

43. Thiboutot DM, Weiss J, Bucko A, et al.; Adapalene-BPO Study Group. Adapalene-benzoyl peroxide, a fixed-dose combination for the treatment of acne vulgaris: results of a multicenter, randomized double-blind, controlled study. J Am Acad Dermatol 2007; 57(5):791–799; [Epub July 26, 2007].
44. Pariser DM, Westmoreland P, Morris A, et al. Long-term safety and efficacy of a unique fixed-dose combination gel of adapalene 0.1% and benzoyl peroxide 2.5% for the treatment of acne vulgaris. J Drugs Dermatol 2007; 6(9):899–905.
45. Eichenfield LF, Wortzman M. A novel gel formulation of 0.25% tretinoin and 1.2% clindamycin phosphate: efficacy in acne vulgaris patients aged 12 to 18 years. Pediatr Dermatol 2009; 26(3):257–261.

3.2

Topical antibiotics

James Q. Del Rosso

INTRODUCTION

Topical antibiotics have been an integral component of the topical armamentarium for the treatment of acne vulgaris for approximately four decades and remain commonly prescribed by dermatologists in clinical practice (1,2). Over time, the most common topical antibiotics used for acne treatment have been erythromycin and clindamycin, with the latter being favored over the past several years, primarily due to widespread emergence globally of *Propionibacterium acnes* strains resistant to erythromycin (3–7). Although clindamycin-resistant *P. acnes* are also relatively prevalent due to its common use, the clinical efficacy of topical clindamycin in the treatment of acne vulgaris has sustained over several years of usage as compared with topical erythromycin on the basis of review of data from several studies (4–7).

In addition to topical erythromycin and clindamycin, sulfacetamide with or without sulfur has also been used topically for treatment of acne vulgaris; however, data on mechanism and efficacy for this indication are very limited (8). Azelaic acid has also been used for treatment of acne and is discussed later in this chapter (1).

RATIONALE FOR USE OF TOPICAL ANTIBIOTICS IN ACNE THERAPY

Data on the pharmacologic and antibiotic properties of topical antibiotics related to treatment of acne vulgaris have been evaluated predominantly with erythromycin and clindamycin. The principal mechanism of action of these topical antibiotics appears to be through reduction in *P. acnes* organisms, which reduces the subsequent triggering of inflammatory activities and pathways believed to relate to acne lesion pathogenesis (1–3,6–8). The use of benzoyl peroxide in combination with erythromycin or clindamycin augments reduction in *P. acnes*, reduces the emergence of resistant *P. acnes* strains, and may improve efficacy over use of either agent alone (1,2,6). Although a variety of anti-inflammatory properties have been reported with both erythromycin and clindamycin, the relevance of these effects to acne treatment is not definitively known (9).

TOPICAL ANTIBIOTIC USE IN ACNE AND CHANGES IN CUTANEOUS FLORA

Concerns regarding emergence of clinically significant antibiotic-resistant bacteria primarily focus on systemic antibiotic use. Importantly, topical antibiotic use can also change the cutaneous flora (6,7,10–16).

As application of topical antibiotics for treatment of acne is usually continued over several months to years, the issues of alteration of cutaneous flora, antibiotic selection pressure, and increase in antibiotic resistance are clinically relevant. In fact, changes in cutaneous flora have been reported with both topical and oral antibiotic use (6,17–23). Antibiotics commonly used for the treatment of acne vulgaris have been correlated with the progressive emergence of normal bacterial flora that are less antibiotic sensitive. These include macrolide-resistant *Staphylococcus epidermidis* and erythromycin- and tetracycline-resistant *P. acnes* strains, the latter increasing by an estimated prevalence of 40% globally over approximately three decades (6,17–25). Additionally, antibiotic-resistant *P. acnes* strains have been demonstrated on skin of untreated contacts of acne patients treated with topical antibiotic therapy, supporting interpersonal spread (20). In another study, facial application of topical erythromycin over three months has been shown to affect the bacterial flora of both treated and untreated skin (22). This study confirmed an increase in coagulase-negative staphylococci on treated facial skin, and also at untreated sites such as the back and nares (22).

The clinically relevant effects of the aforementioned changes in normal bacterial flora secondary to antibiotic use are not entirely clear. However, there is evidence for a correlation between antibiotic-resistant *P. acnes* and a reduction in efficacy with antibiotic therapy (10–12,17,24–27).

COMPARISON OF TOPICAL ANTIBIOTICS IN THE TREATMENT OF ACNE

Erythromycin, a macrolide antibiotic, and clindamycin, a lincosamide antibiotic, have been widely used for the treatment of acne for approximately four decades and represent the vast majority of topical antibiotic prescriptions written by dermatologists for acne. Since 2003, prescribing data indicate that clindamycin is the predominant topical antibiotic used by dermatologists to treat acne in clinical practice, with approximately half of prescriptions written for benzoyl peroxide–clindamycin combination formulations (6,17).

An important concern related to use of topical antibiotics, especially with chronic administration for acne, is the emergence of antibiotic-resistant bacterial strains. Potential issues of concern that have been raised in the literature include increased prevalence of *P. acnes* strains less responsive to antibiotics, alterations in cutaneous flora, decreased therapeutic responsiveness to antibiotic therapy, and promotion of other clinical infections among treated patients and/or their close contacts (6,17,18,21–24,26,27). Although in vitro antibiotic cross-resistance between erythromycin and clindamycin has been reported, a difference in clinical efficacy between these two agents used for acne has been noted over time (5). A report analyzing several monotherapy studies using either topical erythromycin or topical clindamycin for acne vulgaris demonstrated that the efficacy of topical erythromycin in reducing acne lesions has markedly decreased over time; however, the efficacy of topical clindamycin has not diminished on the basis of the same parameters of acne lesion reduction (5). Subsequent studies not analyzed in this report, inclusive of approximately 2000 subjects treated with topical clindamycin in the monotherapy study groups, have demonstrated consistent reduction of inflammatory acne lesions ranging from 45% to 49% and noninflammatory acne lesions ranging from 30% to 41% (4,28–31). Overall, these results support the sustained efficacy of topical clindamycin for acne, at least on the basis of clinical trials. Factors that may explain the efficacy differences between topical clindamycin and topical erythromycin observed over time may include inherent differences in pharmacologic properties, nonantibiotic activities such as possible anti-inflammatory effects, tissue concentrations achieved by topical administration, which may overcome in vitro resistance, and differences in antibiotic resistance genes. Available data, including well-designed studies or analyses, comparing topical erythromycin and/or clindamycin with other topical antibiotics used to treat acne vulgaris are limited.

ECOLOGIC MISCHIEF AND TOPICAL ANTIBIOTIC USE FOR ACNE

Chronic facial application of antibiotics used to treat acne does alter cutaneous and anterior nasal flora (6,15,17). Topical erythromycin or clindamycin application does promote emergence of less sensitive strains of *P. acnes*, with concomitant use of benzoyl peroxide reducing both the emergence of less sensitive *P. acnes* strains and the proliferation of preexistent antibiotic-resistant strains (17,23,32).

Pharyngeal colonization with *Streptococcus pyogenes* has been associated with chronic use of antibiotics for acne, including topical agents. A cross-sectional study evaluated 39 subjects with acne treated chronically with oral and/ or topical antibiotics versus 63 control subjects not treated with antibiotic therapy (18). The results demonstrated that 33% of antibiotic-treated subjects exhibited *S. pyogenes* on oropharyngeal culture, as compared with 10% in the control group (18). Importantly, 85% of *S. pyogenes* cultures obtained from antibiotic-treated subjects demonstrated resistance to at least one tetracycline antibiotic as compared with 20% in control subjects. In this same study, 10 subjects used only topical therapy without an oral antibiotic for acne. Four of these 10 subjects who were treated only with a topical antibiotic exhibited a positive oropharyngeal culture for *S. pyogenes*, with resistance to at least one tetracycline antibiotic observed in 3 of the 4 subjects. Despite the small study size, these results raise questions regarding the potential clinical significance of oropharyngeal carriage of pathogenic streptococci related to antibiotic use for acne, including topical agents.

In an additional study using retrospective cohort analysis of a large patient database, potential clinical implications of chronic oral and/or topical antibiotic therapy for acne vulgaris were analyzed (26). The topical antibiotics included in the evaluation were erythromycin and clindamycin. Antibiotic therapy needed to be used for a duration of at least six weeks. Among the antibiotic-treated group, 6.1% used topical therapy only and 92.6% used a combination of oral and topical agents. The United Kingdom General Practice Research Database was used, identifying 118,496 patients with a diagnosis of acne vulgaris between the ages of 15 and 35 years. Among this acne patient group, 71.7% ($n = 84,977$) received an oral and/or topical antibiotic, with 28.3% ($n = 33,519$) not receiving antibiotic therapy. It was shown within the first observation year on the basis of chart review that the odds of an antibiotic-treated patient developing an upper respiratory tract infection (URTI) was 2.15 times greater than patients not treated with antibiotic therapy. Individually, the odds ratios were 2.37, 1.88, and 2.75 for topical therapy only, combined use of topical and oral agents, and oral antibiotic therapy only, respectively. Identified limitations of this analysis include retrospective evaluation based on diagnosis coding, lack of exclusion of other antibiotics for disorders other than acne vulgaris, dependence on diagnosis codes only for documentation of URTI, and failure to differentiate the etiology of URTI. Despite the questions raised by this report, further study is needed to determine clinical relevance.

INTEGRATION OF TOPICAL ANTIBIOTICS IN ACNE TREATMENT

Topical antibiotics have long been an integral component of the combination therapy approach to acne therapy, including use with benzoyl peroxide and/or a topical retinoid (1–6,17,28–34). Importantly, topical antibiotics are best combined with benzoyl peroxide to optimize acne lesion reduction and reduce emergence of antibiotic-resistant *P. acnes* strains (7,17,23,32–35). Benzoyl peroxide may be used concurrently as either a "leave-on" formulation or a wash/cleanser (35,36). Data supporting the therapeutic benefits of the combination use of benzoyl peroxide with antibiotics are based on studies using specific brand vehicle formulations, including both leave-on and wash/cleanser products (37,38). As vehicle formulation can influence several factors such as percutaneous drug penetration and tolerability, results from a given study cannot be automatically assumed to apply to unstudied formulations, including generic products.

OTHER TOPICAL ANTIBIOTICS AND ACNE TREATMENT

As mentioned above, despite availability for several years, data on the use of topical sodium sulfacetamide, with or without sulfur, for the treatment of acne vulgaris are limited. One study ($n = 60$) demonstrated a marked decrease in total acne lesion count, primarily a reduction in inflammatory lesions, in women with acne vulgaris treated with sulfacetamide 10% and sulfur 5% lotion for 12 weeks (8).

Azelaic acid has been shown to exhibit antibiotic properties and has been used for the treatment of acne vulgaris, primarily as a 20% cream formulation (1,34). The use of the 15% gel formulation for acne treatment has also been studied with reductions in acne lesions reported to be comparable to benzoyl peroxide or topical clindamycin (39). Overall, the position of azelaic acid in the treatment algorithm of acne vulgaris has been as an alternative to other topical agents (1,34). Initial improvement in acne with topical azelaic acid has been reported to be observed in 4 to 8 weeks, with maximum benefit generally noted after approximately 16 weeks of use (40–42). Symptoms of tingling, stinging, or burning have been reported to occur in 10% to 20% of patients treated with azelaic acid, usually within the first one to two weeks, with most cases noted as transient and without necessitation of discontinuation of therapy (40–42).

Topical metronidazole is well established as a therapeutic option for papulopustular rosacea. A study evaluating the use of topical metronidazole 0.75% gel for the treatment of acne vulgaris did not demonstrate therapeutic benefit (43).

SAFETY CONSIDERATIONS WITH TOPICAL ANTIBIOTICS USE FOR ACNE

Overall, the safety profile related to the use of topical antibiotics for treatment of acne vulgaris has been very favorable (1–4,8,17,28–31,34,39–42). The majority of adverse events reported in association with topical antibiotic use for acne have been signs and/or symptoms of cutaneous intolerability at sites of application, such as erythema, scaling, stinging, burning, and/or pruritus in some patients; true allergy to the conventional topical antibiotics used to treat acne vulgaris are rare (44). The frequency and intensity of local cutaneous side effects have been relatively infrequent overall and are often dependent on the vehicle formulation.

Importantly, there has been a conspicuous absence of significant systemic safety signals associated with topical antibiotic use for acne, especially considering the plethora of clinical trials and the extensive clinical use worldwide over several years (44). A warning regarding possible association of topical clindamycin use and development of pseudomembranous colitis has been noted on the basis of a few older case reports, with only one involving proprietary formulations (44–46). Considering the availability of this agent for approximately four decades and its widespread use over long durations of time, the risk of association with pseudomembranous colitis appears to be very small (44). Although the actual risk is unclear, it is prudent to avoid topical application of a formulation containing sulfacetamide in patients with a true sulfonamide allergy (47).

With regard to the safety of topical antibiotics during pregnancy, it is very difficult to make definitive statements as recommendations are determined indirectly on the basis of clinical observation, results from animal studies, limited data in humans from clinical trials, sporadic reports from community experience, and information collected from pregnancy exposure databases. Overall, the topical use of erythromycin, clindamycin, sulfacetamide, and azelaic acid appears to be safe; there are no formal contraindications during pregnancy mandated with these agents; teratogenicity does not appear to be associated with their use; and topical erythromycin is generally considered safe in a pregnant female patient (48). However, absolute safety of topical antibiotic use during pregnancy cannot be definitively stated, especially as application is typically for a prolonged duration. Because of the risk of kernicterus potentially associated with sulfonamide exposure in pregnancy, especially during the third trimester, it appears prudent to avoid application of a formulation containing sodium sulfacetamide in a pregnant female patient. It is important for clinicians to recognize that despite apparent and anticipated safety during pregnancy based on published general guidelines and Pregnancy Category listings (classified as B or C depending on the topical agent), some product monographs of topical antibiotics contain pregnancy "disclaimers" stated by the manufacturer (48). Such disclaimers typically imply that data may be too limited to assess safety in pregnancy and/or that the true risk is unknown.

The potential concerns related to emergence of antibiotic-resistant bacterial strains or changes in microbial flora have been discussed above. Although these concerns are valid and of likely clinical relevance, their true clinical significance remains somewhat controversial. Additional study and dedicated surveillance are definitely warranted in this very important area related to antibiotic use for acne.

CONCLUSION

Topical antibiotics remain an important part of acne treatment and are recommended as a component of combination topical therapy; monotherapy with a topical antibiotic for acne is not recommended (1,7,17,34). At present, topical clindamycin remains the predominant topical antibiotic used for acne treatment; however, other agents such as erythromycin, sulfacetamide with or without sulfur, and azelaic acid are also options (1,6,7,17,34). Importantly, data suggest that the efficacy of topical erythromycin in acne has diminished over time since its inception (5). Concerns regarding development of antibiotic resistance and changes in cutaneous flora associated with topical antibiotic use, especially chronic application, may be clinically relevant and warrant additional study. Overall, the tolerability and safety profiles of topical antibiotics discussed in this chapter are very favorable.

REFERENCES

1. Gollnick H, Cunliffe W, Berson D, et al. Management of acne: a report from the global alliance to improve outcomes in acne. J Am Acad Dermatol 2003; 49(suppl 1):S1–S38.
2. Leyden JJ. The evolving role of *Propionibacterium acnes* in acne. Semin Cutan Med Surg 2001; 20:139–143.
3. Rosen T, Waisman M. Topically administered clindamycin in the treatment of acne vulgaris and other dermatologic disorders. Pharmacotherapy 1981; 1:201–205.
4. Shalita AR, Myers JA, Krochmal L, et al. The safety and efficacy of clindamycin phosphate foam 1% versus clindamycin phosphate topical gel 1% for the treatment of acne vulgaris. J Drugs Dermatol 2005; 4:48–46.
5. Simonart T, Dramaix M. Treatment of acne with topical antibiotics: lessons from clinical studies. Br J Dermatol 2005; 153:395–403.
6. Del Rosso JQ, Leyden JJ, Thiboutot D, et al. Antibiotic use in acne vulgaris and rosacea: clinical considerations and resistance issues of significance to dermatologist. Cutis 2008; 82(2S[ii]):5–12.
7. Del Rosso JQ, Leyden JJ. Status report on antibiotic resistance: implications for the dermatologist. Dermatol Clin 2007; 25:127–132.
8. Breneman DL, Ariano MC. Successful treatment of acne vulgaris in women with a new topical sulfacetamide/sulfur lotion. Int J Dermatol 1993; 32:365–367.
9. Del Rosso JQ, Schmidt NF. A review of the anti-inflammatory properties of clindamycin in the treatment of acne vulgaris. Cutis 2010; 85:15–24.

10. Levy SB. The challenge of antibiotic resistance. Sci Am 1998; 278:46–53.
11. Esperson F. Resistance to antibiotics used in dermatologic practice. Br J Dermatol 1998; 139:4–8.
12. Leyden JJ, McGinley KJ, Cavalieri S, et al. *Propionibacterium acnes* resistance to antibiotics in acne patients. J Am Acad Dermatol 1983; 8:41–45.
13. Eady AH, Cove JH, Layton AM. Is antibiotic resistance in cutaneous propionibacteria clinically relevant? Implications of resistance for acne patients and prescribers. Am J Clin Dermatol 2003; 12:813–831.
14. Finkelstein JA, Stille C, Nordin J, et al. Reduction in antibiotic use among US children 1996-2000. Pediatrics 2003; 139:467–471.
15. Eady EA, Gloor M, Leyden JJ. Propionibacterium acnes resistance: a worldwide problem. Dermatology 2003; 206:54–56.
16. Bojar RA, Eady EA, Jones CE, et al. Inhibition of erythromycin-resistant propionibacteria on the skin of acne patients by topical erythromycin with and without zinc. Br J Dermatol 1990; 130:329–336.
17. Leyden JJ, Del Rosso JQ, Webster GF. Clinical considerations in the treatment of acne vulgaris and other inflammatory skin disorders: focus on antibiotic resistance. Cutis 2007; 79(suppl 6):9–25.
18. Levy RM, Huang EY, Rolling D, et al. Effect of antibiotics on the oropharyngeal flora in patients with acne. Arch Dermatol 2003; 139:467–471.
19. Dreno B, Reynaud A, Moyse D, et al. Erythromycin-resistance of cutaneous bacterial flora in acne. Eur J Dermatol 2001; 11:549–553.
20. Ross JL, Snelling AM, Carnegie E, et al. Antibiotic-resistant acne: lessons from Europe. Br J Dermatol 2003; 148:467–478.
21. Vowels BR, Feingold DS, Sloughfy C, et al. Effects of topical erythromycin on ecology of aerobic cutaneous bacterial flora. Antimicrob Agents Chemother 1996; 40:2598–2604.
22. Mills O Jr., Thornsberry C, Cardin CW, et al. Bacterial resistance and therapeutic outcome following three months of topical acne therapy with 2% erythromycin gel versus its vehicle. Acta Derm Venereol 2002; 82:260–265.
23. Harkaway KS, McGinley KJ, Foglia AN, et al. Antibiotic resistance patterns in coagulase-negative staphylococci after treatment with topical erythromycin, benzoyl peroxide, and combination therapy. Br J Dermatol 1992; 126:585–590.
24. Eady EA, Cove JH, Holland KT, et al. Erythromycin resistant propionibacteria in antibiotic treated acne patients: association with therapeutic failure. Br J Dermatol 1989; 121:51–57.
25. Cooper AJ. Systematic review of Propionibacterium acnes resistance to systemic antibiotics. Med J Austral 1998; 169:259–261.
26. Margolis DJ, Bowe WP, Hoffstad O, et al. Antibiotic treatment of acne may be associated with upper respiratory tract infections. Arch Dermatol 2005; 141:1132–1136.
27. Bowe WP, Hoffstad O, Margolis DJ. Upper respiratory tract infection in household contacts of acne patients. Dermatology 2007; 215:213–218.
28. Schlessinger J, Menter A, Gold M, et al. Clinical safety and efficacy studies of a novel formulation combining 1.2% clindamycin phosphate and 0.025% tretinoin for the treatment of acne vulgaris. J Drugs Dermatol 2007; 6:607–615.

29. Leyden JJ, Krochmal L, Yaroshinsky A. Two randomized, double-blind, controlled trials of 2219 subjects to compare the combination clindamycin/tretinoin hydrogel with each agent alone and vehicle for the treatment of acne vulgaris. J Am Acad Dermatol 2006; 54:73–81.

30. Thiboutot D, Zaenglein A, Weiss J, et al. An aqueous gel fixed combination of clindamycin phosphate 1.2% and benzoyl peroxide 2.5% for the once-daily treatment of moderate to severe acne vulgaris: assessment of efficacy and safety in 2813 patients. J Am Acad Dermatol 2008; 59:792–800.

31. Zouboulis CC, Derumeaux L, Decroix J, et al. A multicentre, single-blind, randomized comparison of a fixed clindamycin phosphate/tretinoin gel formulation applied once daily and a combination lotion formulation applied twice daily in the topical treatment of acne vulgaris. Br J Dermatol 2000; 143:498–505.

32. Cunliffe WJ, Holland KT, Bojar R, et al. A randomized, double-blind comparison of a clindamycin phosphate/benzoyl peroxide gel formulation and a matching clindamycin gel with respect to microbiologic activity and clinical efficacy in the topical treatment of acne vulgaris. Clin Ther 2002; 24:1117–1133.

33. Tanghetti EA, Popp KF. A current review of topical benzoyl peroxide: new perspectives on formulation and utilization. Dermatol Clin 2009; 27:17–24.

34. Thiboutot D, Gollnick H, Bettoli V, et al. New insights into the management of acne: an update from the global alliance to improve outcomes in acne group. J Am Acad Dermatol 2009; 60(suppl 5):S1–S50.

35. Leyden JJ, Wortzman M, Baldwin EK. Antibiotic-resistant *Propionibacterium acnes* suppressed by a benzoyl peroxide cleanser 6%. Cutis 2008; 82:417–421.

36. Shalita AR, Rafal ES, Anderson D, et al. Compared efficacy and safety of tretinoin 0.1% microsphere gel alone and in combination with benzoyl peroxide 6% cleanser for the treatment of acne vulgaris. Cutis 2003; 72:167–172.

37. Del Rosso JQ. What is the role of benzoyl peroxide cleansers in acne management? J Clin Aesthet Dermatol 2008; 41:48–51.

38. Del Rosso JQ. Benzoyl peroxide cleansers for the treatment of acne vulgaris: status report on available data. Cutis 2008; 82:336–342.

39. Thiboutot D. Versatility of azelaic acid 15% gel in the treatment of inflammatory acne vulgaris. J Drugs Dermatol 2008; 7:13–16.

40. Cunliffe WJ, Holland KT. Clinical and laboratory studies on treatment with 20% azelaic acid cream for acne. Acta Derm Venereol Suppl (Stockh) 1989; 143:31–34.

41. Katsambas A, Graupe K, Stratigos J. Clinical studies of 20% azelaic acid cream in the treatment of acne vulgaris—comparison with vehicle and topical tretinoin. Acta Derm Venereol Suppl (Stockh) 1989; 143:35–39.

42. Hjorth N, Graupe K. Azelaic acid for the treatment of acne vulgaris—a clinical comparison with oral tetracycline. Acta Derm Venereol Suppl (Stockh) 1989; 143:45–48.

43. Tong D, Peters W, Barnetson RS. Evaluation of 0.75% metronidazole gel in acne—a double-blind study. Clin Exp Dermatol 1994; 19:221–223.

44. Yang DJ, Quan LT, Hsu S. Topical antibacterial agents. In: Wolvterton SE, ed. Comprehensive Dermatologic Drug Therapy. 2nd ed. Philadelphia: Saunders-Elsevier, 2007; 525–546.

45. Milstone EB, McDonald AJ, Scholhamer CF Jr. Pseudomembranous colitis after topical application of clindamycin. Arch Dermatol 1981; 117:154–155.
46. Parry MF, Rha CK. Pseudomembranous colitis caused by topical clindamycin phosphate. Arch Dermatol 1986; 122:583–584.
47. Aronson PJ. Systemic adverse effects due to topical medications. In: Wolverton SE, ed. Comprehensive Dermatologic Drug Therapy. 2nd ed. Philadelphia: Saunders-Elsevier, 2007; 807.
48. Reed BR. Dermatologic drugs during pregnancy and lactation. In: Wolverton SE, ed. Comprehensive Dermatologic Drug Therapy. 2nd ed. Philadelphia: Saunders-Elsevier, 2007; 925–947.

3.3

Combination therapy

Jennifer Villasenor, Diane S. Berson, and Daniela Kroshinsky

INTRODUCTION

Successful treatment for acne vulgaris is guided by the severity of the acne and is aimed at correcting the altered pattern of follicular keratinization, decreasing sebaceous gland activity, decreasing the follicular bacterial population, and providing an anti-inflammatory effect (1). In many cases, management of acne vulgaris should be approached as a chronic disease with a prolonged course and a pattern of recurrence or relapse that manifests as acute or gradual outbreaks (2,3). Early and aggressive treatment of acne vulgaris is encouraged to limit the occurrence of physical scarring, persistent hyperpigmentation, and psychological sequelae (4).

Treatment modalities include both local and systemic therapies and may include combinations of both types of therapies. Selection of single versus combination treatment should be made following the determination of the severity of disease, the types of lesions present, the psychological impact of the disease, and the patient's treatment history (5). Several guidelines have been proposed for the assessment of acne severity; however, currently, there is no single standardized and reproducible grading system. In general, acne severity is determined by the number of lesions, the number and presence of non-inflammatory (e.g., open and closed comedones) versus inflammatory lesions (e.g., papules, pustules, nodules/nodulocystic lesions), and the extent of disease. Cunliffe et al. have proposed a severity scale based on the number and types of lesions (6). Mild acne is characterized by the predominance of comedones with less than 10 small papules and pustules. The presence of 10 to 40 papules and pustules and 10 to 40 comedones define moderate acne. Mild disease on the trunk may also be present. In moderately severe disease, numerous papules and pustules (40–100), several comedones (40–100), and up to five large and deep nodular inflamed lesions are present with widespread involvement of the face, chest, and back. Severe acne is characterized by the presence of nodulocystic acne and acne conglobata with many large and painful nodular or pustular lesions including several smaller papules, pustules, and comedones.

FIRST-LINE THERAPY

The pathogenesis of acne occurs as a result of four major factors: (*i*) excess sebum production, (*ii*) bacterial colonization of the pilosebaceous duct and release of inflammatory mediators, (*iii*) inflammation, and (*iv*) abnormal keratinization within the follicle. Current treatment modalities are formulated to simultaneously affect these pathogenic factors. The use of topical retinoids is based on their comedolytic and anticomedogenic activity, anti-inflammatory effects, and their ability to normalize desquamation to allow penetration of other topical agents (7). Although the combination of antimicrobials with benzoyl peroxide has been shown to have some effectiveness in the treatment of acne, antibiotics and benzoyl peroxide have only minimal comedolytic or anticomedogenic effects (7). The anti-inflammatory and antimicrobial properties of antimicrobials and benzoyl peroxide complement the properties of topical retinoids and have been more effective in combination compared to monotherapy with either antimicrobials or topical retinoids (8). Moreover, the combination of antimicrobials with benzoyl peroxide may help prevent the emergence of resistant strains of *Propionibacterium acnes* (7,9). No single therapy is able to counter the growth of *P. acnes* inflammation and comedogenesis as effectively as antibiotics and retinoids in combination (7,9). For most patients, first-line therapy using the combination of a topical retinoid and antimicrobial agent results in faster and more complete clearing of acne lesions compared with monotherapy (4).

TOPICAL RETINOIDS WITH TOPICAL ANTIMICROBIALS

Combination therapy using topical retinoids and topical antibiotics (e.g., clindamycin and erythromycin) and benzoyl peroxide are most effective in the treatment of patients with mild-to-moderate acne with an inflammatory component (10–13). A 12-week, randomized study comparing the combination of adapalene gel 0.1% and clindamycin 1% gel versus clindamycin 1% with the adapalene vehicle revealed faster and significantly greater clearance of acne lesions using the combination of adapalene gel with clindamycin (13). In addition, tretinoin gel 0.025% plus clindamycin gel 1% was more effective compared with either treatment alone in an eight-week study involving 64 patients (14). A randomized, parallel-group, investigator-blinded study of clindamycin 1% gel in combination with either tazarotene 0.1% cream or tretinoin 0.025% gel in 135 patients with mild-to-moderate acne showed that the tazarotene regimen was associated in greater improvements in overall disease severity and better global assessments (15). Studies comparing the cumulative skin tolerance of topical retinoids (adapalene gel 0.1%, tretinoin cream 0.025%, and tretinoin microsphere gel 0.1% and 0.4%) in combination with topical microbials (clindamycin 1%, erythromycin 2%, benzoyl peroxide 5%, and erythromycin/BPO gel) have demonstrated minimal erythema, dryness, or burning/stinging with adapalene gel compared to other retinoids (15–18). In general, retinoid-based combination therapy with an antimicrobial agent is recommended as first-line therapy for most patients with acne because the combination decreases abnormal desquamation, *P. acnes* colonization, and inflammation (4).

TOPICAL RETINOIDS WITH ORAL ANTIBIOTICS

The use of topical retinoids in combination with oral antibiotics is very effective for the treatment of moderate-to-severe or persistent acne. Two multicenter, randomized, investigator-blinded studies comparing the efficacy and tolerability of oral antibiotics (lymecycline, doxycycline) in combination with topical retinoids (adapalene) demonstrated significant decreases in the total number of inflammatory and noninflammatory lesions in a short amount of time compared to monotherapy (6,19). Topical tretinoin in combination with oral tetracycline also has increased efficacy and faster therapeutic response in reducing *P. acnes* than with either agent alone (8,12). The Global Alliance cautions against prolonged antibiotic treatment to prevent the emergence of resistant strains of *P. acnes* and recommends no more than three to four months of antibiotic treatment in combination with retinoids followed by maintenance therapy with a topical retinoid (4). If inflammatory lesions are still present, then the use of benzoyl peroxide or a benzoyl peroxide/antibiotic combination should be used in addition to a topical retinoid.

FIXED-DOSE COMBINATION PRODUCTS

Fixed-dose combination products were developed with the goal of increasing patient compliance and have shown enhanced efficacy and speed of treatment of acne. Studies comparing fixed-dose combination products with BPO (adapalene 0.1%/BPO 2.5%) or topical antibiotics (tretinoin 0.025%/clindamycin 1.2% gel, tretinoin 0.025%/clindamycin 1% hydrogel, and erythromycin 4%/tretinoin 0.025% gel) have also shown increased effectiveness of fixed-dose combination products compared to treatment without topical retinoids (20–22). Adapalene gel

0.1% combined with BPO 2.5% in a fixed-dose product has been carefully studied in a multicenter, randomized, double-blind study in 517 patients with moderate to moderately severe acne (23). The 12-month study consisted of 452 patients with acne using the once-daily fixed-dose combination of adapalene/ BPO and showed sustained reduction of inflammatory and noninflammatory lesions and improved cutaneous tolerability (24). Use of adapalene treatment in combination with a clindamycin/BPO fixed-dose product was evaluated in a randomized, multicenter, parallel group study and showed the greatest reduction in lesion counts in patients treated with adapalene in combination with the fixed-dose clindamycin/BPO product (25). Moreover, the combination of tazarotene plus a clindamycin/BPO fixed-dose product in the treatment of moderate-to-severe inflammatory acne showed significant global improvement, reduced number of inflammatory lesions, and reduced skin irritation (26,27). A multi-center case series evaluated efficacy and tolerability of the fixed-dose combination of tretinoin 0.025%/erythromycin 4% product and showed improvement with rapid onset and good tolerability in 85% of patients with acne (28). Comparison of tretinoin 0.025%/erythromycin 4% with erythromycin 3%/BPO 5% in patients with moderate acne showed comparable efficacy; however, the erythromycin 3%/BPO 5% product was preferred and had better cutaneous tolerability (21). Additionally, two randomized, double-blind, active-drug and vehicle-controlled studies of tretinoin/clindamycin fixed combination product in 2219 patients with mild-to-moderate acne showed greater reductions in the number of inflammatory and noninflammatory lesions and there were a greater number of patients at the end of the study with clear or almost clear skin on Investigator Global Assessment in patients who received the combination treatment (22). The irritancy potential of various fixed-dose combinations has also been studied. Comparisons between adapalene gel 0.1%, tazarotene cream 0.05%, and tretinoin microsphere 0.04% in combination with clindamycin/ benzoyl peroxide products have shown that adapalene resulted in the least amount of irritation compared to tretinoin and tazarotene (29).

Combining BPO or antibiotics with retinoids is guided by the bactericidal properties of BPO and antimicrobials and the comedolytic and anticomedogenic properties of retinoids. Moreover, retinoids have been shown to downregulate the expression of TLR-2, thereby decreasing cytokine production and blocking the AP-1 inflammatory pathway. Retinoids have also been shown to increase CD-1d expression and decrease IL-10 expression on keratinocytes, which may enhance dendritic and T-cell interaction and antimicrobial activity against *P. acnes* (30). However, it should be noted that combination formulations consisting of topical antibiotics without benzoyl peroxide (e.g., fixed-dose retinoid/ antibiotic formulations) may increase the prevalence of resistant strains of *P. acnes*. According to the Global Alliance, any retinoid/antibiotic combination should also include benzoyl peroxide or should be changed to a retinoid with or without benzoyl peroxide to decrease the incidence of resistant strains of *P. acnes* (4).

MAINTENANCE THERAPY

The chronic nature of acne merits continued therapy, as this disease tends to recur when treatment is withdrawn following successful initial therapy (31,32). For most types of acne, topical retinoids are recommended because of their anticomedogenic and comedolytic properties. There have been many studies evaluating the efficacy of topical retinoids as maintenance therapy, usually following initial treatment with a topical retinoid and topical antimicrobial. In a study involving patients with moderate to moderately severe acne following combination therapy, patients continued on adapalene maintenance therapy had a significant reduction in lesion counts and had less rebound of acne lesion compared to those who did not receive maintenance therapy (33). Similarly, in a randomized, vehicle-controlled maintenance study of patients who showed improvement following combination treatment, more than half of patients were able to maintain 90% of their clearing while on their adapalene maintenance therapy compared to those using the vehicle control (34). In both studies, patients who were untreated or treated with vehicle eventually developed rebound of acne lesions, whereas those treated with adapalene maintenance therapy had stable or decreased lesion counts. Using patients who showed improvement after combination treatment, a randomized, parallel-group, double-blind, 12-week study assessed the efficacy of three different maintenance therapy regimens including tazarotene gel, minocycline, and tazarotene gel with minocycline. All three groups showed no significant differences in mean overall disease score, reductions in acne lesions from baseline, or percent of patients with good or excellent maintenance (35). This study not only indicates that topical retinoids are effective but also indicates that the use of antibiotics does not provide additional benefit. In general, long-term use of topical or oral antibiotics should be discouraged to reduce the potential for antimicrobial resistance (4,5).

The anticomedogenic property of topical retinoids is the basis for use of these agents as maintenance therapy. An assessment of microcomedone formation in patients with mild-to-moderate acne treated with adapalene maintenance therapy was done using cyanoacrylate stripping. Using computer-assisted densitometric analysis, cyanoacrylate stripping allows for analysis of the lipid composition in the sebaceous follicular infundibulum and surface lipids. Patients treated with topical retinoids show increased ceramide subfractions, and this is correlated with decreased microcomedone formation (32). At baseline, week 8 and week 20, cyanoacrylate strip analysis showed a significant decrease in microcomedone formation in patients treated with adapalene maintenance therapy compared to the vehicle (36).

CONCLUSIONS

Several treatment algorithms have been proposed based on acne severity. The use of combination therapies as first-line treatment of acne has been shown to have the most significant effect with faster onset than other treatment modalities. In general, mild acne can be treated with topical retinoids with the addition of antibiotics or benzoyl peroxide–containing products if inflammatory lesions are present. Mild-to-moderate acne (e.g., mild-to-moderate popular/pustular acne) can best be treated with combination therapy composed of the following regimens: (*i*) a topical retinoid combined with a topical or oral antibiotic, (*ii*) a topical retinoid combined with benzoyl peroxide or benzoyl peroxide/antibiotic fixed-dose product, or (*iii*) a fixed-dose topical retinoid/benzoyl peroxide in combination with a topical antibiotic. Moderate-to-severe acne (e.g., severe nodulocystic) can also be treated with combination therapy composed of topical retinoids combined topical or oral antibiotics. Additional benefit can be achieved using systemic isotretinoin alone; however, the side effects profile of oral isotretinoin may prohibit its use in some patients. Following successful treatment with combination therapy, maintenance therapy with topical retinoids can be initiated.

REFERENCES

1. Gong P, Gasparrini P, Rho D, et al. An in situ respirometric technique to measure pollution-induced microbial community tolerance in soils contaminated with 2,4,6-trinitrotoluene. Ecotoxicol Environ Saf 2000; 47(1):96–103.
2. Heidrich JP, Niemeier A, Seyfarth M. Continuous analysis in extracorporeally circulating blood—a rat model applying flow-through ion-selective electrodes for the measurement of Ca2+, K+, Na+ and pH. Clin Chem Lab Med 1998; 36(11): 847–854.
3. James WD. Acne. N Engl J Med 2005; 352(14):1463–1472.
4. Thiboutot D, Gollnick H, Bettoli V, et al. New insights into the management of acne: an update from the Global Alliance to Improve Outcomes in Acne Group. J Am Acad Dermatol 2009; 60(5 suppl 1):S1–S50.
5. Gollnick H, Cunliffe W, Berson D, et al. Management of acne: a report from a Global Alliance to Improve Outcomes in Acne. J Am Acad Dermatol 2003; 49(1 suppl):S1–S37.
6. Cunliffe WJ, Meynadier J, Alirezai M, et al. Is combined oral and topical therapy better than oral therapy alone in patients with moderate to moderately severe acne vulgaris? A comparison of the efficacy and safety of lymecycline plus adapalene gel 0.1%, versus lymecycline plus gel vehicle. J Am Acad Dermatol 2003; 49(3 suppl 1): S218–S226.
7. Leyden JJ. A review of the use of combination therapies for the treatment of acne vulgaris. J Am Acad Dermatol 2003; 49(3 suppl 1):S200–S210.

8. Mills OH Jr., Marples RR, Kligman AM. Acne vulgaris. Oral therapy with tetra-cycline and topical therapy with vitamin A. Arch Dermatol 1972; 106(2):200–203.
9. Webster GF. Topical tretinoin in acne therapy. J Am Acad Dermatol 1998; 39(2 pt 3):S38–S44.
10. Shalita AR, Rafal ES, Anderson DN, et al. Compared efficacy and safety of tretinoin 0.1% microsphere gel alone and in combination with benzoyl peroxide 6% cleanser for the treatment of acne vulgaris. Cutis 2003; 72(2):167–172.
11. Handojo I. The combined use of topical benzoyl peroxide and tretinoin in the treatment of acne vulgaris. Int J Dermatol 1979; 18(6):489–496.
12. Kligman AM, Mills OH, McGinley KJ, et al. Acne therapy with tretinoin in com-bination with antibiotics. Acta Derm Venereol Suppl (Stockh) 1975; 74:111–115.
13. Wolf JE, Kaplan D, Kraus SJ, et al. Efficacy and tolerability of combined topical treatment of acne vulgaris with adapalene and clindamycin: a multicenter, randomized, investigator-blinded study. J Am Acad Dermatol 2003; 49(3 suppl 1): S211–S217.
14. Rietschel RL, Duncan SH. Clindamycin phosphate used in combination with treti-noin in the treatment of acne. Int J Dermatol 1983; 22(1):41–43.
15. Tanghetti E, Dhawan S, Torok H, et al. Tazarotene 0.1 percent cream plus clinda-mycin 1 percent gel versus tretinoin 0.025 percent gel plus clindamycin 1 percent gel in the treatment of facial acne vulgaris. Dermatol Online J 2007; 13(3):1.
16. Brand B, Gilbert R, Baker MD, et al. Cumulative irritancy comparison of adapalene gel 0.1% versus other retinoid products when applied in combination with topical antimicrobial agents. J Am Acad Dermatol 2003; 49(3 suppl 1):S227–S232.
17. Leyden J. New developments in topical antimicrobial therapy for acne. J Drugs Dermatol 2008; 7(2 suppl):s8–s11.
18. Capizzi R, Landi F, Milani M, et al. Skin tolerability and efficacy of combination therapy with hydrogen peroxide stabilized cream and adapalene gel in comparison with benzoyl peroxide cream and adapalene gel in common acne. A randomized, investigator-masked, controlled trial. Br J Dermatol 2004; 151(2):481–484.
19. Thiboutot DM, Shalita AR, Yamauchi PS, et al. Combination therapy with adapalene gel 0.1% and doxycycline for severe acne vulgaris: a multicenter, investigator-blind, randomized, controlled study. Skinmed 2005; 4(3):138–146.
20. Zouboulis CC, Derumeaux L, Decroix J, et al. A multicentre, single-blind, randomized comparison of a fixed clindamycin phosphate/tretinoin gel formulation (Velac) applied once daily and a clindamycin lotion formulation (Dalacin T) applied twice daily in the topical treatment of acne vulgaris. Br J Dermatol 2000; 143(3):498–505.
21. Gupta AK, Lynde CW, Kunynetz RA, et al. A randomized, double-blind, multi-center, parallel group study to compare relative efficacies of the topical gels 3% erythromycin/5% benzoyl peroxide and 0.025% tretinoin/erythromycin 4% in the treatment of moderate acne vulgaris of the face. J Cutan Med Surg 2003; 7(1):31–37.
22. Leyden JJ, Krochmal L, Yaroshinsky A. Two randomized, double-blind, controlled trials of 2219 subjects to compare the combination clindamycin/tretinoin hydrogel with each agent alone and vehicle for the treatment of acne vulgaris. J Am Acad Dermatol 2006; 54(1):73–81.

23. Thiboutot DM, Weiss J, Bucko A, et al. Adapalene-benzoyl peroxide, a fixed-dose combination for the treatment of acne vulgaris: results of a multicenter, randomized double-blind, controlled study. J Am Acad Dermatol 2007; 57(5):791–799.

24. Pariser DM, Westmoreland P, Morris A, et al. Long-term safety and efficacy of a unique fixed-dose combination gel of adapalene 0.1% and benzoyl peroxide 2.5% for the treatment of acne vulgaris. J Drugs Dermatol 2007; 6(9):899–905.

25. Del Rosso JQ. Study results of benzoyl peroxide 5%/clindamycin 1% topical gel, adapalene 0.1% gel, and use in combination for acne vulgaris. J Drugs Dermatol 2007; 6(6):616–622.

26. Draelos ZD, Tanghetti EA. Optimizing the use of tazarotene for the treatment of facial acne vulgaris through combination therapy. Cutis 2002; 69(2 suppl):20–29.

27. Tanghetti E, Abramovits W, Solomon B, et al. Tazarotene versus tazarotene plus clindamycin/benzoyl peroxide in the treatment of acne vulgaris: a multicenter, double-blind, randomized parallel-group trial. J Drugs Dermatol 2006; 5(3): 256–261.

28. Amblard P, Bazex A, Beylot C, et al. [The association tretinoin-erythromycin base: a new topical treatment for acne. Results of a multicentric trial on 347 cases (authors transl)]. Sem Hop 1980; 56(17–18):911–915.

29. Dosik JS, Gilbert RD, Arsonnaud S. Cumulative irritancy comparison of topical retinoid and antimicrobial combination therapies. Skinmed 2006; 5(5):219–223.

30. Tenaud I, Khammari A, Dreno B. In vitro modulation of TLR-2, CD1d and IL-10 by adapalene on normal human skin and acne inflammatory lesions. Exp Dermatol 2007; 16(6):500–506.

31. Ropke EM, Augustin W, Gollnick H. Improved method for studying skin lipid samples from cyanoacrylate strips by high-performance thin-layer chromatography. Skin Pharmacol 1996; 9(6):381–387.

32. Thielitz A, Helmdach M, Ropke EM, et al. Lipid analysis of follicular casts from cyanoacrylate strips as a new method for studying therapeutic effects of antiacne agents. Br J Dermatol 2001; 145(1):19–27.

33. Zhang JZ, Li LF, Tu YT, et al. A successful maintenance approach in inflammatory acne with adapalene gel 0.1% after an initial treatment in combination with clindamycin topical solution 1% or after monotherapy with clindamycin topical solution 1%. J Dermatolog Treat 2004; 15(6):372–378.

34. Thiboutot DM, Shalita AR, Yamauchi PS, et al. Adapalene gel, 0.1%, as maintenance therapy for acne vulgaris: a randomized, controlled, investigator-blind follow-up of a recent combination study. Arch Dermatol 2006; 142(5):597–602.

35. Leyden J, Thiboutot DM, Shalita AR, et al. Comparison of tazarotene and minocycline maintenance therapies in acne vulgaris: a multicenter, double-blind, randomized, parallel-group study. Arch Dermatol 2006; 142(5):605–612.

36. Thielitz A, Sidou F, Gollnick H. Control of microcomedone formation throughout a maintenance treatment with adapalene gel, 0.1%. J Eur Acad Dermatol Venereol 2007; 21(6):747–753.

4.1

Oral antibiotics

James Q. Del Rosso

INTRODUCTION

Acne vulgaris is one of the most common disorders encountered in dermatology practice accounting for approximately 8.8% of total visits to office-based dermatologists in the United States in 2006 (1). Treatment of acne in teenage patients accounts for greater than 2 million visits annually (2). Although peripubertal onset is most common, prepubertal onset is not uncommon, and several acne patients present after the teenage years, with approximately 10% of visits noted in patients 35 to 44 years of age (2,3). The negative psychosocial impact of acne in many affected patients is well documented (4,5).

Despite the multifactorial pathogenesis of acne vulgaris, *Propionibacterium acnes*, a component of the normal bacterial flora of sebaceous gland-rich skin of the face and upper trunk, appears to play a major role in the development of inflammatory acne lesions, and very likely comedonal lesions (6–8). *P. acnes* has been identified as a trigger of innate immune response and exhibits other proinflammatory properties that are believed to be operative in the development and progression of acne vulgaris (9,10). Current basic science and clinical research including identification of the *P. acnes* genome, analysis of innate immune response in acne inflammation, evaluation of the role of inflammation in comedogenesis, and microbiologic studies correlating *P. acnes* with specific treatments and therapeutic benefit, all support the goal of *P. acnes* suppression with antimicrobial therapy as a component of acne management (6–12). In addition to *P. acnes* suppression, some antibiotics such as the tetracycline derivatives also exhibit anti-inflammatory properties that appear to contribute to their therapeutic benefit in acne vulgaris (11,13,14).

USAGE PATTERNS WITH ORAL ANTIBIOTICS
IN ACNE MANAGEMENT

Prescribing data from 2001 to 2006 in the United States show that office-based dermatologists prescribe 8 to 9 million oral antibiotic prescriptions annually, with two-thirds of prescriptions inclusive of tetracycline derivatives, primarily minocycline and doxycycline, used for therapy of acne and rosacea (15,16). Prior to approval of the extended-release tablet formulation of minocycline by the US Food and Drug Administration (FDA) in 2006, oral antibiotics have been utilized for acne based on widespread anecdotal experience and a collection of small clinical studies (17–19). Conventionally, the predominant oral antibiotics used for treatment of acne vulgaris in most countries have been tetracycline, doxycycline, minocycline, and erythromycin, with some locations outside of the United States also incorporating trimethoprim, primarily due to low cost (2,11,19–22). At present, doxycycline and minocycline are used more frequently than tetracycline and erythromycin by dermatologists in the United States, likely due to the marked emergence of *P. acnes* strains that exhibit decreased sensitivity to the latter two agents (11). Over time there has been a trend toward an increase in *P. acnes* strains becoming less sensitive to doxycycline and minocycline, which has been correlated with the frequency of their usage (11,23–25).

Tetracycline derivatives represent the predominant oral antibiotic agents used to treat acne vulgaris. Oral tetracycline and oxytetracycline have been available since the mid-1950s, doxycycline since 1967, and minocycline since 1972 (13). Reviews of acne treatment studies that incorporated use of tetracycline, doxycycline, and immediate-release minocycline formulations found a total of 12 studies (N = 953) completed between 1969 and 2001 (19–21). The studies, which assessed extended-release minocycline tablets, were completed prior to FDA approval and included one phase II dose-finding study and two phase III pivotal trials. These studies evaluated the efficacy and safety of weight-based dosing with once-daily administration of the extended-release minocycline tablet formulation (N = 1038) (18). The recommended dose of extended-release minocycline based on the completed studies is 1 mg/kg once a day (17–19). Alternative oral antibiotics, such as trimethoprim-sulfamethoxazole and azithromycin, have also been reported to be of benefit for acne treatment (26–28).

RATIONALE FOR USE OF ORAL ANTIBIOTIC THERAPY
IN ACNE TREATMENT

Reduction of *P. acnes* organisms, with an ensuing decrease in inflammatory lesion development and possibly comedogenesis, is the primary objective of oral antibiotic therapy in acne (2,16,29). The greatest decrease in *P. acnes* colony counts has been demonstrated with minocycline, followed in order of magnitude by doxycycline, tetracycline, trimethoprim-sulfamethoxazole, and erythromycin (29). The clinical efficacy of oral antibiotic therapy for acne vulgaris is well established and recognized as a conventional component of rational acne treatment (2,11,12,17,18,20–22,29,30).

INDICATIONS AND RECOMMENDED DOSING OF ORAL ANTIBIOTICS USED IN ACNE THERAPY

The main indication for oral antibiotic therapy in acne vulgaris is moderate-to-severe inflammatory involvement on the face and/or trunk (12). Table 4.1.1 depicts the recommended dosing schedule with oral antibiotics currently used most commonly for acne therapy by dermatologists in the United States. Antibiotic monotherapy should be avoided due to promotion of antibiotic-resistant bacterial strains, with oral antibiotic therapy best utilized in combination with a topical regimen (11,12,29–31). In patients with moderate-to-severe acne vulgaris, combination therapy using a topical regimen inclusive of benzoyl peroxide and a topical retinoid concurrently with an oral antibiotic is rational and

Table 4.1.1 Major Oral Antibiotics Used for Treatment of Acne Vulgaris by Dermatologists in the United States

Drug	Usual dosage range	Comments	Refs
Minocycline (immediate-release)	50–100 mg once or twice daily	Vestibular reactions may be dose related and may be more common with immediate-release formulations (especially generic formulations with rapid release properties)	11, 19–22, 26
Minocycline (extended-release)	1 mg/kg/day (45–135 mg once daily)	Efficacy comparable to 2 mg/kg/day and 3 mg/kg/day; potential for vestibular reactions appear to be lower than with immediate-release formulations	17, 18
Doxycycline	75–100 mg once or twice daily 150 mg once daily	Photosensitivity reported to be dose related (higher potential at 100 mg/day)	19–22, 26

optimizes efficacy (11,30–33). It is most rational to include a benzoyl peroxide–containing formulation as part of the combination therapy regimen with an oral antibiotic, as benzoyl peroxide reduces the emergence of *P. acnes* antibiotic-resistant strains to multiple antibiotics including erythromycin, tetracycline, doxycycline, and minocycline (11–35). It has also been suggested that a short course of benzoyl peroxide therapy prior to initiating antibiotic therapy assists in the eradication of antibiotic-resistant *P. acnes* strains, thus enhancing the overall efficacy of antibiotic treatment (12,35–37).

If not enterically coated, doxycline, especially the hyclate salt, is best administered with food and a large glass of water to reduce the risk of gastro-intestinal (GI) side effects such as esophagitis (12,22). Both doxycycline and minocycline may be administered with food; however, concomitant adminis-tration with iron supplements may decrease GI absorption of both agents (12,22). Concurrent ingestion of metal ions such as calcium, magnesium, and aluminum, found in many vitamin-mineral supplements and antacids, may significantly decrease absorption of tetracycline from the GI tract (12,22).

Among the macrolide antibiotic derivatives, oral erythromycin is best administered with food to reduce GI side effects. Azithromycin differs from erythromycin as it does not as commonly cause GI upset, and is best taken on an empty stomach to maximize GI absorption (12,22,26). Oral antibiotics that are commonly associated with GI side effects and esophagitis are best ingested with a large glass of water when the patient is upright and not prior to anticipated reclining for at least a few hours.

ORAL ANTIBIOTIC THERAPY IN ACNE VULGARIS AND ANTIBIOTIC RESISTANCE

Antibiotic resistance patterns develop over time due to selection pressure and transfer of antibiotic resistance genes resulting in the emergence of bacterial organisms that are less sensitive to previously effective antibiotics (23,24,36,38). Approximately three decades ago, it was shown that long-term oral antibiotic therapy administered over a mean duration of 21 months increased the minimum inhibitory concentration (MIC) for *P. acnes* up to 5-fold for tetracycline and 100-fold for erythromycin as compared to acne-free control subjects and those not receiving antibiotics (39). Several other reports have addressed the concern regarding emergence of *P. acnes* strains less sensitive to multiple topical and oral antibiotic agents used to treat acne vulgaris (23–25,36,40–43). Additionally, reports from the United Kingdom demonstrate a progressively increasing trend in *P. acnes* resistance to erythromycin, clindamycin, and/or tetracycline, noted to be 20%, 38%, 49%, and 62%, in 1988, 1993, 1995, and 1996, respectively (43).

Focused initiatives to alter how antibiotics are prescribed for acne vulgaris due to concerns regarding antibiotic resistance emerged in the early 1990s in the

United Kingdom, with emphasis continuing into the millennium (38–40). A similar trend may have also occurred in the United States based on prescribing trends of acne medications reported in the 1990 to 2002 National Ambulatory Medical Care Survey (44). A substantial decline in several antimicrobial drug classes, such as benzoyl peroxide, topical clindamycin, oral erythromycin, and oral tetracycline agents, was noted, coupled with an increase in non-antimicrobial therapies, such as topical retinoids and oral isotretinoin. From 1995 to 2000, antibiotic prescriptions in the United Kingdom declined by 33%, with the majority of the decrease comprising oral antibiotic agents (25,45).

PROPIONIBACTERIUM ACNES ANTIBIOTIC RESISTANCE AND EFFICACY OF ORAL ANTIBIOTIC USE IN ACNE

Some studies have noted a poor therapeutic response of acne to antibiotics in patients with confirmed substantial quantities of *P. acnes* that demonstrate high MIC levels to macrolides and tetracyclines (25,36,39,46). It is important to recognize, however, that a direct correlation between prevalence of *P. acnes* resistance and poor therapeutic response to antibiotic therapy has not always been consistent (11). Factors potentially associated with a reduced response to antibiotic therapy may include preexisting antibiotic resistance, the quantity of antibiotic-resistant *P. acnes* strains in the individual patient, resistance to multiple antibiotics, use of antibiotics without concomitant use of benzoyl peroxide, repeated courses of antibiotic therapy especially without concomitant use of benzoyl peroxide, unnecessary switching of oral antibiotic agents despite previous efficacy, individual drug characteristics such as GI absorption and lipophilicity, relative effects on serum and tissue levels due to interference of GI absorption by coadministered chelating metal ions, and existence of *P. acnes* in a protective extracellular biofilm in vivo (11,12,17,18,22,36,39,47).

Although the prevalence of antibiotic-resistant *P. acnes* has been shown to be increasing globally over time, oral antibiotics, which have been used extensively over several years, continue to demonstrate efficacy in acne vulgaris, including doxycycline and minocycline (11,18,48–51). Importantly, some of the most recent data evaluating the efficacy of a commonly used oral antibiotic in acne may be culled from phase II and phase III studies, which evaluated extended-release minocycline as monotherapy for moderate and severe acne vulgaris for FDA approval ($N = 1038$) (18,51). The study results demonstrated a significantly greater inflammatory lesion reduction in actively treated subjects as compared to the placebo group and suggested a once-daily dose of 1 mg/kg ($p < 0.001$) (51). Properties other than antibiotic activity, which leads to reduction in *P. acnes*, may also be operative in acne treatment as some antibiotics demonstrate biologic activities unrelated to their antibiotic effects (13,14). For example, tetracycline derivatives such as minocycline and doxycycline exhibit multiple direct anti-inflammatory properties that appear to contribute to their therapeutic benefit in acne vulgaris (11,13,14,19,52).

ALTERNATIVE ORAL ANTIBIOTICS IN ACNE THERAPY

Among the alternative oral antibiotics reported for treatment of acne vulgaris, trimethoprim-sulfamethoxazole and azithromycin have been mentioned most frequently in the literature (12,22–28,53). In some patients with acne who are refractory to conventionally used oral antibiotics, trimethoprim-sulfamethoxazole has been reported to be effective (26,27). However, the frequent need for use of trimethoprim-sulfamethoxazole for treatment of cutaneous and systemic infections caused by community-acquired *Staphylococcus aureus* (CA-MRSA) and the possible risk of major side effects associated with its use, both support the recommendation that trimethoprim-sulfamethoxazole is best reserved for selected cases of refractory acne vulgaris (27).

Oral azithromycin has been reported to be effective in the treatment of acne vulgaris in four open studies ($N = 187$) and two investigator-blinded clinical trials ($N = 241$) with a variety of treatment regimens utilized (26,28). Most regimens have incorporated intermittent dosing schedules due to a long terminal half-life (68 hours) and the propensity of azithromycin to achieve high tissue level without the need for persistently high serum concentrations (26). Azithromycin is a commonly prescribed antibiotic in the general medical community, which is used to treat a variety of systemic infections in both adult and pediatric populations. This agent is also of benefit for therapy of intracellular pathogens such as *Chlamydia* spp. and atypical *Mycobacterium* spp. Therefore, use of azithromycin for treatment of acne is best reserved for selected cases, primarily to avoid widespread use that is likely to promote the increased emergence of antibiotic-resistant organisms (26).

Other alternative oral antibiotics that have been sporadically and randomly reported to be effective for acne treatment are cephalosporins and fluoroquinolones (26). The heavy dependence on these agents within the general medical community for both ambulatory and hospital-based treatment of a variety of systemic infections discourages their use for treatment of acne; however, exceptions may include short-term use for selected refractory cases and gram-negative acne/folliculitis.

DURATION OF ORAL ANTIBIOTIC USE IN ACNE THERAPY

As the vast majority of clinical trials evaluating acne therapies typically assess treatment over a relatively short duration of two to four months, scientific data on the long-term management of acne is sparse. The literature does strongly support that an oral antibiotic be used in combination with a rational topical regimen, preferably composed of a benzoyl peroxide–containing formulation and a topical retinoid (11,12,22,30). This may allow for better ability to discontinue the oral antibiotic at some point based on response to treatment, and hopefully allow the topical regimen alone to maintain control of acne.

When oral antibiotic therapy is incorporated with a topical regimen for acne, it has been suggested that it be administered over a minimum period of 6 to 8 weeks and a maximum of 12 weeks to 6 months (11,12,22,30). Hard-and-fast rules on treatment duration with an oral antibiotic are not justifiable as treatment response among patients may be highly variable. At initial follow-up six to eight weeks after the start of therapy, if a substantial lack of efficacy is observed despite adequate compliance, a change in oral antibiotic therapy is reasonable (22,47). If partial improvement is observed, it may be reasonable to continue with the current therapy for an additional six to eight weeks to evaluate if further progress is achieved. Changing a regimen too frequently often results in suboptimal outcomes as a given regimen is never afforded a true opportunity to initiate its therapeutic effect.

Once control of acne is felt to be stable, which is usually achieved over a duration of three to six months assuming compliance is adequate, discontinuation of the oral antibiotic therapy may be suggested, with continuation of the topical regimen for long-term maintenance (12,22). Stabilized control of acne does not necessarily imply complete clearance, but may be defined as the observation that new inflammatory lesions have stopped or markedly decreased (12). As there is no consensus opinion on whether oral antibiotic therapy should be discontinued abruptly or tapered, clinical judgment is warranted. The author prefers abrupt discontinuation of the oral antibiotic once new inflammatory lesions have stopped or markedly decreased *and* most flat foci of residual inflammation secondary to resolving lesions have substantially faded.

Despite the alleged use of a topical maintenance regimen, some patients return with an acne flare within a few weeks to months after discontinuation of the oral antibiotic. In such cases, it is suggested to reinitiate therapy with the same oral antibiotic that was previously effective. Additionally, it is very important to incorporate use of benzoyl peroxide to suppress the presence and emergence of less antibiotic-sensitive *P. acnes* organisms (11,12,22,34,35,45,47). It is very important to reemphasize patient adherence to the topical therapy regimen, which has been shown to be optimized by incorporating a topical retinoid both initially and for long-term maintenance therapy (12,54).

ADVERSE REACTIONS OF ORAL ANTIBIOTICS USED FOR ACNE TREATMENT

All oral antibiotics may be associated with "nuisance" side effects such as GI upset, with the latter most commonly observed with erythromycin and doxycycline (12,22). Doxycycline is associated with dose-related phototoxicity, with appropriate photoprotection recommended (12,19,22).

The available literature regarding major side effects associated with minocycline, other than acute vestibular adverse events, relate to the use of immediate-release minocycline formulations, available since 1972. As extended-release minocycline has only been available since July 2006, and only in the US, it remains to be seen if the unique pharmacokinetic profile of this formulation, and weight-based dosing (1 mg/kg once daily), will alter the potential risk of other minocycline-induced side effects, beyond the reduction in acute vestibular adverse events discussed earlier.

Minocycline has been associated with cutaneous and/or mucosal hyper-pigmentation, including brown, gray, or blue pigmentation of skin and/or mucosa and blue discoloration of acne scars (12,22). A suggested correlation between hyperpigmentation and cumulative exposure to minocycline has been reported, with the time course of onset and resolution variable (55). If hyperpigmentation is noted, it is recommended that minocycline be discontinued for acne treatment. As cumulative minocycline exposure appears to correlate with risk of hyper-pigmentation, extended-release minocycline, dosed at 1 mg/kg/day, may be less likely to induce this side effect, however, further pharmacosurveillance is needed.

Drug hypersensitivity syndrome (DHS) has been reported with both min-ocycline and trimethoprim-sulfamethoxazole, and much less likely, doxycycline (56). The clinical presentation of DHS is fever, a diffuse exanthem-like skin eruption, and systemic abnormalities, including hepatitis and interstitial pneu-monitis. The onset of DHS is typically within two to six weeks after first exposure to the inciting drug, with the most important component in manage-ment being early recognition and discontinuation of the offending agent. Despite the relative lack of association between doxycycline and tetracycline with DHS, it is not absolutely certain that these agents are safe in patients who have a history of DHS due to minocycline (56).

A lupus-like syndrome has been reported in association with minocycline use, especially with prolonged administration (56). Although any patient may be potentially affected, young females treated chronically over one to two years represent the majority of cases (56). Characteristic clinical findings include fever, malaise, and polyarthralgias, with a cutaneous eruption rarely noted. Associated laboratory abnormalities may include a positive antinuclear antibody (ANA) test, elevation of hepatic enzymes, and positivity for perinuclear anti-neutrophilic cytoplasmic antibodies (p-anca) directed against elastase or myeloperoxidase (56). The lupus-like syndrome due to minocycline is typically reversible after drug discontinuation, serologic positivity may be persistent for several months after stopping minocycline, and rechallenge with minocycline is not recommended.

A variety of relatively uncommon but potentially severe adverse reactions may be caused by trimethoprim-sulfamethoxazole, including DHS, toxic epi-dermal necrolysis (TEN), Stevens–Johnson syndrome (SJS), and hematologic reactions (26,27,57). The onset of TEN and SJS is usually within the first one to two months after starting therapy (27). Although relatively uncommon, hematologic reactions reported in association with trimethoprim-sulfamethoxazole have included agranulocytosis, thrombocytopenia, and pancytopenia (27,57). The potential for hematologic toxicity related to either short-term or long-term ($\geq$3 months) administration of trimethoprim-sulfamethoxazole may be increased in patients receiving higher than conventional doses, and in those with preexisting folic acid deficiency and/or megaloblastic hematopoiesis (57).

There are no specific recommendations to routinely perform baseline or periodic laboratory testing with oral antibiotics used to treat acne vulgaris. A complete blood cell (CBC) with platelet count performed at baseline and periodically in patients treated with trimethoprim-sulfamethoxazole may be prudent (57). Routine baseline or periodic laboratory monitoring is not generally recommended in patients treated with minocycline (56). Although routine laboratory monitoring recommendations may not be suggested with an oral antibiotic used for acne treatment, the medical history of the individual patient may prompt the clinician to avoid use of a specific oral antibiotic or to incorporate baseline and/or periodic laboratory monitoring.

Some adverse events related to oral antibiotic use result from drug-drug interaction. Erythromycin may inhibit hepatic cytochrome 3A4 enzymes responsible for the metabolism of other drugs, such as carbamazepine, cyclosporine, and some cholesterol-lowering agents, such as lovastatin, simvastatin, and atorvastatin, potentially leading to toxicity due to accumulation of the inhibited drug (22). Trimethoprim-sulfamethoxazole should be avoided in patients on methotrexate due to an increased risk of hematologic reactions (27,57).

Use of an oral antibiotic for acne during pregnancy is not recommended (12,22,26). Importantly, the suggestion that oral erythromycin is safe during pregnancy is not based on data evaluating prolonged administration over several months during pregnancy (26).

CONCLUSION

Oral antibiotic therapy is indicated for treatment of moderate-to-severe acne vulgaris and is recommended for use in combination with a rational topical therapy regimen. Overall, the efficacy and safety of conventional oral antibiotic therapy used for acne have been very favorable based on available studies and extensive clinical experience over many years. In general, the usual duration of treatment is three to six months if clinically feasible, with long-term maintenance achieved with topical therapy if possible. The progressive increase in antibiotic-resistant *P. acnes* strains over time has prompted suggested methods to reduce the risk of antibiotic resistance. Oral antibiotics used to treat acne vulgaris differ in their pharmacologic properties and adverse reaction profiles. In addition, clinicians need to remain cognizant of potential adverse reactions associated with individual oral antibiotics, especially those with more serious implications.

REFERENCES

1. Weinstock MA, Boyle MM. Statistics of interest to the dermatologist. In: Thiers BH, Lang PG, eds. Year Book of Dermatology. Philadelphia: Elsevier Mosby, 2009:63.
2. James WD. Acne. N Engl J Med 2005; 352(14):1463–1472.
3. Krakowski A, Eichenfield LF. Pediatric acne: clinical presentations, evaluation, and management. J Drugs Dermatol 2007; 6(6):589–593.
4. Tan JKL. Psychosocial impact of acne vulgaris: evaluating the evidence. Skin Therapy Lett 2004; 9(7):1–3.
5. Rapp DA, Brenes GA, Feldman SR, et al. Anger and acne: implications for quality of life, patient satisfaction and clinical care. Br J Dermatol 2004; 151(1):183–189.
6. Bruggemann H. Insights in the pathogenic potential of Propionibacterium acnes from its complete genome. Semin Cut Med Surg 2005; 24(2):63–72.
7. Harper JC. An update on the pathogenesis and management of acne vulgaris. J Am Acad Dermatol 2004; 51(1):S36–S38.
8. Rosen T. The Propionibacterium acnes genome: from the laboratory to the clinic. J Drugs Dermatol 2007; 6(6):582–586.
9. McInturff JE, Kim J. The role of toll like receptors in the pathophysiology of acne. Semin Cut Med Surg 2005; 24(2):73–78.
10. Holland DB, Jeremy AHT. The role of inflammation in the pathogenesis of acne and acne scarring. Semin Cut Med Surg 2005; 24(2):79–83.
11. Leyden JJ, Del Rosso JQ, Webster GF. Clinical considerations in the treatment of acne vulgaris and other inflammatory skin disorders. Cutis 2007; 79(6S):9–25.
12. Gollnick H, Cunliffe W, Berson D, et al. Management of acne: report from a global alliance to improve outcomes in acne. J Am Acad Dermatol 2003; 49(1):S1–S37.
13. Del Rosso JQ. A status report on the use of subantimicrobial-dose doxycycline: a review of the biologic and antimicrobial effects of the tetracyclines. Cutis 2004; 74:118–122.
14. Webster GW, Del Rosso JQ. Anti-inflammatory activity of tetracyclines. Dermatol Clin 2007; 25(2):133–135.
15. Del Rosso JQ. Report from the scientific panel on antibiotic use in dermatology: introduction. Cutis 2007; 79(6S):6–8.
16. Del Rosso JQ, Leyden JJ, Thiboutot D, et al. Antibiotic use in acne and rosacea: clinical considerations and resistance issues of significance to dermatologists. Cutis 2008; 82(suppl 2[ii]):5–12.
17. Leyden JJ. Extended-release minocycline—first systemic antibiotic approved for the treatment of acne: introduction. Cutis 2006; 78(4S):4–5.
18. Del Rosso JQ. Recently approved systemic therapies for acne vulgaris and rosacea. Cutis 2007; 80(2):113–120.
19. Bikowski JB. Subantimicrobial dose doxycycline for acne and rosacea. Skin Med 2003; July–August:234–245.

20. Feldman S, Carrecia R, Barham KL, et al. Diagnosis and treatment of acne. Am Fam Physician 2004; 69(9):2123–2130.
21. Haider A, Shaw JC. Treatment of acne vulgaris. JAMA 2004; 292(6):726–735.
22. Tan AW, Tan HH. Acne vulgaris: a review of antibiotic therapy. Expert Opin Pharmacother 2005; 6(3):409–418.
23. Ross JI, Snelling AM, Eady EA, et al. Phenotypic and genotypic characterization of antibiotic-resistant Propionibacterium acnes isolated from acne patients attending dermatologic clinics in Europe, the USA, Japan and Australia. Br J Dermatol 2001; 144:339–346.
24. Ross JI, Snelling AM, Carnegie E, et al. Antibiotic-resistant acne: lessons from Europe. Br J Dermatol 2003; 148(3):467–478.
25. Eady AE, Cove JH, Layton AM. Is antibiotic resistance in cutaneous propionibacteria clinically relevant? Implications of resistance for acne patients and prescribers. Am J Clin Dermatol 2003; 4:813–831.
26. Amin K, Riddle CC, Aires DJ, et al. Common and alternative oral therapies for acne vulgaris: a review. J Drugs Dermatol 2007; 6(9):873–880.
27. Bhambri S, Del Rosso JQ, Desai A. Oral trimethoprim-sulfamethoxazole in the treatment of acne vulgaris. Cutis 2007; 79(6):430–434.
28. Rafiei R, Yaghoobi R. Azithromycin versus tetracycline in the treatment of acne vulgaris. J Drugs Dermatol 2006; 17(14):217–221.
29. Leyden JJ. The evolving role of *Propionibacterium acnes* in acne. Semin Cutan Med Surg 2001; 20:139–143.
30. Leyden JJ. A review of the use of combination therapies for the treatment of acne vulgaris. J Am Acad Dermatol 2003; 49(3):S206–S210.
31. Tanghetti E. The impact and importance of resistance. Cutis 2007; 80(1S):5–9.
32. Del Rosso JQ. Study results of benzoyl peroxide 5%/clindamycin 1% topical gel, adapalene 0.1% gel, and use in combination for acne vulgaris. J Drugs Dermatol 2007; 6(6):616–622.
33. Lookingbill DP, Dhalker DK, Lindholm JS. Treatment of acne with a combination clindamycin/benzoyl peroxide gel compared with clindamycin gel, benzoyl peroxide gel and vehicle gel: combined results of two double-blind investigations. J Am Acad Dermatol 1997; 37:590–595.
34. Leyden J, Kaidbey K, Levy S, et al. The combination formulation of clindamycin 1% plus benzoyl peroxide 5% versus 3 different formulations of topical clindamycin alone in the reduction of *Propionibacterium acnes*. Am J Clin Dermatol 2001; 2:263–266.
35. Leyden JJ, Wortzman M. Baldwin EK. Antibiotic-resistant *Propionibacterium acnes* suppressed by benzoyl peroxide 6% cleanser. Cutis 2008; 82:417–421.
36. Leyden JJ. Antibiotic resistance in the topical treatment of acne vulgaris. Cutis 2004; 73(6S):6–9.
37. Eady EA, Farmery MR, Ross JL, et al. Effects of benzoyl peroxide and erythromycin alone and in combination against antibiotic-sensitive and—resistant skin bacteria from acne patients. Br J Dermatol 1994; 131(3):331–336.
38. Del Rosso JQ, Leyden JJ. Status report on antibiotic resistance: implications for the dermatologist. Dermatol Clin 2007; 25(2):127–132.

39. Leyden JJ, McGinley KJ, Cavalieri S, et al. *Propionibacterium acnes* resistance to antibiotics in acne patients. J Am Acad Dermatol 1983; 8(1):41–45.

40. Eady EA, Jones CE, Tipper JL, et al. Antibiotic resistant propionibacteria in acne: need for policies to modify antibiotic use. Br Med J 1993; 306(6877):555–556.

41. Eady EA, Gloor M. Leyden JJ. Propionibacterium acnes resistance: a worldwide problem. Dermatology 2003; 206(1):54–56.

42. Simpson N. Antibiotics in acne: time for a rethink. Br J Dermatol 2001; 144(2): 225–228.

43. Cooper AJ. Systematic review of *Propionibacterium acnes* resistance to systemic antibiotics. Med J Aust 1998; 169(5):259–261.

44. Thevarajah S, Balkrishnan R, Camacho F, et al. Trends in prescription of acne medication in the US: shift from antibiotic to non-antibiotic treatment. J Dermatol Treat 2005; 16:224–228.

45. Tanghetti E. Antibiotic resistance and the role of combination acne therapy: introduction. Cutis 2007; 80(1S):3.

46. Eady EA, Cove JH, Holland KT. Erythromycin resistant propionibacteria in antibiotic treated acne patients: association with therapeutic failure. Br J Dermatol 1989; 121:51–57.

47. Ozolins M, Eady EA, Avery AJ, et al. Comparison of five antimicrobial regimens for treatment of mild to moderate facial acne vulgaris in the community: randomised controlled trial. Lancet 2004; 364(9452):2188–2195.

48. Simonart T, Dramaix M. Treatment of acne with topical antibiotics: lessons from clinical studies. Br J Dermatol 2005; 153:395–403.

49. Schlessinger J, Menter A, Gold M, et al. Clinical safety and efficacy studies of a novel formulation combining 1.2% clindamycin phosphate and 0.025% tretinoin for the treatment of acne vulgaris. J Drugs Dermatol 2007; 6(6):607–615.

50. Shalita AR, Myers JA, Krochmal L, et al. The safety and efficacy of clindamycin phosphate foam 1% versus clindamycin topical gel 1% for the treatment of acne vulgaris. J Drugs Dermatol 2005; 4:48–56.

51. Fleischer AB, Dinehart S, Stowe D, et al. Safety and efficacy of a new extended-release formulation of minocycline. Cutis 2006; 78(4S):21–31.

52. Skidmore R, Kovach R, Walker C, et al. Effects of subantimicrobial-dose doxycycline in the treatment of moderate acne. Arch Dermatol 2003; 139:459–464.

53. Cunliffe WJ, Aldana OL, Goulden V. Oral trimethoprim: a relatively safe and successful third-line treatment for acne vulgaris. Br J Dermatol 1999; 141(4):757–758.

54. Campbell JL. A comparative review of the efficacy and tolerability of retinoid-containing combination regimens for the treatment of acne vulgaris. J Drugs Dermatol 2007; 6(6):625–629.

55. Del Rosso JQ. Systemic therapy for rosacea: focus on oral antibiotic therapy and safety. Cutis 2000; 66(4S):7–13.

56. Knowles SR, Shear SR. Cutaneous drug reactions associated with systemic features. In: Wolverton SE, ed. Comprehensive Dermatologic Drug Therapy. 2nd ed. Philadelphia: Saunders Elsevier, 2007:977–981, 982–983.

57. Remlinger KA. Hematologic toxicity of drug therapy. In: Wolverton SE, ed. Comprehensive Dermatologic Drug Therapy. 2nd ed. Philadelphia: Saunders Elsevier, 2007:901–903.

4.2

Clinical implications of antibiotic resistance: risk of systemic infection from *Staphylococcus* and *Streptococcus*

Whitney P. Bowe and James J. Leyden

INTRODUCTION

Antibiotic use has been associated with the emergence of resistant organisms, increased exposure to and colonization with pathogenic organisms, and increased risk of infectious illness. The growing prevalence of antibiotic resistance is rapidly eroding one of our most formidable forces against bacterial pathogens. The pervasive and indiscriminate use of antibiotics is considered one of the most important inciting agents in this globally developing crisis. However, even what was thought to be the appropriate use of antibiotics for acne and rosacea has led to problems with resistance because of the chronic nature of these conditions.

Antibiotic-resistant *Propionibacterium acnes* is on the rise. Although the effects of antibiotic use on cutaneous microbial environments have been well studied, the effects on noncutaneous surfaces such as the nose and throat have recently come to the attention of the medical community. Recent studies are forcing dermatologists to ask the following questions:

1. Are acne patients on long-term antibiotics more likely to harbor potential pathogens in their nose/throat?
2. Are these organisms more likely to be resistant?
3. Are these patients at an increased risk for systemic infection?

The impact of acne antibiotics on *P. acnes* and coagulase-negative *Staphylococcus* sp. has been extensively documented in the past (1–5). This chapter focuses on recent advances in our knowledge relating to the influence of acne antibiotic use on two serious potential pathogens: *Staphylococcus aureus* and *Streptococcus pyogenes*.

STAPHYLOCOCCUS AUREUS

S. aureus is a facultatively aerobic, coagulase-positive, and gram-positive coccus, which appears as grapelike clusters on microscopy. Although some strains of *S. aureus* can be human commensals in the perineum and axilla, other strains of *S. aureus* produce toxins, for example, the toxin associated with bullous impetigo, the leukocidin of methicillin-resistant *S. aureus* (MRSA), toxic shock toxin, etc., making it a frequent cause of infections in both the hospital and the community (6,7). *S. aureus* primarily leads to skin and soft tissue infections such as impetigo, furuncles, carbuncles, cellulitis, and abscesses, but it is also capable of causing life-threatening diseases such as pneumonia, meningitis, osteomyelitis, endocarditis, and toxic shock syndrome. *S. aureus* does not depend on a human host for survival; it can survive for extended periods of time on dry environmental surfaces increasing its ability to infect new hosts (7).

Since the discovery of *S. aureus* in 1880 by Alexander Ogston, it has become a significant organism across the field of medicine. As early as 1931, an association between *S. aureus* nasal carriage and increased risk of staphylococcal skin disease was reported. With the introduction of penicillin in 1943, *S. aureus* infections and mortality were briefly abated, but resistant strains developed quickly. The first reported case of penicillin-resistant *S. aureus* (PRSA) producing β-lactamase was in 1947, and within a decade, 90% of hospital-acquired *S. aureus* was resistant to penicillin (6,8). Then in the 1950s, methicillin, a β-lactamase-insensitive β-lactam, was used to effectively treat PRSA, but by 1961, *S. aureus* had evolved again forming resistance to methicillin. MRSA was first identified in the hospital setting, and the rate increased slowly and steadily until the late 1990s when there was spike in the incidence of MRSA, which correlated with evidence of community-acquired MRSA (CA-MRSA). Patients with no hospital-associated risk factors were developing MRSA infections, and by 2001 increasing numbers of outbreaks of CA-MRSA were occurring worldwide (6,7).

Just in the last decade, there has been a dramatic rise in the incidence of reported CA-MRSA infections. A seminal study conducted by Moran and his colleagues in 2006 demonstrated that MRSA has become the most common identifiable cause of skin and soft tissue infections among patients presenting to emergency departments across the United States. They examined 422 patients presenting to 11 university-affiliated emergency departments with acute skin and soft tissue infections. *S. aureus* was isolated from 76% of the patients, making it the most common cause of community-acquired skin and soft tissue infections.

Seventy-eight percent of the *S. aureus* isolates were methicillin resistant, establishing the overall prevalence of MRSA at 59%. It is essential that isolates that are resistant to erythromycin but susceptible to clindamycin on initial testing be further evaluated using D-zone disk diffusion testing. This assay is capable of identifying *S. aureus* strains that are capable of clindamycin resistance under certain circumstances, and therefore must not be treated with clindamycin monotherapy (9).

As a consequence of studies such as Moran's, clindamycin, trimethoprim-sulfamethoxazole, and doxycycline have been recommended as first-line outpatient treatment for community-acquired MRSA (9). Ironically, these antibiotics are commonly prescribed as long-term therapy for acne vulgaris.

Coagulase-negative *Staphylococcus* resistance develops within weeks of usage. Less is known about how quickly *S. aureus* is capable of acquiring resistance to these drugs. Even if the *S. aureus* genome itself is not directly altered by antibiotic treatment, resistance genes can be transferred from coagulase-negative staphylococci to coagulase-positive staphylococci as described by Naidoo (10). This potential for horizontal transfer of resistance genes further emphasizes the concern that dermatologists might induce resistance against our main arsenal for MRSA, putting not only patients but potentially the whole community at risk for infection (10).

There are several plausible mechanisms that might account for why antibiotic treatment predisposes to MRSA infection and/or colonization. Antibiotics can partially suppress the normal, protective flora, leaving cell surface receptors open to colonization with pathogens such as MRSA. Additionally, antibiotics can directly select for preexisting MRSA in carriers, allowing these strains to proliferate and even disseminate. Furthermore, the use of antibiotics can change low-level intermittent carriers to persistent carriers (discussed later in the chapter), allowing for increased transmission (11).

There is strong evidence to suggest that people colonized with MRSA in their anterior nares are at an increased risk for MRSA infection. Although there are multiple sites on the body that can be colonized with *S. aureus*, the anterior nares remain the most common reservoir. Cross-sectional surveys have estimated nasal carriage rates of 27% in the general population. It should be noted that longitudinal studies have shown there are three main patterns of *S. aureus* nasal carriage: persistent carriage, intermittent carriage, and noncarriage. Persistent carriers are likely to be carrying higher loads of bacteria increasing their risk of infection and ability to disseminate bacteria into the environment (12–14). Persistent carriers typically carry the same strain of *S. aureus* at all times, while intermittent carriers are more likely to shift between various strains of *S. aureus* (15–17). Approximately 20% (12–30%) of individuals are considered persistent *S. aureus* carriers, roughly 30% (16–70%) are intermittent carriers, and 50% (16–69%) of individuals are noncarriers (14–16,18).

A central concept integral to host colonization with pathogens such as *S. aureus* is known as "bacterial interference." In a healthy nose, the ecological niche is already occupied with normal, protective flora. However, patients on antibiotic therapy have significant changes in their flora that could allow virulent organisms to take hold of epithelial receptors and proliferate.

Mills et al. followed 208 acne patients treated either with topical erythromycin or with vehicle. He noted an increase in the incidence of *S. aureus* nasal carriage, and the rates of erythromycin-resistant *S. aureus* among previous carriers increased from 15% to 40% during the course of treatment. These changes persisted for up to four weeks after the cessation of treatment before returning to baseline (19). A few years later, Levy et al. set out to study the effects of antibiotics on the carriage of *S. aureus* in the oropharynx, another area that commonly serves as a reservoir for *S. aureus*. In this study, 105 acne patients at the Dermatology Department of the University of Pennsylvania who had either been taking antibiotic therapy (oral, topical, or both) for at least three months or had not taken antibiotic therapy within the past six months were enrolled. The oropharynx of each patient was swabbed and cultured and the growing bacteria were tested for antibiotic resistance by agar disk diffusion. Although they found similar prevalence rates of *S. aureus* colonization between the two populations, 44% of *S. aureus* cultures from antibiotic users were resistant to at least one tetracycline compared to 18% of cultures from nonantibiotic users (20). This finding did not reach statistical significance. Similar effects on nasal *S. aureus* had been seen in prior studies (21).

GROUP A STREPTOCOCCUS

Str. pyogenes, also known as group A streptococcus (GAS), is a gram-positive coccus and an exclusively human pathogen. As a highly adhesive extracellular organism, its virulence is dependent on the presence of specific surface components as well as the production of exotoxins (22). GAS causes many human diseases ranging from mild superficial skin infections to life-threatening systemic diseases. Pharyngitis and impetigo are the most common infections attributed to GAS today, but it can also occasionally lead to purulent and non-purulent skin infections including cellulitis. It accounts for 15% to 30% of childhood cases of acute pharyngitis and 10% of adult cases (23). Therapy for these infections is primarily aimed to prevent both suppurative (tonsillopharyngeal cellulitis or abscess, otitis media, sinusitis, and necrotizing fasciitis) and nonsuppurative sequelae (acute rheumatic fever, poststreptococcal glomerulonephritis, and streptococcal toxic shock syndrome).

The oropharynx is the most common location for asymptomatic colonization of GAS. The asymptomatic carrier state, as evidenced by positive throat cultures in the absence of symptoms, is typically not treated. However, it can still be easily transmitted from carrier to close contacts via respiratory droplets (24–28). Therefore, asymptomatic GAS carriers represent one of the main GAS reservoirs from which the bacteria can be spread to the general population (22).

Fortunately, GAS still remains, for the most part, susceptible to β-lactam antibiotics. However, clinical failures to penicillin therapy can occur. Penicillin and other β-lactam antibiotics are most effective against rapidly growing bacteria. They have the greatest efficacy when organisms are in the earlier stages of infection or in mild infections. The efficacy of β-lactams may decrease later in infections when bacterial growth slows as higher concentrations of GAS accumulate. Consequently, clindamycin is considered more effective in the treatment of invasive GAS infections (29,30). Unlike penicillin, efficacy of clindamycin is not affected by the size of the inoculums or the stage of bacterial growth. Furthermore, clindamycin is capable of suppressing the production of GAS toxins. Severe GAS infections may lead to shock, multisystem organ failure, and death, making early recognition and effective treatment critical.

We revisit the study of Levy et al., this time focusing on prevalence and resistance patterns of GAS in the oropharynx of acne patients (20). In this study, 105 consecutive acne patients presenting to the Dermatology Department at the University of Pennsylvania were enrolled. The oropharynx of each patient was swabbed and cultured. GAS recovered from the oropharynx were identified and tested for antibiotic resistance by agar disk diffusion. The study demonstrated a threefold increase in the prevalence of GAS in the oropharynx of patients on antibiotic therapy. Eighty-five percent of the GAS in the treated patients were resistant to at least one tetracycline antibiotic. Of note, the association between antibiotic use and GAS carriage was seen with multiple modes of antimicrobial administration (oral alone, topical alone, combination of oral and topical). This finding may lead one to pose the question: how does the topical administration of antibiotic alter a distant site such as the oropharynx? The authors postulated two plausible mechanisms. The first possible explanation involves the direct transfer of antibiotics and/or bacterial organisms to the oropharynx via a person's fingers or by devices such as eating utensils. This theory is supported by the findings of several studies, which demonstrated an increase in erythromycin-resistant coagulase-negative staphylococci at sites (back and anterior nares) where antibiotic was not directly applied (21,31). An alternative less likely (blood levels so low) mechanism is systemic absorption of topically applied antibiotic, leading to hematogenous spread of drug to noncutaneous sites such as the oropharynx.

Given the association between acne antibiotic therapy and increased GAS oropharyngeal carriage, the next logical step was to examine whether antibiotic therapy also placed acne patients at an increased risk for an upper respiratory tract infection (URTI). Although the vast majority of URTIs are not of bacterial origin (in fact, only 10% of URTIs can be attributed to a bacterial cause), recent studies have shown that infections may be polymicrobial. Bacterial colonization with one organism (e.g., GAS) may facilitate the infectious capability of another (e.g., a respiratory virus) by influencing their cell surface receptors (25,32,33).

To address the clinical ramifications of increased GAS oropharyngeal carriage, Margolis and colleagues (including author WPB) designed a follow-up study to investigate the association between acne antibiotic use and URTI. We conducted a retrospective cohort study of 118,496 individuals identified as carrying a diagnosis of acne vulgaris in the General Practice Research Database (GPRD). Of these patients, 71.7% were being treated with topical and/or oral antibiotics (tetracycline, erythromycin, or clindamycin), while 28.3% were not on any antibiotic therapy. All acne patients were followed for one year with the main outcome measure being the onset of a URTI or a urinary tract infection (UTI). The odds of a URTI in a patient receiving long-term antibiotics for acne was 2.15 times greater than those in acne patients not receiving antibiotics (34). As was seen in the precursor study of Levy et al., these effects persisted regardless of the mode of antibiotic administration (oral alone, topical alone, combination). Because of its retrospective design, a correlation can be drawn, but does not necessarily imply causation. Although the true clinical implications need to be further studied in a controlled clinical trial setting, this study raises important considerations for both physicians and patients when choosing a treatment plan for acne.

Our research team then turned to the household contacts of acne patients for two main reasons: first, to better understand the potential mechanism behind this URTI risk, and second, to fully recognize the public health impact resulting from administration of antibiotics. We set out to determine whether household contacts of acne patients with documented UTRIs are at an increased risk of developing a URTI when compared with household contacts of acne patients without documented URTIs. We identified 98,094 household contacts of acne patients and found that a household contact of an acne patient who had a URTI was about 43% more likely to develop a URTI than one without this exposure. However, when exposure to an acne patient with a URTI was controlled for, exposure to an acne patient using antibiotics did not independently increase a contact's risk of URTI. Therefore, the development of URTIs in household contacts is likely due to the direct transmission of the URTI infectious agent and not exposure to another's use of an antibiotic. Consequently, although acne patients on antibiotics are about two times more likely to develop URTIs, they appear to be less likely to transmit these URTIs to their household contacts. While reassuring from a public health perspective, this finding likely supports the hypothesis that antibiotics are immunomodulatory, thus predisposing acne patients to infections from pathogens that are not virulent enough to cause infection in a fully immune competent host. One might hypothesize that the anti-inflammatory properties of antibiotics such as tetracycline's ability to inhibit neutrophil chemotaxis may increase susceptibility to infections (35).

CONCLUSION

Bacterial resistance to antimicrobial treatment has become a significant problem throughout the developed world. Acne vulgaris, the most common dermatological disease, is commonly treated with long-term antibiotics. This chronic use of antibiotics has led to resistance among cutaneous microbes such as *P. acnes*, making the treatment of acne patients more challenging. Of equal importance from a public health perspective, recent evidence suggests that antibiotic use has an effect on colonization rates and resistance patterns of potential pathogens in the nose and throat of acne patients. Although one study has shown an association between acne antibiotic use and systemic infection, future studies are needed to corroborate these findings, and further elucidate the true clinical relevance of the antibiotic-induced shifts in microbial flora.

REFERENCES

1. Leyden JJ, Del Rosso JQ, Webster GF. Clinical considerations in the treatment of acne vulgaris and other inflammatory skin disorders: focus on antibiotic resistance. Cutis 2007; 79(6 suppl):9–25.
2. Leyden JJ. Current issues in antimicrobial therapy for the treatment of acne. J Eur Acad Dermatol Venereol 2001; 15(suppl 3):51–55.
3. Leyden JJ. Antibiotic resistance in the topical treatment of acne vulgaris. Cutis 2004; 73(6 suppl):6–10.
4. Eady EA, Gloor M, Leyden JJ. Propionibacterium acnes resistance: a worldwide problem. Dermatology 2003; 206(1):54–56.
5. Eady AE, Cove JH, Layton AM. Is antibiotic resistance in cutaneous propionibacteria clinically relevant? Implications of resistance for acne patients and prescribers. Am J Clin Dermatol 2003; 4(12):813–831.
6. Boyle-Vavra S, Daum RS. Community-acquired methicillin-resistant Staphylococcus aureus: the role of Panton-Valentine leukocidin. Lab Invest 2007; 87(1):3–9.
7. Wertheim HF, Melles DC, Vos MC, et al. The role of nasal carriage in Staphylococcus aureus infections. Lancet Infect Dis 2005; 5(12):751–762.
8. Roghmann MC, McGrail L. Novel ways of preventing antibiotic-resistant infections: what might the future hold? Am J Infect Control 2006; 34(8):469–475.
9. Moran GJ, Krishnadasan A, Gorwitz RJ, et al. Methicillin-resistant S. aureus infections among patients in the emergency department. N Engl J Med 2006; 355 (7):666–674.
10. Naidoo J. Interspecific co-transfer of antibiotic resistance plasmids in staphylococci in vivo. J Hyg (Lond) 1984; 93(1):59–66.

11. Harbarth S, Samore MH. Interventions to control MRSA: high time for time-series analysis? J Antimicrob Chemother 2008; 62(3):431–433.

12. White A. Increased infection rates in heavy nasal carriers of coagulase-positive Staphylococci. Antimicrob Agents Chemother (Bethesda) 1963; 161:667–670.

13. Nouwen JL, Ott A, Kluytmans-Vandenbergh MF, et al. Predicting the Staphylococcus aureus nasal carrier state: derivation and validation of a "culture rule." Clin Infect Dis 2004; 39(6):806–811.

14. Nouwen JL, Fieren MW, Snijders S, et al. Persistent (not intermittent) nasal carriage of Staphylococcus aureus is the determinant of CPD-related infections. Kidney Int 2005; 67(3):1084–1092.

15. Hu L, Umeda A, Kondo S, et al. Typing of Staphylococcus aureus colonising human nasal carriers by pulsed-field gel electrophoresis. J Med Microbiol 1995; 42(2):127–132.

16. Eriksen NH, Espersen F, Rosdahl VT, et al. Carriage of Staphylococcus aureus among 104 healthy persons during a 19-month period. Epidemiol Infect 1995; 115 (1):51–60.

17. VandenBergh MF, Yzerman EP, van Belkum A, et al. Follow-up of Staphylococcus aureus nasal carriage after 8 years: redefining the persistent carrier state. J Clin Microbiol 1999; 37(10):3133–3140.

18. Kluytmans J, van Belkum A, Verbrugh H. Nasal carriage of Staphylococcus aureus: epidemiology, underlying mechanisms, and associated risks. Clin Microbiol Rev 1997; 10(3):505–520.

19. Mills O Jr., Thornsberry C, Cardin CW, et al. Bacterial resistance and therapeutic outcome following three months of topical acne therapy with 2% erythromycin gel versus its vehicle. Acta Derm Venereol 2002; 82(4):260–265.

20. Levy RM, Huang EY, Roling D, et al. Effect of antibiotics on the oropharyngeal flora in patients with acne. Arch Dermatol 2003; 139(4):467–471.

21. Vowels BR, Feingold DS, Sloughfy C, et al. Effects of topical erythromycin on ecology of aerobic cutaneous bacterial flora. Antimicrob Agents Chemother 1996; 40(11):2598–2604.

22. Passali D, Lauriello M, Passali GC, et al. Group A streptococcus and its antibiotic resistance. Acta Otorhinolaryngol Ital 2007; 27(1):27–32.

23. Cohen-Poradosu R, Kasper DL. Group A streptococcus epidemiology and vaccine implications. Clin Infect Dis 2007; 45(7):863–865.

24. Bisno AL, Gerber MA, Gwaltney JM Jr., et al. Practice guidelines for the diagnosis and management of group A streptococcal pharyngitis. Infectious Diseases Society of America. Clin Infect Dis 2002; 35(2):113–125.

25. Brogden KA, Guthmiller JM, Taylor CE. Human polymicrobial infections. Lancet 2005; 365(9455):253–255.

26. Davies HD, McGeer A, Schwartz B, et al. Invasive group A streptococcal infections in Ontario, Canada. Ontario Group A Streptococcal Study Group. N Engl J Med 1996; 335(8):547–554.

27. Recco RA, Zaman MM, Cortes H, et al. Intra-familial transmission of life-threatening group A streptococcal infection. Epidemiol Infect 2002; 129(2):303–306.

28. Smith A, Lamagni TL, Oliver I, et al. Invasive group A streptococcal disease: should close contacts routinely receive antibiotic prophylaxis? Lancet Infect Dis 2005; 5(8):494–500.

29. Bessen DE. Population biology of the human restricted pathogen, Streptococcus pyogenes. Infect Genet Evol 2009; 9(4):581–593.

30. Stock I. [Streptococcus pyogenes—much more than the aetiological agent of scarlet fever]. Med Monatsschr Pharm 2009; 32(11):408–416; quiz 17–18.

31. Miller YW, Eady EA, Lacey RW, et al. Sequential antibiotic therapy for acne promotes the carriage of resistant staphylococci on the skin of contacts. J Antimicrob Chemother 1996; 38(5):829–837.

32. Gunn GR, Zubair A, Peters C, et al. Two Listeria monocytogenes vaccine vectors that express different molecular forms of humanpapilloma virus-16 (HPV-16) E7 induce qualitatively different T cell immunity that correlates with their ability to induce regression of established tumors immortalized by HPV-16. J Immunol 2001; 167(11):6471–6479.

33. Dietrich G, Kolb-Maurer A, Spreng S, et al. Gram-positive and gram-negative bacteria as carrier systems for DNA vaccines. Vaccine 2001; 19(17–19):2506–2512.

34. Margolis DJ, Bowe WP, Hoffstad O, et al. Antibiotic treatment of acne may be associated with upper respiratory tract infections. Arch Dermatol 2005; 141 (9):1132–1136.

35. Bowe WP, Hoffstad O, Margolis DJ. Upper respiratory tract infection in household contacts of acne patients. Dermatology 2007; 215(3):213–218.

5.1

Isotretinoin

Michael G. Osofsky and John S. Strauss

INTRODUCTION

Currently, isotretinoin is the drug of choice for the management of severe, treatment-resistant acne vulgaris. Treatment with isotretinoin can lead to both marked improvement and long-lasting remission. Essentially, isotretinoin has the capacity to "cure" acne. In a field where physicians are usually resigned to suppressing inflammatory skin disorders until they "burn out," this power of isotretinoin is astounding.

The scientific community has long known that vitamin A significantly impacts proliferation and differentiation of skin (1). Thus, retinoids, or natural and synthetic analogues of vitamin A, have long been studied for the treatment of various dermatologic diseases (2). However, synthesizing an effective, though relatively safe, retinoid proved formidable. From the late 1960s to the 1980s, at least 1500 retinoids were synthesized and tested by Bollag and collaborators (2). The model that they used to test retinoids was chemically induced cutaneous papillomas of mice. These studies were undertaken to find retinoids that were antikeratinizing for the treatment of psoriasis and antineoplastic for the treatment and prevention of skin cancer.

It was not until 1979 when Peck et al. conducted an open label trial in which 13/14 patients with treatment-resistant cystic and conglobate acne achieved complete clearance at four months when administered isotretinoin at an average dose of 2 mg/kg/day (3). A few years later, a randomized placebo control trial was conducted that confirmed the remarkable efficacy of isotretinoin in the treatment of severe acne vulgaris (4). Shortly thereafter in that same year, the Food and Drug Administration (FDA) approved isotretinoin for the treatment of severe nodulocystic acne. Now with 30 years of experience with this drug, our purpose in this chapter is to focus on the basic properties of isotretinoin as well as the principles of its use for acne.

BASIC SCIENCE ASPECTS

Pharmacology

Isotretinoin, though a vitamin A derivative, is a relatively water-soluble molecule. Small amounts are found in the blood naturally, and one month following discontinuation of isotretinoin, levels within the body return to background levels. This rapid clearance from the body is the rationale for prevention of pregnancy for one month after discontinuing isotretinoin in women of childbearing potential.

Peak isotretinoin plasma levels are achieved between 1–4 hours (5). Importantly, the magnitude of this peak level is increased by coadministration with lipids. Thus, patients are instructed to take their doses with a small, fatty meal. Given the half-life of 10 to 20 hours, it is best to take isotretinoin twice a day (5–7). Finally, isotretinoin is metabolized in the liver, where it is oxidized to 4-oxo-isotretinoin via CYP450 3A4 substrate and then excreted in urine and feces.

Mechanism of Action in Acne

The primary mechanism of isotretinoin is its effect on sebaceous glands. Isotretinoin dramatically inhibits sebaceous gland activity, proliferation, differentiation, function, and production of sebum (8–10). In vitro studies conclude that isotretinoin induces apoptosis and cell cycle arrest of human sebocytes (11–13). This effect seems to persist indefinitely upon completion of a full course (120–150 mg/kg) of isotretinoin, and this is thought to be the mode by which treatment with isotretinoin can cure acne.

Precisely how isotretinoin molecularly renders its effect is uncertain. Unlike other retinoids used in dermatology, isotretinoin does not bind retinoic acid receptors (RARs), rather isotretinoin functions via an RAR/RXR-independent mechanism. Secondary mechanisms that contribute to the efficacy of isotretinoin include anti-inflammatory, antibacterial (secondary to sebum reduction/alteration), and antikeratinizing effects.

CLINICAL ASPECTS

Indications

Per FDA guidelines, isotretinoin is indicated for the treatment of severe recalcitrant nodular acne. Its use for less severe acne is often indicated provided such cases are treatment resistant and especially if the disease is leading to scarring, whether physical or emotional. In only the severest cases should it be considered initial therapy.

Dosing

Isotretinoin should be dosed at 0.5 to 1 mg/kg/day divided BID. In the typical acne patient requiring treatment with isotretinoin, we start at 0.5 mg/kg/day for the first month to acclimate the patient to mucocutaneous xerosis, minimize initial inflammatory response, and monitor for any adverse effects. If after the first month the patient is not experiencing excess dryness or other adverse effects, the dose should then be increased to approximately 1 mg/kg/day.

In patients with severe acne in which explosive flares may occur, we often pretreat for one or two weeks with daily prednisone to minimize this risk. After this pretreatment, we initiate isotretinoin at 0.5 mg/kg/day, or even less if necessitated by severity. The prednisone dose should then be gradually decreased as the isotretinoin dose is increased toward a goal of 1 mg/kg/day.

In general, most patients are treated with 1 mg/kg/day. However, more important than the daily dose is achieving a total cumulative dose of 120 to 150 mg/kg, which ensures the greatest likelihood of prolonged remission of acne (14). Calculating this dosage permits flexibility and minimizes adverse reactions.

Relapse

Relapses do occur and most investigators agree that relapses are more common in younger patients, males, and truncal acne. However, acne that recurs after isotretinoin therapy is more responsive to less aggressive acne treatments such as topical agents or oral antibiotics. If still severe, a repeat course of isotretinoin can be tried with success rates similar to that of initial treatments.

Purported relapse rates following treatment of acne with isotretinoin varies between 5.6% and 65.5% (15–26). The most likely reasons for this large discrepancy are small sample size, short follow-up, retrospective design, and/or subtherapeutic cumulative dosage. Perhaps the most convincing study to date showed a relapse rate of 41% and a need for a second course of isotretinoin at 26% (19). We usually communicate to our acne patients that approximately 1/3 will be "cured," 1/3 will be better, and 1/3 will be unimproved following a full course of isotretinoin.

Contraindications

Absolute contraindications include pregnancy, breast-feeding, and hypersensitivity to parabens, soybean oil, or other retinoids.

Relative contraindications include psychiatric disorders, skeletal disorders, seizure disorder, hyperlipidemia, pancreatitis history, diabetes mellitus, hyperuricemia, gout, and anorexia nervosa.

Drug Interactions

Since lists of various drug interactions can easily be obtained from various drug references, we will only comment on the possible interaction of concomitant use of isotretinoin and tetracycline class medications. Both isotretinoin and tetracyclines can cause idiopathic intracranial hypertension (IIH), that is, pseudotumor cerebri. The mechanism of this rare adverse effect is believed to be an idiosyncratic reaction. Therefore, when starting isotretinoin in patients with very severe nodulocystic acne, we occasionally continue/start minocycline or doxycyline and/or systemic corticosteroids to reduce a severe inflammatory response in the patient. After a month or two, we then discontinue the minocycline or doxycycline and continue isotretinoin. Obviously, symptoms of IIH (e.g., headache, visual changes, and tinnitus) should be closely monitored.

Adverse Effects

Treatment with isotretinoin can have various adverse effects since RARs are ubiquitous throughout the body. Many of these adverse effects are common and dose dependent, though some are rare and idiosyncratic. These side effects mimic the effects of hypervitaminosis A, albeit in a much attenuated presentation, and almost all are reversible upon discontinuation of isotretinoin.

The first, and essentially universal, side effect of isotretinoin is cheilitis. Chapped and cracking lips are so expected that its absence is often considered a marker of noncompliance or insufficient dosage. In addition to the lips, any mucocutaneous site can be affected including the skin, conjunctiva, oropharynx, nasopharynx, and genitalia. Treatment for mucocutaneous dryness is straightforward and consists of artificial tears for the eyes, petrolatum for the lips, and bland emollients for the body. In severe cases, topical corticosteroids may also be employed. Other rarely reported cutaneous side effects of isotretinoin include photosensitivity, exuberant granulation tissue, and abnormal wound healing. Telogen effluvium, nail plate fragility, paronychia, and onycholysis are adverse effects that can affect the hair and nails.

Because of xerophthalmia, patients who wear contact lenses should be informed that it may be uncomfortable to wear contact lenses while being treated with isotretinoin. Other reported ocular side effects due to progressive xerophthalmia include night blindness, conjunctivitis, keratitis, corneal opacities, and cataracts.

Reversible alterations in blood lipids are another frequent side effect of isotretinoin. Hypertriglyceridemia is the most common dyslipidemia secondary to isotretinoin and is generally seen in about 20% of acne patients treated with isotretinoin (27–29). LDL may also be increased, while HDL may be decreased. These alterations typically occur early in treatment during the first month or two, stabilize, and then revert to pretreatment levels promptly upon discontinuation of isotretinoin. The long-term effect of relatively brief alterations in lipid levels is thought to be negligible. However, substantially increased triglyceride levels can have immediate risks including pancreatitis and eruptive xanthomas (28). Triglyceride-induced pancreatitis is usually not seen unless triglyceride levels are greater than 800 mg/dL, a level infrequently caused by isotretinoin (30).

Treatment of slight to moderate elevations in triglycerides (300–500 mg/dL) consists of lifestyle changes including weight loss, increased exercise, and incorporation of a healthy diet with increased consumption of fruits, vegetables, whole grains, and lean meat. Decreased consumption of fatty foods, processed foods, carbohydrates, and alcohol should also be emphasized. For triglyceride levels in the 500 to 800 mg/dL range, more immediate intervention may be indicated, particularly if triglyceride levels continue to rise. Since triglyceride elevations are dose related, one can decrease the dose of isotretinoin. If dose reduction is not sufficient, pharmacologic therapy is indicated. The drug of choice for isotretinoin-induced hypertryglyceridemia is gemfibrozil, a fibrate lipid-lowering agent. The standard dose of gemfibrozil is 600 mg twice daily, taken 30 minutes prior to breakfast and dinner. For triglyceride levels greater than 800 mg/dL, discontinuation of isotretinoin is appropriate.

Long-term implications of altered blood lipid levels during treatment with isotretinoin may actually be profound. A relatively recent prospective study makes a strong argument that individuals treated with isotretinoin who develop lipid abnormalities may be at an increased risk for future development of the metabolic syndrome. This is characterized by central obesity, hypertension, hyperglycemia, and dyslipidemia (31). Dermatologists can play a pivotal role in preventing the long-term complications by referring these patients to primary care physicians and specialists for early intervention to prevent obesity, hypertension, hyperlipidemia, and diabetes mellitus. Importantly, this study suggests that treatment with isotretinoin may unmask susceptibility to the metabolic syndrome but in no way suggests causality.

Besides mucocutaneous xerosis and transient dyslipidemia, the incidence of other adverse effects due to isotretinoin is much less frequent. Increased transaminase levels are seen in some 11% to 15% of acne patients treated with isotretinoin (32). However, the development of severe hepatotoxicity is exceedingly rare. Nevertheless, it is a standard of care to check baseline liver enzymes with consideration of foregoing treatment with isotretinoin if levels are substantially elevated. Other occasionally reported gastrointestinal adverse effects of isotretinoin include nausea, diarrhea, abdominal pain, acute gastritis, and acute proctocolitis. Rare reports of decreased white blood cell count, hemoglobin, and platelets compel most physicians to check these levels at baseline.

Idiopathic intracranial hypertension (IIH), or pseudotumor cerebri, is an exceedingly rare idiosyncratic reaction of isotretinoin. It is characterized by severe and persistent headaches, classically worse in the morning, associated with nausea, vomiting, and blurred vision (33). Additional manifestations include pulsatile tinnitus, retrobulbar pain, and focal neurologic deficits. Any of these findings should prompt a fundoscopic exam to evaluate for papilledema, or swelling of the optic disc. Isotretinoin should be immediately discontinued and a neurologist should be consulted for further management. Concurrent treatment with tetracyclines, another class of medications associated with IIH, is generally avoided. However, given that IIH is an idiosyncratic reaction rather than a dose-related side effect, concurrent treatment with isotretinoin and a tetracycline may, on rare instances, be appropriate. Musculoskeletal complaints, such as arthralgias or myalgias, may be reported by some 30% of acne patients treated with iso-tretinoin, though significant elevations in creatine kinase are much rarer (34). It is thought that patients who engage in strenuous physical activity are at greater risk for the development of muscle pains. We recommend patients continue their normal activities and decrease the intensity should they experience myalgias.

Clearly, the most serious side effect of isotretinoin is teratogenicity. Iso-tretinoin affects organogenesis; therefore, its greatest risk to a fetus is early in pregnancy (during the first trimester) (35). However, isotretinoin is contraindicated throughout pregnancy and even one dose is thought to be able to induce congenital defects. Some 18% to 22% of pregnancies exposed to isotretinoin end in spontaneous abortion (35,36). Of those exposed pregnancies not ending in spontaneous abortion or elective abortion, the rate of birth defects ranges from 18% to 28% (35,36). These birth defects include craniofacial, cardiac, central nervous system, thymic, and various other abnormalities (35–37). Furthermore, it is thought that fetal exposure to isotretinoin can also cause impaired neuropsychological functioning and mental retardation, manifesting later in childhood (38).

To minimize the risk of congenital defects, in March 2006, the FDA mandated that all prescribing physicians, patients, and pharmacies distributing isotretinoin must be enrolled in the iPLEDGE program, an Internet-based distribution system that interconnects physicians, patients, and pharmacies. Simply put, iPLEDGE links a monthly negative pregnancy test, conducted at a physician's office or laboratory, to a prescription for a one-month supply of isotretinoin. Prior to starting isotretinoin, a patient must be enrolled in the system, select and adhere to two means of contraception (or may elect for abstinence), and have two negative urine pregnancy tests separated by at least 30 days. If these obligations are met, a patient can then be provided a prescription for a one-month supply of isotretinoin. Every month this process must be repeated with a new negative pregnancy test and counseling on the risks of isotretinoin, both of which must be officially documented in the iPLEDGE program. This program, albeit in a somewhat more lenient form, is also required for women without childbearing potential and males (though there is no evidence of any adverse pregnancies from men treated with isotretinoin). Further details of the iPLEDGE program can be obtained at http://www.ipledgeprogram.com.

Altered bone mineralization is another controversial aspect of isotretinoin. Long-term treatment with isotretinoin can affect bone mineral density (BMD) (39–41). However, these effects probably do not apply to the short-term treatment of acne with a standard course of isotretinoin. At least four studies have demonstrated that short courses of isotretinoin for treatment of acne do not decrease BMD (34,42–44), though two of the four studies did find a decreased BMD at Ward's Triangle (34,43). Still, measurements at this site are notoriously unreliable and should not be used to determine, or monitor, BMD (45,46). Rather, the preferred site to measure BMD is the lumbar spine and, if not feasible there, then the total hip region should be used (34,35).

The development of hyperostosis, or osteophytes, and diffuse idiopathic skeletal hyperostosis (DISH) (calcification of interosseous tendons and ligaments), is another controversial possible toxicity of isotretinoin. Whether brief courses of isotretinoin for the treatment of acne do cause hyperostosis or DISH-like changes is debatable. Further uncertain is the consequences of hyperostosis and DISH-like changes.

There are two putative adverse effects of isotretinoin treatment that are currently the topic of courtroom battles. We feel that the verdicts of these legal proceedings are not founded by evidence-based medicine. The first of these concerns psychiatrics events. The first case report suggesting a relationship between the use of isotretinoin and the development of depression was in 1983 (47). Since that time, perhaps no other issue in dermatology has been more controversial and divisive. Nevertheless, there is no evidence that there is a causal relationship between mood disturbances such as depression, anxiety, or suicidal ideation and the use of isotretinoin.

To date, numerous large, valid studies have demonstrated that there is no increased risk of depression in patients treated with isotretinoin (48–51). On the contrary, there have actually been numerous studies showing improved mood or reduced anxiety in patients treated with isotretinoin (52–56). In 2008, a study was published alleging an association between isotretinoin and depression (57). However, this study was flawed for many reasons and has been disproven (58). Confounding factors included the similar age of onset of acne and depression and that acne itself is a well-established cause of depression (59,60).

Given the serious nature of depression and suicidal ideation, we do recommend close psychological monitoring of patients treated with isotretinoin. At this time, there does not appear to be a causal relationship between the use of isotretinoin and depression. However, this does not mean that some patients may not develop an idiosyncratic reaction to isotretinoin.

The second adverse effect to be considered is the alleged relationship between treatment of acne with isotretinoin and the development of inflammatory bowel disease (IBD). The two major diseases of IBD are Crohn's disease and ulcerative colitis. Since the approval of isotretinoin for the treatment of acne in the 1980s, there have been scattered case reports and case series that associate isotretinoin use and onset or flaring of IBD (61,62). A systematic review was conducted evaluating whether isotretinoin may trigger IBD (63). Using the Naranjo adverse drug reaction probability scale, they determined that of the 85 cases reported to the FDA MedWatch program from 1997 to 2002, 4 cases (5%) scored in the "highly probable" range for isotretinoin as the cause of IBD, 58 cases (68%) were "probable," 23 cases (27%) were "possible," and no cases were "doubtful" (63).

There is just as much evidence that suggests there is no causal link between isotretinoin and IBD. Similar to the study cited above, though using different criteria of causality, it was concluded that there is insufficient evidence to confirm or refute a causal association between isotretinoin and IBD (64). In the most powerful study to date examining isotretinoin and IBD, a population-based, matched case-control study showed that IBD patients were no more likely to use isotretinoin than the general population (65). Patients with known IBD have been treated with isotretinoin for acne. In one study, only one of the four patients with IBD developed a flare in IBD when his/her acne was treated with isotretinoin, further supporting the concept that there is no casual link between isotretinoin and IBD (66).

It is our opinion at this time that there is insufficient evidence to conclude that isotretinoin can cause IBD. Perhaps the greatest confounding factor that leads to this erroneous conclusion is the overlap between the age of onset of acne and IBD. Similar to acne, the age of onset of IBD begins in the second decade and peaks in the third decade (65,67). Acne vulgaris similarly rises in incidence and peaks at the same time. Thus, it seems to be more of an incidental occurrence, rather than causal, that patients treated with isotretinoin develop IBD.

Nevertheless, it would be foolish to ignore the case reports suggesting a link between the use of isotretinoin and the development of mental disturbances or IBD. However, coassociation does not equal causation. Larger studies investigating these occurrences have failed to establish any increased incidence of either of these problems in patients treated with isotretinoin. Therefore, it is our opinion that isotretinoin should continue to be employed, albeit with caution and informed consent, when appropriately necessary.

Monitoring Guidelines

At time of publication, the isotretinoin package insert recommends checking fasting lipids and liver function tests (LFTs) at baseline, then every one to two weeks until stable. Given the minimal immediate risk of elevated lipid levels and the exceedingly rare incidence of dangerously high LFTs, in our practice we check lipids and LFTs at baseline and then lipids monthly for the first two months. If no abnormalities are found and the dose unchanged, we do not check any further labs unless there are reasons to be concerned based on history of rising or unstable laboratory values. Of course, one should check labs more frequently if abnormalities are encountered.

As per iPLEDGE requirements, women of child bearing potential require two negative in-office urine or serum pregnancy tests separated by at least 28 days before starting therapy. Thereafter, they will need monthly in-office negative urine or serum pregnancy tests throughout therapy and for one month after treatment is finished.

Finally, it is recommended that all patients receiving isotretinoin be evaluated for signs or symptoms of suicidality or any unusual behavior changes every month. If any concerns arise, psychiatric consultation should be immediately obtained and discontinuing isotretinoin should be considered.

REFERENCES

1. Wolbach SB, Howe PR. Tissue changes following deprivation of fat-soluble a vitamin. J Exp Med 1925; 42:753–777.
2. Bollag W. The development of retinoids in experimental and clinical oncology and dermatology. J Am Acad Dermatol 1983; 9:797–805.
3. Peck GL, Olsen TG, Yoder FW, et al. Prolonged remissions of cystic and conglobate acne with 13-cis-retinoic acid. N Engl J Med 1979; 300:329–333.
4. Peck GL, Olsen TG, Butkus D, et al. Isotretinoin versus placebo in the treatment of cystic acne. A randomized double-blind study. J Am Acad Dermatol 1982; 6:735–745.
5. Khoo KC, Reik D, Colburn WA. Pharmacokinetics of isotretinoin following a single oral dose. J Clin Pharmacol 1982; 22:395–402.
6. Brazzell RK, Vane FM, Ehmann CW, et al. Pharmacokinetics of isotretinoin during repetitive dosing to patients. Eur J Clin Pharmacol 1983; 24:695–702.
7. Colburn WA, Gibson DM, Wiens RE, et al. Food increases the bioavailability of isotretinoin. J Clin Pharmacol 1983; 23:534–539.
8. Strauss JS, Stewart ME, Downing DT. The effect of 13-cis-retinoic acid on sebaceous glands. Arch Dermatol 1987; 123:1538a–1541a.
9. Strauss JS, Stranieri AM. Changes in long-term sebum production from isotretinoin therapy. J Am Acad Dermatol 1982; 6:751–756.
10. Strauss JS, Stranieri AM, Farrell LN, et al. The effect of marked inhibition of sebum production with 13cis-retinoic acid on skin surface lipid composition. J Invest Dermatol 1980; 74:66–67.
11. Nelson AM, Gilliland KL, Cong Z, et al. 13-cis Retinoic acid induces apoptosis and cell cycle arrest in human SEB-1 sebocytes. J Invest Dermatol 2006; 126: 2178–2189.
12. Nelson AM, Zhao W, Gilliland KL, et al. Temporal changes in gene expression in the skin of patients treated with isotretinoin provide insight into its mechanism of action. Dermatoendocrinol 2009; 1:177–187.

13. Nelson AM, Zhao W, Gilliland KL, et al. Early gene changes induced by isotretinoin in the skin provide clues to its mechanism of action. Dermatoendocrinol 2009; 1:100–101.

14. Strauss JS, Rapini RP, Shalita AR, et al. Isotretinoin therapy for acne: results of a multicenter dose-response study. J Am Acad Dermatol 1984; 10:490–496.

15. Al-Mutairi N, Manchanda Y, Nour-Eldin O, et al. Isotretinoin in acne vulgaris: a prospective analysis of 160 cases from Kuwait. J Drugs Dermatol 2005; 4:369–373.

16. Chivot M, Midoun H. Isotretinoin and acne—a study of relapses. Dermatologica 1990; 180:240–243.

17. Harms M, Masouye I, Radeff B. The relapses of cystic acne after isotretinoin treatment are age-related: a long-term follow-up study. Dermatologica 1986; 172:148–153.

18. Haryati I, Jacinto SS. Profile of acne patients in the Philippines requiring a second course of oral isotretinoin. Int J Dermatol 2005; 44:999–1001.

19. Azoulay L, Oraichi D, Bérard A. Isotretinoin therapy and the incidence of acne relapse: a nested case-control study. Br J Dermatol 2007; 157(6):1240–1248.

20. Lehucher-Ceyrac D, de La Salmoniere P, Chastang C, et al. Predictive factors for failure of isotretinoin treatment in acne patients: results from a cohort of 237 patients. Dermatology 1999; 198:278–283.

21. Lehucher-Ceyrac D, Weber-Buisset MJ. Isotretinoin and acne in practice: a prospective analysis of 188 cases over 9 years. Dermatology 1993; 186:123–128.

22. Ng PP, Goh CL. Treatment outcome of acne vulgaris with oral isotretinoin in 89 patients. Int J Dermatol 1999; 38:213–216.

23. Quereux G, Volteau C, N'Guyen JM, et al. Prospective study of risk factors of relapse after treatment of acne with oral isotretinoin. Dermatology 2006; 212:168–176.

24. Shahidullah M, Tham SN, Goh CL. Isotretinoin therapy in acne vulgaris: a 10-year retrospective study in Singapore. Int J Dermatol 1994; 33:60–63.

25. Stainforth JM, Layton AM, Taylor JP, et al. Isotretinoin for the treatment of acne vulgaris: which factors may predict the need for more than one course? Br J Dermatol 1993; 129:297–301.

26. White GM, Chen W, Yao J, et al. Recurrence rates after the first course of isotretinoin. Arch Dermatol 1998; 134:376–378.

27. Bershad S, Rubinstein A, Paterniti JR, et al. Changes in plasma lipids and lipoproteins during isotretinoin therapy for acne. N Engl J Med 1985; 313:981–985.

28. McCarter TL, Chen YK. Marked hyperlipidemia and pancreatitis associated with isotretinoin therapy. Am J Gastroenterol 1992; 87:1855–1858.

29. Zech LA, Gross EG, Peck GL, et al. Changes in plasma cholesterol and triglyceride levels after treatment with oral isotretinoin. A prospective study. Arch Dermatol 1983; 119:987–993.

30. Fortson MR, Freedman SN, Webster PD 3rd. Clinical assessment of hyperlipidemic pancreatitis. Am J Gastroenterol 1995; 90:2134–2139.

31. Rodondi N, Darioli R, Ramelet A, et al. High risk for hyperlipidemia and the metabolic syndrome after an episode of hypertriglyceridemia during 13-cis retinoic acid therapy for acne: a pharmacogenetic study. Ann Int Med 2002; 136:582–589.

32. Zane LT, Leyden WA, Marqueling AL, et al. A population-based analysis of laboratory abnormalities during isotretinoin therapy for acne vulgaris. Arch Dermatol 2006; 142:1016–1022.
33. Wall M, George D. Idiopathic intracranial hypertension. A prospective study of 50 patients. Brain 1991; 114(pt 1A):155–180.
34. DiGiovanna JJ, Langman CB, Tschen EH, et al. Effect of a single course of isotretinoin therapy on bone mineral density in adolescent patients with severe, recalcitrant, nodular acne. J Am Acad Dermatol 2004; 51:709–717.
35. Lammer EJ, Chen DT, Hoar RM, et al. Retinoic acid embryopathy. N Engl J Med 1985; 313:837–841.
36. Dai WS, LaBraico JM, Stern RS. Epidemiology of isotretinoin exposure during pregnancy. J Am Acad Dermatol 1992; 26:599–606.
37. Lynberg MC, Khoury MJ, Lammer EJ, et al. Sensitivity, specificity, and positive predictive value of multiple malformations in isotretinoin embryopathy surveillance. Teratology 1990; 42:513–519.
38. Adams J, Lammer EJ. Neurobehavioral teratology of isotretinoin. Reprod Toxicol 1993; 7:175–177.
39. Pennes DR, Ellis CN, Madison KC, et al. Early skeletal hyperostoses secondary to 13-cis-retinoic acid. AJR Am J Roentgenol 1984; 142:979–983.
40. Ellis CN, Pennes DR, Martel W, et al. Radiographic bone surveys after isotretinoin therapy for cystic acne. Acta Derm Venereol 1985; 65:83–85.
41. Ellis CN, Madison KC, Pennes DR, et al. Isotretinoin therapy is associated with early skeletal radiographic changes. J Am Acad Dermatol 1984; 10:1024–1029.
42. Kocijancic M. 13-Cis-Retinoic acid and bone density. Int J Dermatol 1995; 34: 733–734.
43. Leachman SA, Insogna KL, Katz L, et al. Bone densities in patients receiving isotretinoin for cystic acne. Arch Dermatol 1999; 135:961–965.
44. Margolis DJ, Attie M, Leyden JJ. Effects of isotretinoin on bone mineralization during routine therapy with isotretinoin for acne vulgaris. Arch Dermatol 1996; 132:769–774.
45. Lenchik L, Leib ES, Hamdy RC, et al. Executive summary International Society for Clinical Densitometry position development conference Denver, Colorado July 20–22, 2001. J Clin Densitom 2002; 5(suppl):S1–S3.
46. Hamdy RC, Petak SM, Lenchik L, International Society for Clinical Densitometry Position Development Panel and Scientific Advisory Committee. Which central dual X-ray absorptiometry skeletal sites and regions of interest should be used to determine the diagnosis of osteoporosis? J Clin Densitom 2002; 5(suppl):S11–S18.
47. Hazen PG, Carney JF, Walker AE, et al. Depression—a side effect of 13-cis-retinoic acid therapy. J Am Acad Dermatol 1983; 9:278–279.
48. Jick SS, Kremers HM, Vasilakis-Scaramozza C. Isotretinoin use and risk of depression, psychotic symptoms, suicide, and attempted suicide. Arch Dermatol 2000; 136:1231–1236.
49. Hersom K, Neary MP, Levaux HP, et al. Isotretinoin and antidepressant pharmacotherapy: a prescription sequence symmetry analysis. J Am Acad Dermatol 2003; 49:424–432.

50. Chia CY, Lane W, Chibnall J, et al. Isotretinoin therapy and mood changes in adolescents with moderate to severe acne: a cohort study. Arch Dermatol 2005; 141:557–560.

51. Marqueling AL, Zane LT. Depression and suicidal behavior in acne patients treated with isotretinoin: a systematic review. Semin Cutan Med Surg 2007; 26:210–220.

52. Rubinow DR, Peck GL, Squillace KM, et al. Reduced anxiety and depression in cystic acne patients after successful treatment with oral isotretinoin. J Am Acad Dermatol 1987; 17:25–32.

53. Hahm BJ, Min SU, Yoon MY, et al. Changes of psychiatric parameters and their relationships by oral isotretinoin in acne patients. J Dermatol 2009; 36:255–261.

54. Kaymak Y, Kalay M, Ilter N, et al. Incidence of depression related to isotretinoin treatment in 100 acne vulgaris patients. Psychol Rep 2006; 99:897–906.

55. Kellett SC, Gawkrodger DJ. A prospective study of the responsiveness of depression and suicidal ideation in acne patients to different phases of isotretinoin therapy. Eur J Dermatol 2005; 15:484–488.

56. Kaymak Y, Taner E, Taner Y. Comparison of depression, anxiety and life quality in acne vulgaris patients who were treated with either isotretinoin or topical agents. Int J Dermatol 2009; 48:41–46.

57. Azoulay L, Blais L, Koren G, et al. Isotretinoin and the risk of depression in patients with acne vulgaris: a case-crossover study. J Clin Psychiatry 2008; 69:526–532.

58. Bigby M. Does isotretinoin increase the risk of depression? Arch Dermatol 2008; 144:1197–1199; discussion 1234–1235.

59. Lasek RJ, Chren MM. Acne vulgaris and the quality of life of adult dermatology patients. Arch Dermatol 1998; 134:454–458.

60. Newton JN, Mallon E, Klassen A, et al. The effectiveness of acne treatment: an assessment by patients of the outcome of therapy. Br J Dermatol 1997; 137:563–567.

61. Reniers DE, Howard JM. Isotretinoin-induced inflammatory bowel disease in an adolescent. Ann Pharmacother 2001; 35:1214–1216.

62. Passier JL, Srivastava N, van Puijenbroek EP. Isotretinoin-induced inflammatory bowel disease. Neth J Med 2006; 64:52–54.

63. Reddy D, Siegel CA, Sands BE, et al. Possible association between isotretinoin and inflammatory bowel disease. Am J Gastroenterol 2006; 101:1569–1573.

64. Crockett SD, Gulati A, Sandler RS, et al. A causal association between isotretinoin and inflammatory bowel disease has yet to be established. Am J Gastroenterol 2009; 104:2387–2393.

65. Bernstein CN, Nugent Z, Longobardi T, et al. Isotretinoin is not associated with inflammatory bowel disease: a population-based case-control study. Am J Gastroenterol 2009; 104:2774–2778.

66. Godfrey KM, James MP. Treatment of severe acne with isotretinoin in patients with inflammatory bowel disease. Br J Dermatol 1990; 123:653–655.

67. Loftus CG, Loftus EV Jr., Harmsen WS, et al. Update on the incidence and prevalence of Crohn's disease and ulcerative colitis in Olmsted County, Minnesota, 1940–2000. Inflamm Bowel Dis 2007; 13:254–261.

6.1

Hormonal treatment of acne in women

Jonette Keri, Diane S. Berson, and Diane M. Thiboutot

INTRODUCTION

Acne is a common skin condition affecting most people in their lifetime and in most in a mild to moderate degree. Although traditionally thought of as a disease of teenagers and a "rite of passage," we know acne can affect from infancy well into the adult years. Studies show 79% to 95% of teenagers are affected (1). In addition, acne may begin in the twenties and thirties, with persistence into adulthood. In one review, up to 12% of female patients had symptoms of acne until the age of 44 (1). This percentage appears to be less for men, around 3% in the same study had acne until the age of 44. In a more recent study, surveyed patients reported an increased prevalence of acne into adulthood (2). In this study, over 1013 patients were divided into four age groups: 20 to 29 years, 30 to 39 years, 40 to 49 years, and over 50 years. In each adult age group, women reported more acne than men and the percentages were striking. In the 20- to 29-year-olds, 50.9% of women versus 42.5% of men reported acne. This trend continued in each age group, with the 35.2%, 26.3%, and 15.3% of women aged 30 to 39, 40 to 49, and over 50 years, respectively, reporting acne. The percentages for men with acne in the same age groups of increasing years were 20.1%, 12%, and 7.3%. It is these female patients whom we most often refer to when discussing hormonal treatment of acne.

However, when discussing the hormonal treatment of acne, it is important to remember age groups other than teenagers/young adults, and these will be discussed below.

REVIEW OF PATHOGENESIS OF ACNE

For acne to occur, basically four steps are required: (*i*) follicular plugging and excessive sebum production, (*ii*) enlargement of sebaceous glands and development of microcomedones, (*iii*) inflammatory processes triggered by *Propionibacterium acnes* in microcomedones, and (*iv*) release of cytotoxic and chemotactic agents that leads to further inflammation. The purpose of this chapter is to review the hormonal influences in the development of acne and evaluate therapy.

In general, it can be thought that acne begins with the action of androgens. Androgens act at the level of the pilosebaceous unit by increasing the size and secretion of the sebaceous gland and possibly affecting follicular hyperkeratinization. The androgens can come from the adrenal glands, the gonads, and also can be converted at the level of the sebaceous gland from steroid precursors (3). When evaluating a patient, it is helpful to think of the sources of their androgens. In the following section, a guide for initial evaluation of these patients will help define the source of androgens.

HORMONAL EVALUATION OF THE ACNE PATIENT

Infantile Acne

Infantile acne, in children beyond the neonatal period, can present with comedones, papules, and pustules. It can persist through early childhood and be associated with scarring. Boys tend to be affected more commonly than girls. This is thought to be because females have a rapid drop-off in testosterone by 2 weeks of age (4), whereas boys persist with testosterone and luteinizing hormone (LH) until around 6 to 12 months (5).

During the first year of life, conditions not to be missed include congenital adrenal hyperplasia (CAH), virilizing tumors, and endocrinopathies. A good evaluation of these patients would include the screening tests of dehydroepiandrosterone sulfate (DHEAS), follicle-stimulating hormone (FSH), LH, prolactin, 17-hydroxyprogesterone, free and total testosterone (6) (Krakowski), and androstenedione (Table 6.1.1). In addition, assessing for accelerated bone age as a sign of androgen excess can be done by performing a wrist radiograph.

Early Childhood Acne

Acne from the ages of one to seven years, after the infantile androgen abates, should be viewed with caution, and a source of hyperandrogenism should be considered, again with similar laboratory examinations as those listed above (7). Diagnoses that should be excluded include Cushing's syndrome; CAH; premature adrenarche; true precocious puberty; polycystic ovarian syndrome (PCOS); and gonadal, adrenal, and ovarian tumors (6).

Table 6.1.1 Recommeded Laboratory Evaluations for Patients with Acne and Possible Hormonal Abnormalities

Labs to be considered when evaluating a patient with androgen excess
Dehydroepiandrosterone sulfate (DHEAS)
Follicle-stimulating hormone (FSH)
Luteinizing hormone (LH)
Prolactin
17-Hydroxyprogesterone
Androstenedione
Free and total testosterone
Sex hormone–binding globulin
In a patient where polycystic ovarian syndrome (PCOS) is a consideration, add
Fasting insulin
Fasting lipids
In a patient where Cushing's syndrome is considered, add
Midnight salivary cortisol level (new test approved by FDA)

Prepubertal Acne

Acne in the prepubertal phase, meaning after approximately age 7 in girls and around age 7 to 8 in boys, is considered normal and is correlated with an increase in DHEAS by the adrenal cortex in both sexes (8). However, if severe acne or other concerning physical characteristics such as increased amounts of pubic hair, early breast development, or clitoral enlargement are present, then laboratory screening for androgen excess should be performed.

Pubescent Acne

As we enter the teenage years, acne becomes commonplace and the concern for rare diagnoses decreases. However, the role of the hormonal abnormalities in acne pathogenesis should always be considered.

Adult Acne

Most frequently, androgen excess is considered in female acne patients. However, we must remember that androgen secreting tumors can occur in all ages, including older patients with sudden onset acne. In addition, young men with resistant acne may have CAH or Cushing's syndrome. This can be evaluated in such patients with the same labs listed above and a midnight salivary cortisol.

The largest group to benefit from hormonal therapy in the treatment of acne will be young women. As noted above, the percentage of young adult women with acne appears to be rising or at the minimum, becoming more reported. Therefore, hormonal treatment is a valuable adjuvant in an acne regimen.

History and Physical Examination of Female Acne Patients

Upon initial patient examination, it is wise to look for the acne distribution, not only facial but also truncal. Androgen excess in female patients is often characterized by large nodulocystic papules along the jawline and a multitude of small comedones over the forehead. Inspection for other signs of hyperandrogenism is a must. This would include hirsutism, with evaluation not only of the face and neck but also of the lower back and abdomen. Examination of the breasts may also reveal signs of hirsutism, but may be an uncomfortable examination for unsuspecting young women in the dermatologists' office. Seborrhea and alopecia are also signs of possible hyperandrogenism. During the examination, the patient can be questioned about menses regularity. This question should be asked in an open ended manner, namely, how often do you get your periods/menses? If the clinician asks whether menses/periods are regular, many will say yes because it may be regular for them. It is important to note that many women with androgen excess can still have normal menstrual periods.

It is important to question patients regarding medications that may exacerbate acne. Contraceptives that contain progestins only such as intramuscular progesterone or intrauterine devices that release progestins can exacerbate acne. For example, recently in a letter to the editor, five patients with new-onset acne after using levonorgestrel-releasing intrauterine system were reported (9). The authors suggest this finding is underreported and suggest dermatologists be aware of the association, although it had been reported in a large open study in the past (10).

Laboratory Examination of Female Acne Patients

If signs, on examination, point to hyperandrogenism, it is best to draw some baseline labs while the patient is free of external hormonal influences, namely, that they are not on oral contraceptive pills (OCPs). It is important to avoid drawing the labs during the middle of the patient's menstrual cycle when estrogen surges with ovulation. Labs can be drawn within the one to two weeks prior to the menstrual period or within the first few days of the menstrual period. Difficulty in the timing of such blood draws occurs in young women with very irregular periods, and in such a setting, labs drawn on day 3 of menses will suffice. Patients currently on OCP should discontinue them for four to six weeks prior to hormonal laboratory examination as hyperandrogenism may be masked by the OCP (11). When evaluating the labs, look for elevations of DHEAS, which can be associated with CAH, PCOS, or Cushing's syndrome. Very large elevations (>7000–8000 ng/mL) in DHEAS can mean an adrenal tumor. To differentiate between the diseases, also compare the LH/FSH ratio, and if this is greater than 2:1, then consider a diagnosis of PCOS and refer to an endocrinologist or gynecologist for medical management of PCOS including drugs such as insulin sensitizers: metformin or thiazolidinediones, nutrition counseling, and lifestyle modification. To exclude CAH, review the 17-hydroxyprogesterone and the dehydroepiandrostenedione levels, where increases in both represent deficiencies in 11- or 21-hydroxylase.

Referral to Endocrinologist Is Appropriate When Such Abnormalities Are Uncovered

PCOS is the most common endocrinologic abnormality that occurs in the acne patient. In the United States, the incidence of PCOS can range from 5% to 10% of women. PCOS is a defined syndrome with significant morbidity. PCOS patients can have other important abnormalities including insulin resistance, diabetes, cardiovascular disease, and infertility. Thus, their identification is essential for the general well being of the patient. Sex hormone–binding globulin (SHBG), fasting insulin, and fasting lipid levels are required in addition to the hormonal labs listed above.

Specifically, SHBG levels are getting more attention. SHBG is known to be increased with the use of OCPs. Previously, SHBG has been shown to be decreased in some patients with acne. In postpubertal acne, there appears to be a negative relationship between acne severity and serum SHBG (12). Interestingly, SHBG may be more important than once thought. Recently, it was found to be inversely related to the development of diabetes in women over 45 years of age, so a higher plasma level of SHBG was associated with a lower risk of type 2 diabetes (13). Thus, identifying such women at younger ages can have an impact on their future health.

Most young women do not have true laboratory abnormalities or physical symptoms associated with PCOS or other endocrinopathy. However, many more will have acne that is responsive to an OCP.

HORMONAL THERAPY OF ACNE

Oral Contraceptive Pills

In the United States, there are currently three Food and Drug Administration (FDA)-approved oral contraceptives for acne: (*i*) ethinyl estradiol and norgestimate (Ortho Tri-Cyclen), (*ii*) ethinyl estradiol and norethindrone (Estrostep), and (*iii*) ethinyl estradiol and drospirenone (Yaz); although many others have been reported to be beneficial in acne.

When asked which oral contraceptive will work better, it is sometimes difficult for the clinician to make a choice. Patients have multiple concerns from weight gain to medicine cost, thus starting points are necessary as a reference point. A Cochrane database review was done in 2009 (14). The search yielded 25 trials. There were 7 placebo controlled trials that made 4 different comparisons; 17 trials that made 13 comparisons between 2 different combination oral contraceptives; and 1 trial that compared an oral contraceptive versus an antibiotic. The conclusions reached were that combined OCPs worked better than placebo at controlling acne. Differences between pills containing various progestins and dosages were less clear. However, limited data suggested chlormadinone and cyproterone acetate (neither of which is available in the United States) resulted in greater improvement in acne than levonorgestrel. In addition, levonorgestrel was a little better in reducing acne than desogestrel in one trial, but a second trial found them the same (14).

Recently, the safety of the newer contraceptives containing drospirenone has been called into question. A large study to evaluate the safety of the lower estrogen containing 24 active day pill has been launched to study patients over a five-year period. It will engage over 2000 gynecologists and take place in the United States and five European countries (Austria, Germany, Italy, Poland, and Sweden). The main goal of this study is to provide data to assess the concern of increased risks for the patient, including deep vein thrombosis, pulmonary embolism, acute myocardial infarction, and cerebrovascular accidents (15).

Thus, the initial choice of OCPs may include those approved by FDA. Other OCPs may be helpful, and if choosing outside of these three, it is best to use medications that have been studied and shown some success (16). These include combination pills with levonorgestrel, desogestrel, norgestimate, and desogestrel. In general, these later generation progestins have lower androgenic activity, although in practice all OCPs reduce serum androgens and have the potential to improve acne. In conclusion, we know that such combination OCPs work better than placebo, but there is little data to compare these pills to other acne treatments and limited data evaluating them head to head.

Antiandrogens

Antiandrogens for the use in treating acne come into play in the adult acne patient more commonly than the younger female and can be utilized with great success in the patient with PCOS.

Spironolactone

Spironolactone is an aldosterone antagonist and an antiandrogen that works both by blocking the androgen receptor and by inhibiting androgen biosynthesis. It also influences the ratio of LH to FSH by decreasing the response of LH to gonadotropin-releasing hormone (GnRH) (17). It is a pregnancy category C drug due to its risk of feminization effects on male fetuses, thus it is a good agent to be used in combination with OCP. Spironolactone absorption is increased with food (18). The main concern with its use is the risk of hyperkalemia. Patients with a history of adrenal, renal, or cardiac disease should avoid this drug. In addition to medications such as angiotensin-converting enzyme inhibitors, which decrease aldosterone production and increase the likely hood of hyperkalemia, chronic nonsteroidal anti-inflammatory use can lead to hyperkalemia in patients taking spironolactone. Younger healthy women patients taking this medication do not appear to have the consequence of hyperkalemia. However, in older women or those with cardiac disease or renal insufficiency, it is prudent to advise the patient of signs/symptoms of hyperkalemia (paresthesia, muscle weakness, fatigue, flaccid paralysis of the extremities, and bradycardia). A potassium level should be taken during the first month and after increasing the dose. Some practitioners recommend taking blood pressure measurements and caution young women on the possibility of orthostatic hypotension. Finally, patients should be advised of the potassium connection and avoid potassium supplements and foods/salt substitutes high in potassium. In addition to the above adverse effects, another long-debated concern is the development of hormonally sensitive cancers in patients on spironolactone. Although there is no conclusive evidence in humans and no documented cases of breast carcinomas related to spironolactone, some recommend avoidance in patients with a genetic predisposition to breast cancer (19). Other side effects include gynecomastia, menstrual irregularities, lethargy, headache, and reduced libido. A Cochrane database review of spironolactone showed there was evidence that it worked for hirsutism but not for acne, although the data was limited (20).

Flutamide

Flutamide is a nonsteroidal antiandrogen devoid of other hormonal activity. As a drug, it acts after conversion to 2-hydroxyflutamide, a potent competitive inhibitor of dihydrotestosterone (DHT) binding to the androgen receptor. It is indicated for use in prostate cancer. It has also been used in the treatment of acne and hirsutism. It cannot be given to pregnant females as it crosses the placenta and can produce a pseudohermaphrodite condition of a male fetus. It can also cause breast tenderness, decreased libido, diarrhea, nausea, and hot flashes. Serious adverse events include hepatotoxicity and the hematologic conditions of anemia, leucopenia and thrombocytopenia. The most severe adverse is a drug-induced hepatitis. Flutamide has been used alone and in combination with metformin and OCP in patients with PCOS to improve the hyperandrogenic findings in these patients (21).

Cyproterone Acetate

Cyproterone acetate (not available in the United States) is a progestin with antiandrogen properties. The primary action is competition with DHT for the androgen receptor, and like other antiandrogens will induce pseudohermaphrodism in a male fetus exposed to this medication. Cyproterone has been used to treat prostate cancer, benign prostatic hypertrophy, virilizing syndromes, androgenetic alopecia, hirsutism, and acne. The most concerning side effect is hepatotoxicity, which appears to be related to other hepatic disease and also to be dose dependent (22). Other adverse events appear to be similar to other antiandrogens. In Europe and Latin America, great success has occurred in the treatment of acne when combined with ethinyl estradiol as a contraceptive (Diane-35 and Dianette).

Other Hormonal Therapies

Low-dose glucocorticoids, generally dexamethasone and prednisone, can be used to treat patients with CAH. This condition can be divided into early onset or late onset. Most of the time in dermatology practices, we see late-onset CAH. These patients lack the enzymes 21-hydroxylase or 11-hydroxylase and get a buildup of androgen precursors. Laboratory evidence for this includes elevated levels of androstenedione, 17-hydroxyprogesterone, and DHEAS. In such patients, monitoring for adrenal suppression is necessary given the use of possible long-term use of glucocorticoids. Doses to treat the condition and the acne associated with it are usually low, from 2.5 to 5 mg of prednisone daily are standard.

Other Androgen Blockers

Other androgen blockers include buserelin (23), nafarelin, and leuprolide, which can be used to block ovarian androgen production but are associated with various side effects that often preclude their use in the acne patient.

To conclude, it is important for physicians to recognize, diagnose, and treat acne in patients with hormonal abnormalities and to assure that patients are appropriately referred and followed for management of the underlying problem and its comorbidities. In the case of PCOS, the most common cause of androgen-induced acne, a holistic approach that often involves medical management and counseling regarding nutrition and lifestyle changes may be most effective. It is also important to recognize that hormonal therapy, when added to an acne regimen, cannot only improve the patient's acne but in many cases can also obviate the need for chronic antibiotic therapy or repeat courses of iso-tretinoin.

REFERENCES

1. Cordain L, Lindeberg S, Hurtado M, et al. Acne vulgaris: a disease of Western civilization. Arch Dermatol 2002; 138:1584–1590.
2. Collier CN, Harper JC, Cafardi JA, et al. The prevalence of acne in adults 20 years and older. J Am Acad Dermatol 2008; 58(1):56–59.
3. Chen W, Thiboutot D, Zouboulis CC. Cutaneous androgen metabolism: basic research and clinical perspectives. J Invest Dermatol 2002; 119(5):992–1007.
4. Herane MI, Ando I. Acne is infancy and acne genetics. Dermatology 2003; 206 (1):24–28.
5. Katsambas AD, Katoulis AC, Stavropoulos P. Acne neonatorum: acne neonatorum: a study of 22 cases. Int J Dermatol 1999; 38(2):128–130.
6. Krakowski AD, Eichenfield LF. Pediatric acne: clinical presentations, evaluation, and management. J Drugs Dermatol 2007; 6:589–593.
7. Lucky AW. Hormonal correlates of acne and hirsutism. Am J Med 1995; 98 (1A):89S–94S.
8. Stewart ME, Downing DT, Cook JS, et al. Sebaceous gland activity and serum dehydroepiandrosterone sulfate levels in boys and girls. Arch Dermatol 1992; 128 (10):1345–1348.
9. Ilse JR, Reenberg HL, Bennett DD. Levonorgestrel-releasing intrauterine system and new-onset acne. Cutis 2008; 82(2):158.
10. Dubuisson JB, Mugnier E. Acceptability of the levonorgestrel-releasing intrauterine system after discontinuation of previous contraception: results of a French clinical study in women aged 35 to 45 years. Contraception 2002; 66(2): 121–128.
11. Ebede TL, Arch EL, Berson D. Hormonal treatment of acne in women. J Clin Aesthetic Dermatol 2009; 2(12):16–22.
12. Borgia F. Correlation between endocrinological parameters and acne severity in adult women. Acta Derm Venereol 2004; 88:201–204.
13. Ding EL, Song Y, Manson JE, et al. Sex hormone-binding globulin and risk of type 2 diabetes in women and men. N Engl J Med 2009; 361:1152–1163.
14. Arowojolu AO. Combines oral contraceptive pills for the treatment of acne. Cochrane Database Syst Rev 2009; 30:CD004425.
15. Dinger JC, Bardenheuer K, Assmann A. International active surveillance study of women taking oral contraceptives (INAS-OC Study). BMC Med Res Methodol 2009; 9:77.
16. Thiboutot D, Archer D, Lemay A, et al. A randomized, controlled trial of a low-dose oral contraceptive containing 20 microg of ethinyl estradiol and 100 microg of levonorgestrel for acne treatment. Fertil Steril 2001; 6:461–468.
17. Young RL, Goldzieher JW, Elking-Hirsch K, et al. The endocrine effects of spironolactone as an antiandrogen. Fertil Steril 1987; 48:223–228.
18. Wolverton SE. Comprehensive Dermatologic Drug Therapy. 2nd ed. Philadelphia: Elsevier, 2007:422.
19. Cumming DC. Use of spironolactone in treatment of hirsutism. Cleve Clin J Med 1990; 57:285–287.

20. Brown J, Farquhar C, Lee O, et al. Spironolactone versus placebo or in combination with steroids for hirsutism and/or acne. Cochrane Database Syst Rev 2009; (2): CD000194.

21. Pizzo A, Borrielli I, Mastroeni MT, et al. Low-dose flutamide in the treatment of hyperandrogenism in adolescents Minerva Pediatr 2008; 60(6):1357–1366.

22. Savidou I, Deutsch M, Soultati AS, et al. Hepatotoxicity induced by cyproterone acetate: a report of three cases. World J Gastroenterol 2006; 12(46):7551–7555.

23. Faloia E, Filipponi S, Mancini V, et al. Treatment with a gonadotropin-releasing hormone agonist in acne or idiopathic hirsutism. J Endocrinol Investig 1993; 16(9):675–677.

7.1

Gram-negative folliculitis

Elizabeth Gaines, Alan R. Shalita, and Guy F. Webster

INTRODUCTION

First described by Fulton et al. in 1968 (1), gram-negative folliculitis (GNF) may occur in several clinical settings. It is seen as a complication of prolonged treatment of acne vulgaris with systemic antibiotics. Acne patients who have sudden flares of pustular or cystic lesions or who have acne that is resistant to standard antimicrobial therapy should be evaluated for the presence of GNF (3). Additionally, GNF may occur following the use of a hot tub and in patients with HIV.

PATHOGENESIS

In many regards, the pathogenesis of GNF is well understood. In most cases, the anterior nares serve as the reservoir for gram-negative organisms. Acne patients who are treated with oral antibiotics have a shift in their normal flora. In the nares, the number of *Staphylococcus aureus* organisms and diphtheroids decreases, while the number of coagulase-negative staphylococcal and enterobacterial organisms increases (2). In patients with GNF, gram-negative flora may constitute up to 4% of the total bacterial flora, as opposed to 1% of flora detected in normal controls (5). In a small number of patients, this increased number of gram-negative organisms results in a transfer of organisms to neighboring areas of the face. The gram-negative bacteria can populate and exacerbate existing acne lesions and create new lesions (4).

Altered immunologic factors may also play a role in the pathogenesis of GNF (6). An assessment of hypersensitivity reactions to various microbial recall antigens and granulocyte functions was performed in 46 patients with GNF. In all patients, deviations in one or more immune parameters were detected, including lowered serum concentrations of immunoglobulin M and α1-antitrypsin and elevated levels of immunoglobulin E. The authors concluded that GNF might not simply be a complication of acne therapy, but rather its own entity as a result of derangements in underlying immunity.

Aside from the nares, other reservoirs, such as the auditory canal and loofah sponges, have been implicated. In 1979, Leyden et al. (7) identified three patients with sudden exacerbation of acne vulgaris who were shown to have GNF from *Pseudomonas aeruginosa* infection. In each patient, the source of the *Pseudomonas* was found to be an otitis externa infection. The anterior nares were not colonized. Unused loofah sponges undergo a shift in bacterial flora from sparse colonies of *Bacillus* spp. and *Staphylococcus epidermidis* to predominantly gram-negative spp. and may serve as a vehicle for the transmission of the pathogenic bacteria to the skin. Regular decontamination of loofah sponges with hypochlorite bleach may mitigate this problem (8).

CLINICAL

The overall incidence of GNF is unclear. A study by Eady et al. (9) found that 15% of acne patients who failed to respond to antibiotic therapy had GNF. Sixty-five percent of nonresponders had no microbiological abnormality and 20% had resistant *P. acnes*. In general, the overall incidence of GNF is likely underestimated due to poor sampling techniques including inadequate sampling, dried-out swabs, and long delays between sampling and arrival of specimen to the laboratory (10). Swabs should be taken from both the pustules and the nasal mucosa with sterile technique.

GNF is most likely to occur after the early teenage years, as this time period correlates with acne vulgaris patients who have been on oral antibiotics for a prolonged period of time. Patients oftentimes present with complaints of an acne flare. Typical acne patients with GNF are men with perioral and perinasal papules and pustules. They often give a history of prolonged treatment with oral and/or topical antibiotics (10).

There are two types of lesions that develop in GNF: superficial papulopustular lesions without comedones, which occur in approximately 80% of patients. Pus is typically very viscous. These lesions are usually associated with a lactose-fermenting, gram-negative rod, including *Klebsiella, Escherichia*, and *Serratia* spp. Nodular lesions, seen in the other 20% of patients, are associated with *Proteus* sp. These species are motile and, thus, have the ability to invade more deeply, producing the large suppurative abscesses that result in deeper cystic lesions (3).

Histological differences between GNF lesions and acne lesions have also been appreciated. In contrast to typical acne lesions, lesions of GNF do not contain an extractable microcomedo. A minimal amount of keratinous material is present in an intrafollicular sea of pus. Segments of the follicular wall may be dissolved. Organisms are typically arranged in nests around clumps of keratinous material, around hairs, and in phagocytes. In contrast to the predominant gram-negative rod recovered on culture, Gram stain of the tissue section may show a mixed flora (i.e., gram-positive rods and cocci, gram-negative rods, budding yeasts) (3). Gram stain and culture are recommended to confirm diagnosis; however, history and physical exam are oftentimes adequate to make the correct diagnosis.

Pseudomonas organisms typically cause hot-tub folliculitis (19). *P. aeruginosa* is a ubiquitous gram-negative rod that is often implicated in this entity. Folliculitis develops in areas covered by swimsuits. *Aeromonas hydrophila* has also been found to cause hot-tub folliculitis and is associated with water sources, including an inflatable pool and poorly maintained home spa baths (11). *Acinetobacter baumannii*, a known important cause of nosocomial infections, has also been implicated in GNF. Bachmeyer et al. (12) described a patient with AIDS who developed *A. baumanii* folliculitis of the face, neck, arms, and upper trunk. The bacterium was not found on healthy skin and the source of the infection remains unknown.

TREATMENT

The mainstay of treatment of acne-related GNF is isotretinoin, which has largely replaced the use of systemic antibiotics. In general, gram-negative infection remits when factors altering the nasal and cutaneous flora are eliminated (6). It has been shown that isotretinoin can reduce sebum levels by up to 90% or more (13). How this affects GNF is not apparent. Isotretinoin is also thought to have anti-inflammatory effects (14). Isotretinoin does not possess antibacterial properties and does not result in the direct killing of gram-negative organisms (18).

Several studies have shown that isotretinoin is the most effective treatment available for GNF, with low rates of recurrence and eradication of gram-negative bacteria from both the skin and the nares (15–17). Treatment may last anywhere from five months to one year, but clearance may be expected within two to three months. Recommended doses are 0.5 to 1.0 mg/kg/day. Follow-up cultures are recommended to ensure species eradication.

Systemic antibiotics were displaced as the treatment of choice for GNF. Topically, therapy is generally ineffective. However, in patients where isotretinoin is contraindicated, appropriate antibiotics may be supplemented. Ampicillin or trimethoprim-sulfamethoxazole for at least two weeks may be considered. Clearance of gram-negative bacteria from the anterior nares can aid in determining therapy duration.

Hot-tub folliculitis is typically self-limited in immunocompetent patients. *A. baumannii* folliculitis in the setting of AIDS has responded to intravenous treatment with ticarcillin-clavulanic acid (12).

REFERENCES

1. Fulton JE, McGinley K, Leyden JJ, et al. Gram-negative folliculitis in acne vulgaris. Arch Dermatol 1968; 98:349–353.
2. Marples RR, Fulton JE, Leyden JJ, et al. Effect of antibiotics on the nasal flora in acne patients. Arch Dermatol 1969; 99:647–651.
3. Leyden JJ, Marples RR, Mills OH, et al. Gram-negative folliculitis—a complication of antibiotic therapy in acne vulgaris. Br J Dermatol 1973; 88:533–583.
4. James WD, Leyden JJ. Gram-negative folliculitis: recognition and treatment. J Am Acad Dermatol 1983; 9:165–166.
5. Blankenship ML. Gram-negative folliculitis: follow-up observation in 20 patients. Arch Dermatol 1984; 120:1301–1303.
6. Neubert U, Jansen T, Plewig G. Bacteriologic and immunologic aspects of Gram-negative folliculitis: a study of 46 patients. Int J Dermatol 1999; 38:270–274.
7. Leyden JJ, McGinley KJ, Mills OH. Pseudomonas aeruginosa gram-negative folliculitis. Arch Dermatol 1979; 115(10):1203–1204.
8. Bottone EJ, Perez AA, Oeser JL. Loofah sponges as reservoirs and vehicles in the transmission of potentially pathogenic bacterial species to human skin. J Clin Microbiol 1994; 32(2):469–472.
9. Eady EA, Cove JH, Blake J, et al. Recalcitrant acne vulgaris. Clinical biochemical and microbiological investigation of patients not responding to antibiotic treatment. Br J Dermatol 1988; 118(3):415–423.
10. Boni R, Nehrhoff B. Treatment of gram-negative folliculitis in patients with acne. Am J Clin Dermatol 2003; 4(4):273–276.
11. Mulholland A, Yong-Gee S. A new possible cause of spa bath folliculitis: Aeromonas hydrophila. Australas J Dermatol 2008; 49(1):39–41.
12. Bachmeyer C, Landgraf N, Cordier F, et al. Acinetobacter baumanii folliculitis in a patient with AIDS. Clin Exp Dermatol 2005; 30(3):256–258.
13. Landthaler M, Kummermehr J, Wagner A, et al. Inhibitory effects of 13-cis-retinoid acid on human sebaceous glands. Arch Dermatol Res 1980; 269:297–309.
14. Plewig G, Nikolowski J, Wolff HH. Action of isotretinoin in acne rosacea and gram-negative folliculitis. J Am Acad Dermatol 1982; 6:766–785.
15. James WD, Leyden JJ. Treatment of gram-negative folliculitis with isotretinoin: positive clinical and microbial response. J Am Acad Dermatol 1985; 12(2):319–324.
16. Jones DH, Cunliffe WJ, King K. Treatment of gram-negative folliculitis with 13-cis-retinoic acid. Br J Dermatol 1979; 107:252–253.

17. Neubert U, Plewig G, Ruhfus A. Treatment of gram-negative folliculitis with iso-tretinoin. Arch Dermatol Res 1986; 278:307–313.
18. Simjee S, Sahm DF, Soltani K, et al. Organisms associated with gram-negative folliculitis: in vitro growth in the presence of isotretinoin. Arch Dermatol Res 1986; 278(4):314–316.
19. Yu Y, Cheng AS, Wang L, et al. Hot tub folliculitis or hot hand-foot syndrome caused by Pseudomonas aeruginosa. J Am Acad Dermatol 2007; 57(4):596–600.

7.2

Acne fulminans

Morgan Rabach and Guy F. Webster

INTRODUCTION

Acne fulminans (AF) is a severe, ulcerative form of acne with an acute onset and systemic symptoms. AF was originally described in 1959 by Burns and Colville (1), who described a 16-year-old student with acute fever and acne conglobata. In 1975, Plewig renamed the syndrome AF to characterize the fast onset, severity, and systemic symptoms. A more common acne fulminans-like syndrome mainly on the trunk may be precipitated by isotretinoin with dramatic ulcerating and granulating lesions and no systemic symptoms.

PATHOPHYSIOLOGY

The pathophysiology of AF is unknown. The combination of fever, arthritis, and leukocytosis point to a primarily immune etiology. The syndrome is mostly seen in those with severe inflammatory acne, that is, those with the greatest anti-*Propionibacterium acnes* immunity, and the disease may be triggered by the response to an antigen from *P. acnes* (2). Additionally, other factors may be involved. Elevated blood levels of testosterone may play an important role in the pathogenesis of AF (3). The mechanism by which isotretinoin precipitates AF is unknown but is associated with high starting doses of the drug in those with the severest acne (4). Identical twins who developed AF have been documented, suggesting a genetic component (5).

FREQUENCY

AF is a rare systemic disease that usually affects men aged 13 to 22 years who have a history of acne. The mean duration of acne before the onset of AF is two years (range 0.5–5) (6). There are approximately 100 patients with AF in the literature.

CLINICAL

Prior to developing AF, most patients have papulopustular or mild nodular acne. Patients experience a sudden onset of severe, ulcerating acne, accompanied by fever and other systemic symptoms. On exam, patients have numerous, highly inflammatory tender nodules with hemorrhagic crusts, distributed more on the upper chest, back, and shoulders than on the face (7). The lesions often ulcerate with gelatinous, necrotic debris, and the healing is slow, leaving severe scars. The systemic symptoms include fatigue, malaise, axial arthralgia, joint swelling, myalgia, and fever.

LABORATORY FINDINGS

AF if often associated with a leukemoid reaction (8). Patients may also have increased erythrocyte sedimentation rate (ESR) or C-reactive protein. Patients with lytic bone lesions may have elevated serum alkaline phosphatase levels (9). Microscopic hematuria, proteinuria, and other kidney abnormalities are sometimes found. Laboratory studies are not helpful in establishing the diagnosis, but may be predictive of therapeutic response (10).

IMAGING STUDIES

Aseptic osteolytic bone lesions have been reported at the clavicle, sternum, and long bones. Approximately 50% of patients have lytic bone lesions demonstrated on radiographs, and 70% of patients show increased uptake using technetium scintigraphy ("hot spots") (11). Destructive lesions resembling osteomyelitis are demonstrated on radiographs in 25% of patients. These frequencies may be elevated, since large studies are lacking and most cases of AF do not have imaging performed.

DIFFERENTIAL DIAGNOSIS

The differential diagnosis of AF includes acne vulgaris, rosacea fulminans/ pyoderma faciale, other acneiform eruptions, folliculitis, pyoderma gangrenosum, and acne conglobata.

PROGNOSIS

Recurrence of AF occurs rarely. Severe scarring and keloid formation is common. Bone lesions usually resolve with treatment but radiographic changes including hyperostosis may remain.

TREATMENT

As with many uncommon dermatoses, there are no large randomized trials to consult for therapy, and we rely on the collective experience of small series and case reports. Topical, high-potency corticosteroids, applied on all ulcerated nodules as well as intralesional corticosteroids, may be beneficial in limited forms of the disease. Systemic steroids are a typically required treatment for AF. Systemic corticosteroids (0.5–1.0 mg/kg of prednisone) are indicated in AF, because they effectively control the skin lesions, reduce fever, and also have a favorable effect on the musculoskeletal symptoms. Symptoms tend to recur when the steroid dose is lowered or discontinued too quickly. Oral steroids should be started and gradually reduced over six weeks to avoid adverse effects of a prolonged course of systemic steroids. The required duration of steroid therapy is determined by symptoms and in rare instances may be as long as three to five months to avoid relapses (10). The relapse usually occurs two to eight weeks after the acute attack when the corticosteroids dosage is reduced or stopped (12). Typically, patients are simultaneously treated with minocycline or doxycycline as a steroid-sparing agent.

The combination of oral steroids and isotretinoin is beneficial. Isotretinoin is started after four weeks of corticosteroid treatment. The delay in starting isotretinoin therapy is necessary not to aggravate the AF (13–16). Isotretinoin should be started at four weeks, initially at 0.25 mg/kg daily and gradually increased to achieve complete clearance. Isotretinoin with a minimum total dose of 120 mg/kg is recommended. If required, a repeat course of isotretinoin (150 mg/kg) may be used. Duration of treatment depends on individual response and usually should not be less than three to five months (17).

Isotretinoin-induced AF typically but infrequently occurs in patients with moderate to severe trunk acne who are treated initially with higher dosages of the drug, for example, >40 mg/day. Acne appears to worsen and then develops ulcerative draining lesions. The isotretinoin should be discontinued or lowered radically, for example, to 10 mg/day and prednisone begun at least 1 mg/kg. Typically, several months of gradually decreasing prednisone and slowly increasing isotretinoin are required before the reaction resolves.

Other options have been reported including azathioprine (18), dapsone (19), methotrexate (20), sulfasalazine (20), cyclosporine A (21), bisphosphonates, and infliximab (22) with varying results. Dapsone has been shown to be effective treatment in patients with AF and erythema nodosum. Dapsone may be substituted for the retinoid if need be. The initial dose is 50 mg/day, which can be increased to 100 or 150 mg/day, rarely 200 mg/day (19,23–25). Pulsed dye laser may be an effective adjuvant treatment for AF–associated granulation tissue (26).

REFERENCES

1. Burns RE, Colville JM. Acne conglobata with septicemia. Arch Dermatol 1959; 79:361–363.
2. Heydenreich G. Testosterone and anabolic steroids and acne fulminans. Arch Dermatol 1989; 125(4):571–572.
3. Wollina U, Gesina H, Koch A, et al. Case reports: acne fulminans in Marfan syndrome. J Drugs Dermatol 2005; 4(4):501–505.
4. Kalbarczyk K, Ciupinska M. Complications during treatment with Roaccutane, acne fulminans 2001. Dermatol Klin (Wroclaw) 2001; 3(suppl 1):130.
5. Palatsi R, Oikarinen A. Hormonal analysis and delayed hypersensitivity reactions in identical twins with severe acne. Acta Derm Venereol 1979; 59(2):157–160.
6. Karvonen SL. Acne fulminans: report of clinical findings and treatment of twenty-four patients. J Am Acad Dermatol 1993; 28:572–579.
7. Mehrany K, Kist JM, Weenig RH, et al. Acne fulminans. Int J Dermatol 2005; 44:132–133.
8. Strom S, Thyresson N, Bostrom H. Acute febrile ulcerative conglobate acne with leukemoid reaction. Acta Derm Venereol (Stockh) 1973; 53:306–312.
9. Knitzer RH, Needleman BW. Musculoskeletal syndromes associated with acne. Semin Arthritis Rheum 1991; 20:247–255.
10. Bolognia JL, Jorizzo JL, Rapini RP. Dermatology: Two Volume Set. Mosby 2007; 498.
11. Jemec GBE, Rasmussen I. Bone lesions of acne fulminans: case report and review of the literature. J Am Acad Dermatol 1989; 20:353–357.
12. Von Den Driesch P, Schell H, Haneke E. Acne fulminans: therapie mit 13-cis-retinsäure und indometazin. Z Hautkr 1986; 61:1145–1151.
13. Hartmann RR, Plewig G. Acne fulminans: tratamento de 11 pacientes com o ácido 13-cis-retinó ico. Ann Bras Dermatol 1983; 58:3–10.
14. Choi EH, Bang D. Acne fulminans and 13-cis-retinoic acid. J Dermatol 1992; 19:378–383.
15. Cavicchini S, Ranza R, Brezzi A, et al. Acne fulminans with sacroiliitis during isotretinoin therapy. Eur J Dermatol 1992; 2:327–328.
16. Leyden JJ. The role of isotretinoin in the treatment of acne: personal observations. J Am Acad Dermatol 1998; 39(2 pt 3):S45–S49.
17. Seukeran DC, Cunliffe WJ. The treatment of acne fulminans: a review of 25 cases. Br J Dermatol 1999; 141(2):307–309.
18. Woolfson H, Road H. Acne fulminans with circulating immune complexes and leukemoid reaction treated with steroids and azathioprine. Clin Exp Dermatol 1987; 12:463–466.

19. Tan B, Lear J, Smith A. Acne fulminans and erythema nodosum during isotretinoin therapy responding to dapsone. Clin Exp Dermatol 1997; 22(1):26–27.

20. Acne fulminans. Available at: http://emedicine.medscape.com/article/1072815-overview.

21. el-Shahawy MA, Gadallah MF, Massry SG. Acne: a potential side effect of cyclosporine A therapy. Nephron 1996; 72(4):679–682.

22. Iqbal M, Kolodney MS. Acne fulminans with synovitis-acne-pustulosis-hyperostosis-osteitis (SAPHO) syndrome treated with infliximab. J Am Acad Dermatol 2005; 52:118–120.

23. Kaminsky A. Less common methods to treat acne. Dermatology 2003; 206(1):68–73.

24. Ismail R. Acne fulminans with dapsone induced haemolysis: a case report. Med J Malaysia 1987; 42(2):124–126.

25. Siegel D, Strosberg JM, Wiese F, et al. Acne fulminans with a lytic bone lesion responsive to dapsone. Rheumatol 1982; 9(2):344–346.

26. Friedlander SF. Effective treatment of acne fulminans-associated granulation tissue with the pulsed dye laser. Pediatr Dermatol 1998; 15(5):396–398.

7.3

Drug and acneiform eruptions

Deeptej Singh, Alan R. Shalita, and Guy F. Webster

INTRODUCTION

Acneiform eruptions are skin conditions that resemble acne. The extent to which an eruption resembles acne depends on the clinician's aptitude and experience. Misclassification of distinct clinical entities such as gram-negative folliculitis, pseudofolliculitis barbae, acne fulminans, and rosacea fulminans, renamed so by Plewig et al. in 1992 (1), is reviewed in other chapters.

Acne medicamentosa, or drug-induced acne, is the prototypic acneiform eruption. Although classical acne treatments may alleviate disease, the presence of a causative agent differentiates acneiform eruptions from garden-variety acne vulgaris as identification and withdrawal of said agents are critical in treatment.

The first documented use of the term acneiform eruption came from Allworthy in 1917. He described young girls who worked as "doffers" or those who cleaned machines and were exposed to dirt, sweat, and sperm oil used in machinery. He rightfully postulated that follicular plugging lead to inflammatory changes that produced the eruptions (2).

Acneiform eruptions originate in the follicles, much like acne vulgaris. Histologically, spongiosis followed by rupture of follicular epithelium and spillage of glandular contents into dermis results in neutrophilic inflammation (3,4). The clinical features of acneiform eruptions are reviewed in Table 7.3.1.

The diagnosis may be confirmed with improvement after discontinuation of offending agent. Many categories of systemic therapies have a long and well-documented history of causing acneiform eruptions, which should assist clinicians in choosing agents to discontinue when possible.

Table 7.3.1 Signs and Symptoms of Acneiform Eruptions

Sudden onset, within days
Monomorphic lesions with papules and pustules in the same stage of development as opposed to acne vulgaris
Involvement of high sebaceous gland density areas, with potential extension to nonclassic areas as well
Development of inflammatory papules prior to comedones
Association with a new oral or topical therapeutic

CHEMOTHERAPEUTICS

Epidermal Growth Factor Receptor Inhibitors

Epidermal growth factor receptor inhibitors (EGFR-I) are the most recently identified and most reported on acneiform eruption. The tyrosine kinase inhibitors include gefitinib, erlotinib, lapatinib, and canertinib, while monoclonal antibodies against the receptor include cetuximab, panitumumab, and matuzumab. Their use has been widespread from glioblastoma, head and neck squamous cell carcinoma, non–small cell lung cancer to pancreatic and colorectal cancer. Many reports have noted that incidence of acneiform eruption on this class of medication actually portends better clinical efficacy. In fact, the association has prompted some to consider a "treatment to rash" approach to therapy. However, the impact on quality of life has also required dose reduction, treatment holidays, and total discontinuation. Recently, an expert consensus group of cutaneous toxicities reported an overall acneiform eruption frequency of 60% to 80% (5).

EGFR-I-induced acneiform eruptions show increased inflammation at the dermoepidermal junction, accompanied by neutrophils and damage to the hair follicles. Further testing reveals high levels of p53 in the basal keratinocytes (6). It has been reported that mild cases of acneiform eruption respond well to topical anti-inflammatory acne therapy, whereas oral tetracyclines are needed to treat moderate to severe cases (7). The pathophysiology of EGFR-I in the development of acneiform eruptions is yet to be elucidated (8); the mechanism is likely to be complicated given the broad range of potential cutaneous side effects reported to EGFR-I: xerosis, eczema, fissures, telangiectasia, hyperpigmentation, hair changes, and paronychia with pyogenic granuloma (7).

Thalidomide and Lenalidomide

Thalidomide and lenalidomide are immunomodulating agents believed to decrease levels of tumor necrosis factor-α. Currently, lenalidomide is used in the treatment of multiple myeloma and myelodysplasic syndromes. Additionally, it may be used as part of a multitherapy regimen for systemic amyloidosis. Thalidomide has the above indications and is also used to treat erythema nodosum leprosum.

Lenalidomide is associated with an overall skin complication rate of 29% in patients with multiple myeloma and 43% in patients with systemic amyloidosis in one study. A relatively low rate of acneiform eruptions, 3% of all patients, was reported (9). Thalidomide has been reported to cause acneiform eruptions as well, although there is no estimate of its incidence (10). Of the two reports cited, no case was biopsied. Although the time of onset after treatment initiation and time of resolution with discontinuing treatment were described for urticarial rashes, the same was not done for acneiform eruptions.

Actinomycin-D

Actinomycin-D binds to deoxyribonucleic acid and inhibits ribonucleic acid transcription. It has been used as chemotherapy against testicular and uterine cancers, Ewing's sarcoma, Wilms' tumor, and rhabdomyosarcoma. Additionally, it has been used as an antibiotic, although mostly in laboratory settings. A single case report of an eight-year-old girl with embryonal rhabdomyosarcoma describes an acneiform eruption within 10 days of treatment initiation. Her physicians monitored and documented rises in androstenedione, dehydroepiandrosterone, and testosterone that coincided with courses of actinomycin-D. The authors concluded that these observations support a relationship between drug, dermatitis, and hormone levels. Further, the authors identified structural similarity between actinomycin-D and amineptine, a tricyclic antidepressant not available in the United States. Amineptine, when in use, was also a causative agent of acneiform eruptions. It is unclear if this can be seen as a general side effect of central dopamine enhancement, due to the inhibitory effect of dopamine on prolactin, with the subsequent increase in testosterone output or through direct simulation of androgen production (11).

CORTICOSTEROIDS

Steroid-induced acne is well documented. Classically, it presents with monomorphic inflammatory papules and pustules. Few to no comedones are apparent. Although short-term use of topical corticosteroids may actually decrease inflammation and shorten the duration to clearance of a single inflammatory papule, extended use has routinely demonstrated the association with subsequent onset and/or worsening of acne. Furthermore, discontinuation of long-standing topical corticosteroid can lead to a severe flare. The situation of steroid-induced acne that flares with discontinuation of the offending agent is a clinical quagmire most dermatologists choose to avoid.

Plewig and Kligman first reported steroid-induced acne in 1973 (12). Kligman and Leyden went on to describe three distinct clinical entities that resulted from months of indiscriminate use of topical steroids: steroid rosacea, perioral dermatitis, and steroid-induced acne. They also reported that occlusive application of fluorinated steroids to the back creates, within three weeks, an acneiform eruption identical to the one that follows systemic corticosteroids. Treatment recommendations included discontinuation of the offending agent and oral tetracycline (13). Beyond causing acneiform eruptions, topical steroids are associated with atrophy, striae, rosacea, perioral dermatitis, and purpura (14).

Kaidbey and Kligman studied the natural history of topical steroid use in a prisoner volunteer population. Fluocinolone acetonide cream 0.01% was applied under occlusion to the upper back three times a week for three weeks. Not all patients developed acneiform eruptions. Patients with a history of acne vulgaris were more likely to develop steroid-induced acne. Serial biopsies revealed that the earliest changes were evident by day 4. A focus of swollen, poorly stained, necrotic epithelial cells with shrunken nuclei appeared deep in the follicle, often localized to one side. The degenerated nests subsequently sloughed and could be found free in the lumen of the follicle at higher levels. By day 6, neutrophils were present in both the spongiotic degenerated zones and in adjacent tissue. The largest sebaceous follicles were the most susceptible, with vellus follicles not being involved at all. At 10 to 15 days of treatment, epithelial disorganization was complete, with neutrophils forming intrafollicular abscesses. At completion of therapy, foreign-body giant cells and comedones were not identified (15).

Both systemic and inhaled corticosteroids (16) have been associated with acneiform eruptions. Often, the illness being treated is associated with such significant morbidity and mortality that using a corticosteroid is indicated in spite of the cutaneous effects.

HORMONES

Anabolic Steroids

Anabolic-androgenic steroids (AAS) cause sebaceous gland hypertrophy along with increased sebum excretion, increased production of skin surface lipids, and an increased population of *Propionibacterium acnes* (17). AAS vary in their affinity to the androgen receptor and their interaction with various steroid-metabolizing enzymes and transport proteins such as sex hormone–binding globulin, thus altering each androgen's specific mechanism of action. Regarding interactions of AAS with intracellular steroid receptor proteins, different binding affinities are known (18).

In 1987, a 12-week strength-training program with self-AAS administration followed the sebum secretion rate and profile. After four weeks of AAS, the sebum excretion rate increased significantly from 0.989 ± 0.191 g/cm^2/min to 1.171 ± 0.076 g/cm^2/min. The relative distribution of the main lipid classes of sebum (free fatty acids, squalene, triglycerides, wax esters) on the forehead showed no statistically significant difference with AAS use. However, a significant increase in cholesterol from the initial level of $2.4 \pm 0.1\%$ to $4.2 \pm 0.7\%$ was reported (19). Beyond effects of androgens on the androgen receptor, other nuclear receptors, specifically the nuclear hormone peroxisome proliferator–activated receptors (PPARs), are involved in development, proliferation, and differentiation of sebocytes. AAS increase sebum synthesis directly by binding to the androgen receptor of the sebocyte and indirectly by induction of the PPAR-γ1 (20,21).

The cutaneous side effects of topical and systemic AAS have been described in both men and women (22). Estimated in 2010 by the National Institute on Drug Abuse at 2.5% of all 12th-grade males (23), use of AAS has been difficult to quantify. Older sources estimate the range to be 11% (24,25). Further, various studies show the incidence of acne in AAS users to be between 43% and 50% (18,26). It has been documented to cause both acne conglobata and acne fulminans (26).

Androgen-induced acne can be difficult to diagnose since the patient rarely reports illicit androgen use voluntarily and the acne is in no way different from normal acne. Treatment involves eliminating the androgen and therapy appropriate to the severity of the acne.

Progestins and Intrauterine Devices

Levonorgestrel-based implants and intrauterine devices are approved for use as a contraceptive and for the treatment of heavy menstrual bleeding. They are promoted as a local source of progestin with minimal systemic adverse effects. However, there is evidence of elevated serum and tissue levels of levonorgestrel. Some have reported high discontinuation and dissatisfaction rate (27,28). Additionally, oily skin and acne have been observed in some, which is postulated to be a direct effect of progestin, although this area of investigation remains controversial (29).

CENTRAL NERVOUS SYSTEM AGENTS

Although used to treat conditions that may have a slightly higher baseline incidence of acne vulgaris, several central nervous system agents have the propensity to induce acneiform eruptions. These agents are difficult to categorize as they have multiple indications. Some are antiepileptics, mood stabilizers, antipsychotics, antidepressants, or any combination thereof.

Lamotrigine

Lamotrigine is used to treat seizure disorders and bipolar disorder. In a report of two cases, two patients developed an acneiform eruption on the back one to two months after starting the medication. Discontinuation of lamotrigine lead to clearance without need for further treatment. Of note, both patients had previously been on lithium but had been discontinued from it one to two months prior to the onset of the eruption. Therefore, lithium as a causative agent could not entirely be excluded (30).

Aripipazole

Aripipazole is used as an antipsychotic and antidepressant. It is a partial agonist of the dopamine-2 and 5-hydroxytryptamine-1A receptors; it acts as an antagonist of the 5-hydroxytryptamine-2A receptor. A single case report of a patient who developed papulopustules with few comedones subsequent to initiation of aripipazole therapy exists. The patient required both discontinuation of the medicine with topical tretinoin therapy to achieve clearance (31).

Valproate

Valproate is a histone deacetylase inhibitor believed to block voltage-gated channels and affect the function of the γ-aminobutyric acid (GABA) receptor. It is used as an antiepileptic, antipsychotic, antidepressant, and as a therapeutic option in the treatment of bipolar disorder and migraine headaches. Although acneiform eruptions have been noted in patients taking valproate, a recent study showed no statistical difference in rates of acne between two cohorts of patients with epilepsy at a tertiary endocrine referral center in Israel. Although the study was not prospective and randomized, data from a total of 88 patients were collected. Even though no increase in acne with valproate was identified, the treated postmenarcheal subgroup had a higher mean testosterone level than the untreated postmenarcheal controls (32).

Lithium

Although previous reports of its cutaneous side effects (33) exist, lithium was first noted to cause acneiform eruptions in the dermatology literature in 1975. Four female patients experienced new-onset acneiform eruptions after initiating lithium treatment. One had worsening of previous acne. All patients improved with discontinuation of medicine (34).

Recent reviews have shown an estimated overall cutaneous reaction rate ranging from 3.4% to 45%, with acne and psoriasis being the most common dermatoses. Lithium tends to exacerbate any skin condition with pathophysiology driven by the action of neutrophils (35). Given that control of mental illness reduces mortality, some continue with therapy in spite of cutaneous side effects. For these patients, oral isotretinoin has been used concomitantly (36).

CHLORACNE

Chloracne is a long-observed cutaneous eruption predominantly of comedones with sparse inflammatory papules on forehead, ears, neck, and genitals. Patients tend to be photosensitive as well. Although seen in laborers and those with exposure to industrial materials, the exact chemicals and route of exposure were debated for over half a century. The causative agents are halogenated aromatic compounds, such as chlorinated dioxins and dibenzofurans; inhalation is sufficient to provoke the eruption, although direct contact is the most common route of exposure. Histopathologic examination reveals either a superficial or a deep cystic structure with complete loss of sebaceous glands (37). Presence of comedones, usually open comedones, after exposure to "toxic chlorine," is what brought about the current terminology. Recently, the recognition that cytochrome p450 enzymes in the skin produce toxic metabolites has lead some to suggest renaming this entity "metabolizing acquired dioxin-induced skin hamartomas" (MADISH) (38); however, this term has not yet gained use.

The most widely known case of chloracne was a poisoning attempt on Ukrainian President, Viktor Yuschenko, during his 2004 campaign (39). Chloracne responds best to discontinuation of exposure. Clearance can be extended, with some cases taking years to decades to respond. Attempts have also been made to increase excretion of the toxic chemical as well. Both topical tretinoin and oral isotretinoin have been used with reasonable efficacy.

Agent Orange is the name given to an herbicide used during the Vietnam War. It was, and continues to be, a source of controversy both politically and medically (40). It is a 1:1 mixture of 2,4-dichlorophenoxyacetic acid and 2,4,5-trichlorophenoxyacetic acid, which contains minute traces of 2,3,7,8-tetrachlorodibenzo-*p*-dioxin (41). The U.S. government, along with the Institutes of Medicine, has shown a positive association between chloracne and dioxin exposure through Agent Orange in reports released in 1994 and updated four times to 2004 (42). The 2004 report concluded it was unlikely, given the environmental dissipation of dioxins, little bioavailability, properties of the herbicides, and application methods, that veterans without direct contact could have experienced clinically meaningful exposure. The report also concluded that those who handled or otherwise had direct contact with the dioxins, as opposed to incidental exposure from spraying under field conditions, could have sustained appreciable accumulation of the toxins (43). Although it has been suggested that there are fewer than 4000 persons with chloracne worldwide (40), there has been considerable debate over the incidence in exposed veterans and even the clinical features of exposure (44–46).

BIOLOGICS AND ANTI–TUMOR NECROSIS FACTOR-α AGENTS

Biologic agents are a relatively new class of medication utilized in the treatment of many inflammatory and autoimmune diseases. A case series of three patients being treated with anti–tumor necrosis factor (anti-TNF)-α therapy for psoriasis developed acneiform eruptions (47). Another case documents the use of different anti-TNF-α products in the same patient. The patient had both psoriasis vulgaris and acne vulgaris. Each disease responded differently to each treatment. Efalizumab, a monoclonal antibody that binds CD11 leukocyte surface antigen and has now been withdrawn from the market, gave mild improvement in the Psoriasis Area and Severity Index (PASI) score with severe worsening of Acne Intensity Score (AIS). Etanercept, which binds and inhibits TNF-α, improved the acne. However, the psoriasis persisted with a high PASI even with a dose of 50 mg subcutaneously twice weekly. After 15 weeks of therapy, the decision was made to switch to infliximab, an intravenous chimeric monoclonal antibody preventing TNF-α from binding its receptor. The PASI reduced rapidly within six weeks, and the AIS continued to improve. It was postulated that since *P. acnes* activates toll-like receptors, therapeutics that either stimulate or inhibit these receptors could cause or treat acne, respectively. Toll-like receptors also stimulate the production of TNF-α, which, through positive feedback, increases the expression of toll-like receptors. The authors further postulated that TNF-α inhibitors decreased activation of mononuclear cells, also implicated in the pathogenesis of acne (48).

In 2006, a single case entered the literature describing a 22-year-old male who had failed years of standard therapies for acne vulgaris. He had been treated unsuccessfully with topical treatments (benzoyl peroxide, erythromycin, azelaic acid, and retinoids), systemic antibiotics (minocyclin: 200 mg/day for 6 months, lymecycline: 300 mg/day for 3 months, and azithromycin: 500 mg/day for 3 consecutive days per month for 3 months), and oral isotretinoin (0.5–1 mg/kg/day for an overall period of 18 months). He was started on etanercept 25 mg subcutaneously twice weekly. The patient and physician noted an improvement within 2 weeks, with complete resolution of disease in 24 weeks. During a 12-week follow-up period when the patient was discontinued from medication, no recurrence was observed (49).

REFERENCES

1. Plewig G, Jansen T, Kligman AM. Pyoderma faciale. A review and report of 20 additional cases: is it rosacea? Arch Dermatol 1992; 128(12):1611–1617.
2. Allworthy SW. Acneiform eruption of "doffers". Proc R Soc Med 1917; 10 (Dermatol Sect):102.
3. Momin SB, Peterson A, Del Rosso JQ. A status report on drug-associated acne and acneiform eruptions. J Drugs Dermatol 2010; 9(6):627–636.
4. Plewig G, Jansen T. Acneiform dermatoses. Dermatology 1998; 196(1):102–107.
5. Thatcher N, Nicolson M, Groves RW, et al. Expert consensus on the management of erlotinib-associated cutaneous toxicity in the U.K. Oncologist 2009; 14(8):840–847.
6. Bernier J, Bonner J, Vermorken JB, et al. Consensus guidelines for the management of radiation dermatitis and coexisting acne-like rash in patients receiving radiotherapy plus EGFR inhibitors for the treatment of squamous cell carcinoma of the head and neck. Ann Oncol 2008; 19(1):142–149.
7. Segaert S, Van Cutsem E. Clinical signs, pathophysiology and management of skin toxicity during therapy with epidermal growth factor receptor inhibitors. Ann Oncol 2005; 16(9):1425–1433.
8. Lacouture ME. Mechanisms of cutaneous toxicities to EGFR inhibitors. Nat Rev Cancer 2006; 6(10):803–812.
9. Sviggum HP, Davis MD, Rajkumar SV, et al. Dermatologic adverse effects of lenalidomide therapy for amyloidosis and multiple myeloma. Arch Dermatol 2006; 142(10):1298–1302.
10. Hall VC, El-Azhary RA, Bouwhuis S, et al. Dermatologic side effects of thalidomide in patients with multiple myeloma. J Am Acad Dermatol 2003; 48(4):548–552.
11. Blatt J, Lee PA. Severe acne and hyperandrogenemia following dactinomycin. Med Pediatr Oncol 1993; 21(5):373–374.
12. Plewig G, Kligman AM. Induction of acne by topical steroids. Arch Dermatol Forsch 1973; 247(1):29–52.
13. Kligman AM, Leyden JJ. Adverse effects of fluorinated steroids applied to the face. JAMA 1974; 229(1):60–62.
14. Hengge UR, Ruzicka T, Schwartz RA, et al. Adverse effects of topical glucocorticosteroids. J Am Acad Dermatol 2006; 54(1):1–15; quiz 16–18.
15. Kaidbey KH, Kligman AM. The pathogenesis of topical steroid acne. J Invest Dermatol 1974; 62(1):31–36.
16. Guillot B. Adverse skin reactions to inhaled corticosteroids. Expert Opin Drug Saf 2002; 1(4):325–329.
17. Scott MJ III, Scott AM. Effects of anabolic-androgenic steroids on the pilosebaceous unit. Cutis 1992; 50(2):113–116.
18. Melnik B, Jansen T, Grabbe S. Abuse of anabolic-androgenic steroids and bodybuilding acne: an underestimated health problem. J Dtsch Dermatol Ges 2007; 5(2):110–117.
19. Kiraly CL, Alén M, Rahkila P, et al. Effect of androgenic and anabolic steroids on the sebaceous gland in power athletes. Acta Derm Venereol 1987; 67(1):36–40.

20. Zouboulis CC. [The sebaceous gland]. Hautarzt 2010; 61(6):467–468, 4704, 476–477.

21. Iwata C, Akimoto N, Sato T, et al. Augmentation of lipogenesis by 15-deoxy-Delta12,14-prostaglandin J2 in hamster sebaceous glands: identification of cytochrome P-450-mediated 15-deoxy-Delta12,14-prostaglandin J2 production. J Invest Dermatol 2005; 125(5):865–872.

22. Wollina U, Pabst F, Schönlebe J, et al. Side-effects of topical androgenic and anabolic substances and steroids. A short review. Acta Dermatovenerol Alp Panonica Adriat 2007; 16(3):117–122.

23. Johnston LD, O'Malley PM, Bachman JG, et al. Monitoring the future national results on adolescent drug use: overview of key findings, 2009, N.I.o.D.A.N.P.N. 10-7583, Editor, 2010, Bethesda, MD.

24. Johnson MD. Anabolic steroid use in adolescent athletes. Pediatr Clin North Am 1990; 37(5):1111–1123.

25. Terney R, McLain LG. The use of anabolic steroids in high school students. Am J Dis Child 1990; 144(1):99–103.

26. O'Sullivan AJ, Kennedy MC, Casey JH, et al. Anabolic-androgenic steroids: medical assessment of present, past and potential users. Med J Aust 2000; 173(6):323–327.

27. Ewies AA. Levonorgestrel-releasing intrauterine system—the discontinuing story. Gynecol Endocrinol 2009; 25(10):668–673.

28. Ilse JR, Greenberg HL, Bennett DD. Levonorgestrel-releasing intrauterine system and new-onset acne. Cutis 2008; 82(2):158.

29. Luukkainen T, Pakarinen P, Toivonen J. Progestin-releasing intrauterine systems. Semin Reprod Med 2001; 19(4):355–363.

30. Nielsen JN, Licht RW, Fogh K. Two cases of acneiform eruption associated with lamotrigine. J Clin Psychiatry 2004; 65(12):1720–1722.

31. Mishra B, Praharaj SK, Prakash R, et al. Aripiprazole-induced acneiform eruption. Gen Hosp Psychiatry 2008; 30(5):479–481.

32. de Vries L, Karasik A, Landau Z, et al. Endocrine effects of valproate in adolescent girls with epilepsy. Epilepsia 2007; 48(3):470–477.

33. Kusumi Y. A cutaneous side effect of lithium: report of two cases. Dis Nerv Syst 1971; 32(12):853–854.

34. Yoder FW. Letter: acneiform eruption due to lithium carbonate. Arch Dermatol 1975; 111(3):396–397.

35. Yeung CK, Chan HH. Cutaneous adverse effects of lithium: epidemiology and management. Am J Clin Dermatol 2004; 5(1):3–8.

36. Lolis MS, Bowe WP, Shalita AR. Acne and systemic disease. Med Clin North Am 2009; 93(6):1161–1181.

37. Suskind RR. Chloracne, "the hallmark of dioxin intoxication." Scand J Work Environ Health 1985; 11(3 spec no):165–171.

38. Saurat JH, Sorg O. Chloracne, a misnomer and its implications. Dermatology 2010; 221(1):23–26.

39. Finkelstein A, Rotman E, Eisenkraft A, et al. [Political poisoning with dioxins—a weapon of chemical "disgracefulness"]. Harefuah 2005; 144(10):729–735, 749.

40. Tindall JP. Chloracne and chloracnegens. J Am Acad Dermatol 1985; 13(4): 539–558.
41. United States Department of Veterans Affairs. Agent orange: about agent orange. Available at: http://www.publichealth.va.gov/exposures/agentorange/basics.asp.
42. United States Department of Veterans Affairs. Agent orange: chloracne or similar acneform disease. Available at: http://www.publichealth.va.gov/exposures/agentorange/conditions/chloracne.asp.
43. Young AL, Giesy JP, Jones PD, et al. Environmental fate and bioavailability of agent orange and its associated dioxin during the Vietnam war. Environ Sci Pollut Res Int 2004; 11(6):359–370.
44. Bogen G. Symptoms in Vietnam veterans exposed to agent Orange. JAMA 1979; 242(22):2391.
45. Weigand DA. Agent Orange and skin rash—a different experience. JAMA 1980; 243(14):1422–1423.
46. Fink DJ. Exposure to agent orange. JAMA 1980; 244(10):1094–1095.
47. Sun G, Wasko CA, Hsu S. Acneiform eruption following anti-TNF-alpha treatment: a report of three cases. J Drugs Dermatol 2008; 7(1):69–71.
48. Colsman A, Sticherling M. Psoriasis vulgaris associated with acne vulgaris: differential effects of biologicals? Acta Derm Venereol 2008; 88(4):418–419.
49. Campione E, Mazzotta AM, Bianchi L, et al. Severe acne successfully treated with etanercept. Acta Derm Venereol 2006; 86(3):256–257.

Acne in pregnancy

Tobechi L. Ebede and Diane S. Berson

INTRODUCTION

Pregnancy can influence the course of acne. In a study of over 400 pregnant women, after delivery, 75% of women reported improvement in acne, 13% reported no change, and 12% reported worsening of their acne (1). Dermatologists will often be consulted for gestational acne, since many physicians are hesitant to prescribe these medications during pregnancy. In some cases, the patient will have been advised to stop their prior acne treatment. But for female patients with severe disease that can lead to scarring, treatment can continue during pregnancy (2). Since 1979, the U.S. Food and Drug Administration (FDA) has categorized drugs that may be used by pregnant women from category A—"controlled studies show no risk" to category X—"contraindicated in pregnancy" (Table 7.4.1). Since controlled studies in pregnant women are usually not available, many drugs are interpreted as category C—"risk cannot be ruled out" (3). The following is a review of the agents used to treat acne in pregnancy.

TOPICAL ANTIMICROBIALS

Topical therapy is the preferred treatment for acne during pregnancy. Topical erythromycin (category B), clindamycin (category B), and benzoyl peroxide (category C) are considered safe in pregnancy (4). When using clindamycin, approximately 5% of topical clindamycin hydrochloride is systemically absorbed and even less topical clindamycin phosphate is absorbed. Although rare, there are reports of pseudomembranous colitis from topical clindamycin formulations (5). Similarly, approximately 5% of topical benzoyl peroxide is absorbed in the skin. The final metabolic product of benzoyl peroxide, benzoate, is excreted

Table 7.4.1 FDA Drug Risk Classification System for Acne Medications

Drug classification	Definition	Medication
A	Controlled studies show no fetal risk	Zinc salts
B	No evidence of risk to human fetus	Azelaic acid, erythromycin, clindamycin, metronidazole
C	Risk to human fetus cannot be ruled out	Adapalene, benzoyl peroxide, salicylic acid, tretinoin,
D	Positive evidence of risk to human fetus; however, potential benefits may outweigh the potential risk	Tetracycline
X	Contraindicated in pregnant	Isotretinoin, tazarotene

unchanged in the urine. Thus, systemic effects in pregnant patients and/or the fetus are not observed (5). Azelaic acid (category B) has not shown mutagenicity, teratogenicity, or embryotoxicity in animals (6). For patients with rosacea, topical metronidazole (category B) is an option. It is minimally absorbed and is also considered safe in pregnancy (4).

TOPICAL RETINOIDS

The three main categories of topical retinoids include tretinoin (category C), adapalene (category C), and tazarotene (category X). Topical retinoids are not recommended for use in pregnant patients despite data suggesting that percutaneous absorption is minimal (1). There have been no reports of infants born with congenital malformation after maternal topical application of tretinoin (5,7). Tretinoin (all-*trans*-retinoic acid) is the isomer of isotretinoin applied topically. There is documented conversion to 13-*cis*-retinoic acid after percutaneous absorption (7). Rothman and Pochi note that, in humans, less than 5% of topical tretinoin is absorbed after one application. They postulate that "if a patient applies 0.1% tretinoin, 1 gm daily, to her skin and one-third is absorbed, it is equivalent to ingesting about 12 IU/kg/day. For a 60 kg woman this amounts to 720 IU/day. Prenatal vitamins contain 5000 IU of vitamin A, that is, seven times the amount of vitamin A expected to be absorbed after topical use of tretinoin. Thus it is highly unlikely that topically applied tretinoin could induce a teratogenic effect" (5). In addition, photodegradation of tretinoin occurs and about 50% of the applied retinoid is recoverable in the subsequent face washing (7). Thus, no elevation in baseline risk for birth defects has been observed with tretinoin. On the other hand, there have been reports of ocular congenital anomaly associated with adapalene use (6). Tazarotene is the only topical retinoid designated category X. In experimental animals, it has been associated with malformations including spina bifida, hydrocephalus, reduced fetal body weight, and skeletal ossification. Since the level of exposure that can lead to teratogenicity is unknown, topical tazarotene is contraindicated in pregnant patients (6).

OTHER TOPICAL TREATMENTS

Topical salicylic acid (category C) is widely used in over-the-counter acne treatment. Although topical salicylic acid penetrates the skin easily, there are no published reports of teratogenicity. Data on possible side effects from topical salicylic acid is taken from information on oral salicylates. Oral salicylates rapidly cross the placenta and are slowly eliminated from the fetus. A large prospective study of over 50,000 pregnant women concluded that there is no increased rate of malformations among babies born to mothers who ingested salicylates during their pregnancy. Thus, topical salicylates are unlikely to be teratogenic (5). Oral salicylates block cyclooxygenase in platelets, which is essential for platelet aggregation. There are reports of decreased platelet aggregation and impaired hemostasis in infants born to mothers who took aspirin during the last weeks of pregnancy. Though no data exists, concerns about possible infant bleeding tendencies from topical salicylic acid have been raised (5).

Because of the hormonal nature of acne, cysts can increase during this time. Intralesional kenalog can be helpful for large inflammatory lesions. To minimize the risk of atrophic scarring, it should be injected into the center of the lesion until the redness blanches (2).

SYSTEMIC TREATMENTS

When systemic therapy for acne is warranted, erythromycin (category B) is the agent of choice (2,3,6). Erythromycin crosses the placenta poorly resulting in low fetal tissue levels, but it can concentrate in the fetal liver (5). Of note, erythromycin estolate has been associated with hepatotoxicity in 10% to 15% of pregnant patients after prolonged use (3). For this reason, erythromycin estolate should be avoided in pregnancy because it appears to cause more liver toxicity than other erythromycin formulations.

Tetracyclines (category D) are not recommended in pregnancy. While they are not known to be teratogenic, they have a negative effect on developing bones and teeth (3). The major concerns related to the use of tetracyclines during pregnancy include development of acute fatty liver of pregnancy in the mother, abnormalities in tooth development, and reversible effects on bone growth in infants. Calcification of the deciduous teeth of children occurs from the fourth month of gestation until 6 to 14 months after birth. Calcification of the permanent teeth begins 4 to 6 months after birth and ends around ages 5 to 12 years. Consequently, maternal tetracycline ingestion does not affect permanent dentition. Overall, tetracycline given during the second or third trimester results in deciduous teeth staining and possible enamel hypoplasia (5). For women of childbearing potential who inadvertently take tetracycline during the first weeks of pregnancy, it is unlikely to be teratogenic, but should be discontinued due to its effect on the developing teeth and bones of the fetus.

Zinc salts (category A) are an alternative systemic treatment for acne in pregnancy. Zinc inhibits chemotaxis, 5α-reductase and tumor necrosis factor-α production, and modulates integrin expression, mainly ICAM-1 and VLA-3 (2,8). These activities play a role in its anti-inflammatory properties. Dreno et al. performed a multicenter, randomized double-blind controlled trial comparing the efficacy of zinc (30 mg) versus minocycline (100 mg). They found that at three months, the efficacy of zinc was 17% lower than minocycline with respect to the mean change in lesion count (8). In clinical trials evaluating zinc salts in acne versus placebo, zinc salts were more effective in six out of nine studies (8). A large retrospective analysis of more than 2500 pregnant women in France evaluating zinc salts for acne found no abnormalities, congenital malformations, harmful effects, or risk to the fetus associated with zinc use (9). Zinc is typically dosed at 200 mg daily without food, and side effects include nausea and gastric pain (2).

In patients with severe inflammatory acne, short courses of oral steroids can be used after the first trimester. Discussion with the patient's obstetrician prior to initiating therapy is essential (2). Oral isotretinoin (13-*cis*-retinoic acid) is a category X medication and is contraindicated in pregnancy. It is a potent teratogen in humans, and female patients must avoid pregnancy for four weeks after stopping isotretinoin (2).

REFERENCES

1. Nussbaum R, Benedetto A. Cosmetic aspects of pregnancy. Clin Dermatol 2006; 24:133–141.
2. Gollnick H, Cunliffe W, Berson D, et al. Management of acne: a report from a global alliance to improve outcomes in acne. J Am Acad Dermatol 2003; 49:S1–S38.
3. Hale EK, Pomeranz MK. Dermatologic agents during pregnancy and lactation: an update and clinical review. Int J Dermatol 2002; 41:197–203.

4. Zip C. A practical guide to dermatological drug use in pregnancy. Skin Therapy Lett 2006; 11(4):1–4.
5. Rothman K, Pochi P. Use of oral and topical agents for acne in pregnancy. J Am Acad Dermatol 1988; 19:431–442.
6. Hammadi A, Al-Haddab M, Sasseville D. Dermatologic treatment during pregnancy: practical overview. J Cutan Med Surg 2006; 10(4):183–192.
7. Bologa M, Pastuszak A, Shear N, et al. Dermatologic drugs in pregnancy. Clin Dermatol 1992; 9:435–451.
8. Dreno B, Moyse D, Alirezai M, et al. Multicenter randomized comparative double-blind controlled clinical trial of the safety and efficacy of zinc gluconate versus minocycline hydrochloride in the treatment of inflammatory acne vulgaris. Dermatology 2001; 203:135–140.
9. Dreno B, Blouin E. Acne, pregnant women and zinc salts: a literature review. Ann Dermatol Venereol 2008; 135(1):27–33.

8.1

Acne in children

Caroline D. S. Piggott, Lawrence F. Eichenfield, and Anne W. Lucky

INTRODUCTION

Acne is one of the most common diseases affecting the pediatric population and a frequent chief complaint for office visits for both pediatricians and dermatologists. While it is primarily a skin disorder of adolescents, acne is also a less studied, but equally important, condition faced by children who have not yet reached puberty. This special group of acne patients may be categorized into the following four clinical entities on the basis of the time of onset and clinical features: neonatal, infantile, mid-childhood, and preadolescent acne (Table 8.1.1). The clinical presentation, pathophysiology, differential diagnosis, workup, and treatment of each of these types of acne differ to varying degrees and will therefore be addressed on an individual basis.

NEONATAL ACNE

Clinical Presentation

Neonatal acne, also known as *acne neonatorum*, presents between the time of birth and approximately the first four to six weeks of life. It has been estimated that neonatal acne affects as many as 20% of newborns (1). "Neonatal acne" may actually be a term used for a heterogeneous set of conditions presenting with papules and pustules, as well as true early acne presenting with comedones. The condition "neonatal cephalic pustulosis" (NCP) has been described as a more distinct entity of superficial pustules without comedones, which may involve the forehead, cheeks, chin, neck, scalp, chest, and back (2,3).

Table 8.1.1   Acne in the Younger Patient

Acne type	Age range
Neonatal acne	0–6 wk
Infantile acne	0–1 yr
Mid-childhood acne	1–8 yr
Preadolescent acne	8–12 yr

Pathophysiology

The pathophysiology of acneiform eruptions in the newborn is only partially understood. Studies have implicated *Pityrosporum* spp., formerly known as *Malassezia* (*M. sympodalis* and *M. globosa*), as a cause of NCP. Some, but not all, neonates with acne are either smear- or culture-positive for a member of the species (2–5). For children with positive smears or cultures, it is likely that the papulopustular lesions are a result of inflammatory reaction to the *Pityrosporum* spp. in the skin.

Both NCP and true acne in neonates may be influenced by a combination of several factors: excess sebum production and hormonal effects on neonatal sebocytes (2,6,7). Neonates have enlarged sebocytes and have an excess of sebum excretion (8). Newborns even excrete more sebum compared with older infants, perhaps due, in part, to placental hormonal transmission from mother to newborn (6,8). One study compared sebum excretion rates (SER) in mothers prenatally, mothers and their neonates immediately after birth, and mothers and their infants between weeks 5 and 12 of age (9). A significant correlation was found between the presence of high maternal SER perinatally and high neonatal SER immediately after birth, whereas infant SER between weeks 5 and 12 was found to be significantly lower compared with the neonatal postpartum SER.

Differential Diagnosis and Evaluation

The presentation of acne in the neonate is similar to that of a number of skin diseases that may appear during the first month of life, including, but not limited to, NCP, transient neonatal pustular melanosis, erythema toxicum neonatorum, and bacterial or *Candida* infection. Similar to neonatal acne, and perhaps synonymous with it, NCP presents during the first weeks of life with erythematous papules and pustules on the face and neck. Smears obtained from pustules may contain *Malassezia* spp. on microscopic examination (5). In the literature, the distinction between NCP and neonatal acne is controversial and unclear. Transient neonatal pustular melanosis can present at delivery or within the first day of life, with pustules on the chin, neck, or trunk, usually in darker-skinned babies. In approximately 24 hours, the pustules will rupture and leave behind light brown macules with a faint white rim of scale.

Occasionally, the baby is born with lesions already transformed into the brown, macular stage. Erythema toxicum neonatorum presents primarily in the first week of life, most often in the first 48 to 72 hours but usually not at delivery. It begins with an erythematous macule that develops a central papule or pustule. Lesions are located primarily on the trunk, face, or extremities and resolve without treatment. The diagnosis may be confirmed with observation of eosinophils in a Gram stain or Tzanck smear of a pustule (10). Signs and symptoms in the newborn that suggest that the pustules may be associated with a significant infection including fever in the mother or infant, skin lesions on the mother during the perinatal period, fussiness, feeding difficulties, or other signs of illness in the newborn, should prompt culture of the pustules for organisms, including bacteria, viruses, and fungi, further infectious disease work-up and medical therapy as appropriate should be undertaken. This is particularly important if the distribution of the lesions is atypical for neonatal acne or other benign transient neonatal pustular disorders.

Treatment

Most neonatal acne is self-limited, lasting from a few days to several weeks. Given this short-lived course, many clinicians elect to reassure parents that neonatal acne will resolve on its own, without scarring, and elect not to treat with any medication (11). If families prefer treatment, a short course of topical azoles, such as 2% ketoconazole cream, is often sufficient to reduce *Pityrosporum* colonization and may improve NCP (5). Some infants with true comedonal and inflammatory acne presenting in the neonatal period may have a prolonged course, overlapping with infantile acne, and may be treated with topical acne therapies, including retinoids, antibiotics, benzoyl peroxide, and combination therapies, rarely requiring systemic therapies.

INFANTILE ACNE

Clinical Presentation

Infantile acne may start in the first month of life or later and can persist for months to years, usually resolves by 24 months of age. It is a relatively rare condition and presents more often in boys than in girls. There may be inflammatory papules, pustules, cysts, and/or nodules, and, unlike in neonatal acne, comedones are usually present (Fig. 8.1.1). Lesions present on the cheeks primarily but can also be found on the forehead, chin, and trunk. A rare subset of infants with acne have refractory, inflammatory cysts, draining sinuses, and nodules—findings more commonly associated with adolescent acne (Fig. 8.1.2) (12). It is believed that the presence of infantile acne, regardless of severity, may predict more severe adolescent acne compared with teenagers who did not have acne as infants (13).

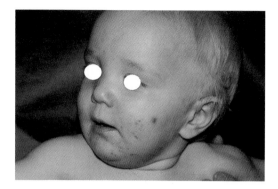

Figure 8.1.1 Infantile acne in a male infant with comedones and papules on the cheeks and chin.

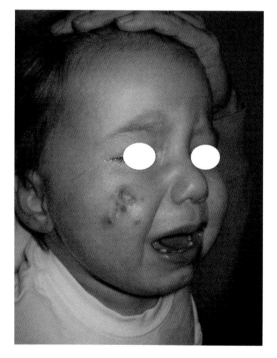

Figure 8.1.2 Severe infantile acne with pustules and nodules on the cheeks. Acne of this severity may warrant consideration of istotretinoin if other modalities such as systemic antibiotics and/or intralesional steroids fail.

Pathophysiology

The pathogenesis of infantile acne is better understood than that of neonatal acne. It is thought to arise because of increased adrenal androgen [dehydroepiandrosterone (DHEA) and dehydroepiandrosterone sulfate (DHEAS)] production by the fetal adrenal gland, the inner zone of the adrenal corresponding to the later zona reticularis (14). This is the androgen-secreting portion of the adrenal, which shrinks after the first year of life and then reappears during adrenarche, usually around ages eight or nine years in girls and boys, respectively. Adrenal androgens stimulate sebaceous glands and, in turn, infants have been shown to have increased sebum production during this period (8). Over the first six months of age, this production of adrenal androgens gradually decreases, as infantile acne shows signs of improvement. In infant boys, during the first six months of life, the testes have been shown to produce androgen levels similar to that of mid-pubertal boys and there appears to be a related increase in the amount of infantile acne in boys compared with girls (15).

Differential Diagnosis and Evaluation

The differential diagnosis of infantile acne is broad and includes periorificial dermatitis, cutaneous infections, seborrhea, and acne secondary to hormonal abnormalities. For the majority of infantile acne cases, clinical findings are typical and no workup is necessary. The exception is hormone abnormality–related infantile acne, whose workup will be discussed later in this section.

The most common conditions mistaken for acne in infants can often be differentiated on the basis of clinical findings. Periorificial dermatitis lacks open and closed comedones and, instead, exhibits inflammatory papules, often with erythema and scale, distributed around the eyes, nose, and mouth, but sparing the oral commissure. It responds to topical antimicrobials, including topical erythromycin and metronidazole, and can be exacerbated, or induced, by, high-potency topical steroid use. Acneiform-like lesions associated with infectious etiologies also lack comedones and are usually pustular, more focally distributed, and may or may not be accompanied by systemic signs such as fever. Culture and/or smear and microscopic examination of pustule contents will usually diagnose the responsible organisms. Most frequent are *Staphylococcus aureus* and *Candida albicans*. Seborrhea can exhibit papules and pustules mimicking acne, but its distribution will favor the scalp, ear, nasolabial folds, eyebrows, and sternum, and lesions may coalesce into plaques accompanied by a greasy, yellow scale. Miliaria pustulosa is a rare cause of infantile pustules in circumstances of excessive heat and or occlusion. Eosinophilic pustular folliculitis is rarely seen on the face but often affects the scalp.

Acne can be the presenting sign infants with hormonal abnormalities. Careful evaluation of the infant should include assesment of linear growth pattern, testicular size, and for pubic or axillary hair. These patients tend to have acne that is severe, persistent, and/or refractory to treatment; it is recommended, therefore, that infants presenting with these acne features undergo endocrine laboratory testing to rule out several rare endocrine diseases. See section "Pre-adolescent Acne: Differential Diagnosis and Evaluation" for recommended laboratory testing.

Treatment

The basic treatment modalities used for infantile acne are similar to conventional acne medications used for teenagers. Medications include topical benzoyl peroxide, retinoids, antibiotics, and combinations of these. For more severe cases requiring oral antibiotic therapy, oral erythromycin can be used. For most cases of infantile acne requiring topical retinoid treatment, milder-strength retinoids such as adapalene or low-potency tretinoin are tolerated best. If irritation is excessive, every-other-day application can be attempted, coupled with liberal moisturizer use. Tetracyclines are contraindicated in this age range because of risk of permanent tooth discoloration. While erythromycin is less effective, its safety profile makes it the oral antibiotic of choice in this population. For cases with erythromycin-resistance, clindamycin and trimethoprim-sulfamethoxazole are alternatives.

Infantile acne is rarely severe enough to warrant consideration of isotretinoin, and the FDA has only approved its use in children aged 12 years and older. However, for severe, scarring infantile acne, aggressive therapy may be needed. There are reports of successful, off-label treatment with isotretinoin (Table 8.1.2) (12,15–22). Isotretinoin may occur at dosages ranging from 0.5 to

Table 8.1.2 Use of Isotretinoin in Infants

Author	Refs	Age (mo)	Sex
Burket and Storrs	22	18	F
Arbegast et al.	21	20	M
Horne et al.	20	20	M
Mengesha et al.	19	20	F
Mengesha et al.	19	37	F
Cunliffe et al.	15	–	M
Sarazin et al.	18	20	F
Barnes et al.	12	14	F
Barnes et al.	12	13	F
Torrelo et al.	17	10	M
Hello, M et al.	(16)	9	M
Hello, M et al.	(16)	16	M

Doses ranged from 0.5 to 2 mg/kg/day for four to seven months.

2 mg/kg/day in toddlers, with treatment duration varying from 5 to 14 months (12,15–22). In addition to requiring off-label usage, the administration of isotretinoin in infants is further complicated by its lack of availability in a liquid or suspension formulation. The drug capsules need to be split and given to children, often in manners requiring some ingenuity. Furthermore, once split, clinicians, pharmacists, and families must also be careful of the high light and oxygen lability of the drug. To overcome these difficulties, one reported clinical pearl is to freeze the isotretinoin capsules, then split them in halves, thirds, or quarters as needed to get the appropriate dose, and place them in a chocolate or a candy bar (12).

MID-CHILDHOOD

Clinical Presentation

The mid-childhood acne category encompasses children presenting with acne beyond roughly one year and before eight years of age. This is the rarest time period in which to encounter a child with acne, probably because there is virtually no adrenal or gonadal source of androgen in this developmental period. The morphology of acne during this period includes open and closed comedones, inflammatory papules, pustules, cysts, and nodules. Distribution is primarily on the face, and less often on the chest and back. Scarring and postinflammatory dyspigmentation can be observed.

Pathophysiology

When present, the pathophysiology of mid-childhood acne is often similar to that of preadolescent acne, to be discussed in section "Preadolescent Acne: Pathophysiology." However, since the adrenal glands normally produce relatively little androgen during this period, mid-childhood acne may be commonly caused by an underlying endocrine abnormality (23).

Differential Diagnosis and Evaluation

There should be strong consideration of an underlying endocrine disorder in mid-childhood acne, and a workup is usually warranted. The most likely causes are congenital adrenal hyperplasia, malignant adrenal or gonadal tumors, true precocious puberty, premature adrenarchy, and polycystic ovary syndrome (PCOS). Evaluation may include a radiologic assessment of bone age, plotting of the child's growth over time (looking for unexpected crossing of percentiles on the growth chart), or abnormal hormone levels, such as high levels of the androgens, testosterone, and DHEAS

Table 8.1.3 Guide for Evaluation of Mid-childhood Acne

Bone age
- Accelerated with androgen excess
- Delayed in Cushing's syndrome

Growth chart
- Height crossing percentiles upward in androgen excess
- Weight crossing percentiles upward and height downward in Cushing's syndrome

Hormone levels
- High levels of androgens such as free testosterone and DHEAS in tumors and PCOS
- High levels of 17-α hydroxyprogesterone in CAH

Abbreviations: DHEAS, dehydroepiandrosterone sulfate; PCOS, polycystic ovary syndrome; CAH, congenital adrenal hyperplasia.

(Table 8.1.3). For a discussion of complete laboratory workup recommendations, see section "Preadolescent Acne: Differential Diagnosis and Evaluation."

Treatment

Treatment is generally very similar to that used for teenagers and adults with acne. The one therapeutic difference is the limitation of use of the tetracycline family of oral antibiotics to children of at least eight years of age when tooth enamel is permanently laid down. Instead, oral erythromycin may be utilized, or antibiotics less commonly used for acne such as trimethoprim-sulfa.

Appropriate indications for the use of isotretinoin in young children include severe, scarring acne, and acne unresponsive to conventional therapy. Family history of severe acne and psychosocial dysfunction may be considered as well. The dosage by weight is similar to that used for young adults. Several concerns regarding potential side effects of isotretinoin in young children have been raised, including the effects of isotretinoin on bone growth, the risk of depression, the potential for relapse upon isotretinoin completion, and a potential increased risk of onset of inflammatory bowel disease (IBD). While the issue of bone growth is particularly important in children because of the risk of premature closure of the epiphyses with isotretinoin (24), this has been reported in cases of high-dose, long-term isotretinoin use for disorders of keratinization, and no strong evidence suggests this to be a problem when using conventional dosages for the treatment of acne (25). A loss of bone density with the use of isotretinoin for cystic acne has also been shown in an older male population, while no specific changes in bone density were noted in a population of adolescents in a prospective study (26,27). There are also rare reports of diffuse idiopathic skeletal hyperostosis (DISH) with isotretinoin use, which most commonly affects the anterior spine; however, these reports are rare, and there is insufficient evidence to support routine radiologic screening for this condition in patients treated with isotretinoin for acne (27). There have been concerns regarding isotretinoin use and IBD stemming from reports of presentation of IBD after use of isotretinoin (28). Given the high rates of development of IBD in the population age groups generally treated with istotretinoin, and conflicting epidemiologic data, it remains uncertain if reports of IBD associated with isotretinoin are chance associations or if a biological relationship is plausible (28–30). The concerns about efficacy and relapse in pre-pubertal children treated with isotretinoin are also unique. While isotretinoin is generally quite effective in this age group, studies have stated that younger age of isotretinoin is a risk factor for more frequent need for further courses of isotretinoin therapy as compared with its use in older patients. This may be due to continued hormonal stimulation in an adolescent pattern that predisposes to acne in this age group. Careful selection of patients and close postisotretinoin follow-up are warranted.

PREADOLESCENT ACNE

Clinical Presentation

What is most unique about preadolescent acne compared with conventional adolescent acne is its distribution on the face—lesions generally occur on the forehead, nose, medial cheeks, and chin, and the trunk is usually unaffected or last to be affected (Fig. 8.1.3). The primary morphology is usually comedonal in early lesions. Inflammatory papules and pustules usually present later and are relatively fewer in number. One distinctive feature of preadolescent acne is the

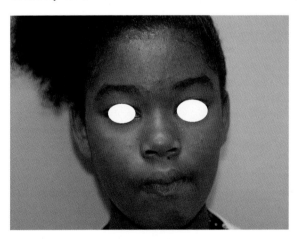

Figure 8.1.3 Preadolescent girl with comedonal acne located primarily in the middle of the face on the forehead and cheeks.

presence of open comedones in the ear, which is often mistaken by parents for poor hygiene/dirt and scrubbed excessively. There may be significant progression in a subgroup of these individuals from noninflammatory comedonal acne to severe, inflammatory disease with scarring.

Pathophysiology

In children from 8 to 12 years, it has been suggested that acne may represent a presenting sign of puberty—sometimes appearing first prior to the development of pubic hair and breasts in girls and pubic hair and testicular enlargement in boys (31,32). The appearance of circulating serum androgens coincides with the onset of sebum production and presentation of acne in boys and girls. These androgens are derived from the adrenal glands, ovaries, and testes. Clinically, adrenarche is the term describing adrenal androgen maturation, and gonadarche is ovarian or testicular maturation. In girls, the prevalence and severity of acne have been associated with early pubertal maturation. In particular, early onset of significant numbers of comedones in females is predictive of the development of severe, inflammatory acne as a teenager (31,33). Increased severity of acne is also associated with earlier onset of menarche. In girls who will eventually develop more severe acne, mean levels of DHEAS and total and free testosterone levels are higher even four years before menarche, although they may still be within the "normal" range (31).

Prepubertal acne is correlated with early and increased sebum output and increased numbers of skin follicles producing acne. With increasing age and pubertal status, the number of sebum-secreting follicles, area of sebum production on the skin, and density of *Propionibacterium acnes* increase in children who have acne (34). In age-matched individuals who did not develop acne, sebaceous gland activity and *P. acnes* counts on the skin did not increase with advancing age. It has been suggested, therefore, that the onset of sebum secretion and the expansion of *P. acnes* flora on the skin occur earlier in children with acne compared with those who do not develop acne. In contrast, *P. acnes* counts obtained from the nares increased proportionate to age, regardless of the status of the acne.

Additional factors thought to play a role in the onset of preadolescent acne include family history of acne and low weight at birth (35,36). Preadolescents with acne often report at least one first relative with a history of acne (35). Additionally, demographic studies on preadolescents with acne have shown a possible association between low birth weight and an increased likelihood of preadolescent acne (36). While explanations for this association are limited, one suggestion is that there may be a correlation between low birth weight and later findings of insulin resistance and PCOS—also known to be related to acne. Further studies are needed to delineate a more detailed causal relationship.

Differential Diagnosis and Evaluation

The differential diagnosis of prepubescent acne includes, but is not limited to, keratosis pilaris, miliaria, drug-induced acne, pediatric rosacea, periorificial dermatitis, sarcoidosis, and cutaneous lupus. Hormone dysregulation due to a variety of etiologies must be considered. When evidence of hormonal irregularities is found on clinical and/or laboratory workup, the more common and concerning etiologies include premature adrenarche, Cushing's disease or syndrome, late-onset congenital adrenal hyperplasia, benign or malignant neoplasms of the gonads or adrenal glands, or true central precocious puberty.

If there is any suspicion of hormonal dysregulation in a preadolescent with acne, it is suggested that a hormonal workup be considered (Table 8.1.3). In particular, children with persistent acne despite treatment, severe acne, and/or clinical evidence of virilization should undergo a more thorough evaluation. It has been recommended that the child's height and weight be plotted on a growth chart, the physician perform a complete physical examination looking, in particular, for signs of virilization such as hirsutism, clitoromegaly, androgenetic alopecia, increased muscle mass, and deepening of the voice, and an assessment be made of his or her Tanner stage of development. Bone age should be determined with radiologic imaging of the left hand and wrist. Laboratory evaluation may include total and free serum testosterone levels, dehydroepiandrosterone sulfate (DHEAS), Δ-4 adrostenedione, leutinizing hormone (LH), follicle stimulating hormone (FSH), prolactin, and 17-α hydroxyprogesterone. If congenital adrenal hyperplasia is suspected, ACTH (Cortrosyn®) stimulation testing with a full range of the androgenic steroids, which are precursors to cortisol, should be measured. If abnormalities are noted, evaluation by a pediatric or gynecologic endocrinologist should be sought.

Treatment

Treatment of preadolescent acne is similar to that of adolescents and adults. From a behavioral perspective, it is important to address the child's own thoughts about his or her acne. In many cases, particularly with only comedonal lesions without an inflammatory component, the child may be unconcerned about the appearance of the acne. Occasionally, there is conflict between the child and parent about treatment. Postponing treatment until the child is more motivated is a valid option as long as there is little risk of scarring. Good skin care practices can be discussed, such as avoiding rigorous facial scrubbing and resisting the urge to "pimple-pop." A basic discussion of acne pathogenesis is often helpful. In particular, discussing the lack of good evidence for a role of dirt or of food in the pathogenesis of acne can help alleviate the tension between parent and child.

If medical intervention is desired, it is best to start with the mildest agents possible while still providing therapeutic efficacy. Benzoyl peroxide may be used for as a first-line agent—it is inexpensive, easy to apply, and available in many formulations (including washes, gels, and pads), and has a long track record of efficacy and safety when used as monotherapy for mild acne (37). From a pathogenic perspective, it also has excellent antimicrobial effects and has minimal tendency to induce antibiotic resistance in the acne-causing organism, *P. acnes* (38,39), as compared to some topical antibiotics. Warnings should be given about bleaching of clothing, towels, and linen, and for leave-on products often nighttime application may be most practical. Topical retinoids remain the cornerstone of treatment for significant comedonal acne and have significant effect on inflammatory lesions (40). Families should be counseled on the proper application of a pea-sized amount to the entire acne-prone areas rather than spot treatment of individual lesions. To avoid excessive dryness of the skin, applications may be initiated several times a week or every other day combined with a noncomedogenic gentle moisturizing agent containing sunscreen. If this is tolerated, slow titration up to daily application is better tolerated. Topical retinoids may be used combined with benzoyl peroxide and/or with topical antibiotics if a multifaceted regimen approach is warranted, and topical retinoid/antibiotic combinations may be utilized. Clindamycin and erythromycin solutions or gels have long been used for cases of mild acne vulgaris. However, with emerging antibiotic resistance patters of *P. acnes*, it is now recommended that they be used in stabilized combination products with benzoyl peroxide (41). In patients unable to tolerate or are allergic to benzoyl peroxide, topical clindamycin or dapsone may be viable alternatives.

Systemic acne treatment, such as antibiotics, isotretinoin, and ocasionally hormonal therapy, antiandrogens, can be added to the patient's regimen for more severe acne. For children of ages eight and above, after their dental enamel has been laid down, drugs of the tetracycline family (tetracycline, doxycycline, or minocycline) are safe options. Similar to treatment of adolescent and adult acne, many practitioners will initiate treatment of moderate to severe acne in this age group with oral antibiotics, in combination with topical benzoyl peroxide and topical retinoids. Hormonal therapy, including estrogen-containing oral contraceptives, is not indicated in girls prior to menarche but can be a very useful adjuvant when more conventional treatment fails. For oral medication, it is also important to determine whether the patient is able to swallow pills; otherwise, liquid preparations, crushed tablets, or sprinkling of capsule contents on food are alternatives to be considered.

Recently, it has been recommended to limit the duration of oral antibiotics to three months (42), in consideration of preadolescents being early in what is commonly a multi-year course of acne, and to minimize bacterial resistance. The rationale behind this recommendation is twofold; first, preadolescents may only be at the cusp of many years of acne, and safeguarding of oral antibiotics and systemic retinoid for later use is best. Additionally, long-term antibiotic use may not be prudent with the emerging concerns about bacterial resistance to antibiotics. Recommended oral antibiotics for preteens (eight years and above) are doxycycline, minocycline and tetracycline. They are no longer contra-indicated by this age because tooth formation, including enamel deposition, is complete and no longer affected by the tetracycline family. If the patient has a tetracycline allergy, other options include erythromycin, clindamycin, trimethoprim-sulfamethoxazole, cephalexin, or amoxicillin. However, these medications are not routinely used for acne and are secondary alternatives because of poorer efficacy, risks of antibiotic resistance, and other associated side effects. It is prudent to restrict use of these drugs because not only *P. acnes* but other microbial flora may develop drug resistance and thus effect drug efficacy for other indications.

When isotretinoin is used in preadolescent acne, the dosage and risk of side effects are similar to those described for mid-childhood acne. It is important to recognize that an additional issue in this age group is the variability of pubertal status, and the need for pregnancy prevention counseling in menarchal girls, and the use of the iPLEDGE program, legally required in the United States. The risk of depression has been proposed as a concern for any individual treated with isotretinoin. Acne itself can be a severe psychosocial stressor and a potential trigger for depression, especially in young people, and successful treatment of acne has been shown to improve depression (43,44). While the increased risk for depression and suicide in patients taking isotretinoin remains controversial, patients and families must be made aware of this concern and be vigilant for signs of mood change (43–45).

An additional treatment option for nodular acne lesions is intralesional injection of low-potency corticosteroids (46). The risks of this procedure are steroid-induced atrophy of the skin, the rare possibility of systemic absorption with subse-quent adrenal suppression, and the fear of injections of many children. To minimize these risks, it is recommended to use low concentrations of steroid, such as tri-amcinolone acetonide 2 mg/mL at low volumes, perform careful and slow injections, and employ standard pediatric techniques to reassure and secure the patient.

How medications are used is important in successful treatment of acne in the young. Studies have shown adherence at all ages to be only 65%, with a negative correlation with age (47). Additionally, many children are unmotivated to treat their acne and are, instead, brought to the office for treatment under duress by their parents. Others have problems adhering to complicated, multidrug regimens, which often take several weeks or months to show signs of efficacy. Therefore, it is often important to simplify the acne therapy as much as possible. Once-daily treatment, even if it means alternating therapies every other day, may be superior to twice-a-day dosing. The formulation of the product may also be important, such as using pumps or pads versus liquids and creams. Additionally, what might be important to each child can vary significantly—some are concerned more with hyper-pigmentation or scarring, whereas others may be more concerned about the texture and smell of products in the treatment regimen. Speaking directly to the patient rather than through the parent and allowing the child to feel that he or she is in partnership with his physician and has some control over the acne regimen is helpful for successful therapy in this age group.

SUMMARY

Acne in the younger patient presents unique challenges. While neonatal acne appears to have a pathophysiology and a morphology that may be unrelated to acne at all, infantile, mid-childhood, and preadolescent acne share in being potential markers for underlying hormonal abnormalities. Once underlying endocrine etiologies are ruled out, however, the basic management principles for these types of acne are similar to those used for older teenagers and adults. These include topical antimicrobials and retinoids, systemic antibiotics, isotretinoin, and hormonal therapy. However, it is vital to employ a pediatric approach to the selection and delivery of acne care in young children to ensure successful therapy and satisfied patients and their families.

REFERENCES

1. Jansen T, Burgdorf WH, Plewig G. Pathogenesis and treatment of acne in childhood. Pediatr Dermatol 1997; 14:17–21.
2. Bergman JN, Eichenfield LF. Neonatal acne and cephalic pustulosis: is *Malassezia* the whole story? Arch Dermatol 2002; 138:255–256.
3. Niamba P, Weill FX, Sarlangue J, et al. Is common neonatal cephalic pustulosis (neonatal acne) triggered by *Malassezia sympodialis*? Arch Dermatol 1998; 134:995–998.
4. Ayhan M, Sancak B, Karaduman A, et al. Colonization of neonate skin by *Malassezia* species relationship with neonatal cephalic pustulosis. J Am Acad Dermatol 2007; 57:1012–1018.
5. Rapelanoro R, Mortureux P, Coupie B, et al. Neonatal *Malassezia* furfur pustulosis. Arch Dermatol 1996; 132:190–193.
6. Antoniou C, Dessinioti C, Stratigos AJ, et al. Clinical and therapeutic approach to childhood acne: an update. Pediatr Dermatol 2009; 26:373–380.
7. Lucky AW. A review of infantile and pediatric acne. Dermatology 1998; 196:95–97.

8. Agache P, Blanc D, Barrand C, et al. Sebum levels during the first year of life. Br J Dermatol 1980; 103:643–649.

9. Henderson CA, Taylor J, Cunliffe WJ. Sebum excretion rates in mothers and neonates. Br J Dermatol 2000; 142:110–111.

10. Morgan AJ, Steen CJ, Schwartz RA, et al. Erythema toxicum neonatorum revisited. Cutis 2009; 83:13–16.

11. Kaminer MS, Gilchrest BA. The many faces of acne. J Am Acad Dermatol 1995; 32: S6–S14.

12. Barnes CJ, Eichenfield LF, Lee J, et al. A practical approach for the use of oral isotretinoin for infantile acne. Pediatr Dermatol 2005; 22:166–169.

13. Herane MI, Ando I. Acne in infancy and acne genetics. Dermatology 2003; 206:24–28.

14. Cantatore-Francis JL, Glick SA. Childhood acne: evaluation and management. Dermatol Ther 2006; 19:202–209.

15. Cunliffe WJ, Baron SE, Coulson IH. A clinical and therapeutic study of 29 patients with infantile acne. Br J Dermatol 2001; 145:463–466.

16. Hello M, Prey S, Leaute-Labreze C, et al. Infantile acne: a retrospective study of 16 cases. Pediatr Dermatol 2008; 25:434–438.

17. Torrelo A, Pastor MA, Zambrano A. Severe acne infantum successfully treated with isotretinoin. Pediatr Dermatol 2005; 22:357–359.

18. Sarazin F, Dompmartin A, Nivot S, et al. Treatment of an infantile acne with oral isotretinoin. Eur J Dermatol 2004; 14:71–72.

19. Mengesha YM, Hansen RC. Toddler-age nodulocystic acne. J Pediatr 1999; 134:644–648.

20. Horne HL, Carmichael AJ. Juvenile nodulocystic acne responding to systemic isotretinoin. Br J Dermatol 1997; 136:796–797.

21. Arbegast KD, Braddock SW, Lamberty LF, et al. Treatment of infantile cystic acne with oral isotretinoin: a case report. Pediatr Dermatol 1991; 8:166–169.

22. Burket JM, Storrs FJ. Nodulocystic acne occurring in a kindred of steatocystoma. Arch Dermatol 1987; 123:432–433.

23. Lucky AW. Hormonal correlates of acne and hirsutism. Am J Med 1995; 16: 89S–94S.

24. DiGiovanna JJ. Isotretinoin effects on bone. J Am Acad Dermatol 2001; 45: S176–S182.

25. Milstone LM, McGuire J, Ablow RC. Premature epiphyseal closure in a child receiving oral 13-cis-retinoic acid. J Am Acad Dermatol 1982; 7:663–666.

26. Leachman SA, Insogna KL, Katz L, et al. Bone densities in patients receiving isotretinoin for cystic acne. Arch Dermatol 1999; 135:961–965.

27. DiGiovanna JJ, Langman CB, Tschen EH, et al. Effect of a single course of isotretinoin therapy on bone mineral density in adolescent patients with severe, recalcitrant, nodular acne. J Am Acad Dermatol 2004; 51:709–717.

28. Reddy D, Siegel CA, Sands BE, et al. Possible association between isotretinoin and inflammatory bowel disease. Am J Gastroenterol 2006; 101:1569–1573.

29. Bernstein CN, Nugent Z, Longobardi T, et al. Isotretinoin is not associated with inflammatory bowel disease: a population-based case-control study. Am J Gastroenterol 2009; 104:2774–2778.

30. Crockett SD, Gulati A, Sandler RS, et al. A causal association between isotretinoin and inflammatory bowel disease has yet to be established. Am J Gastroenterol 2009; 104:2397–2393.

31. Lucky AW, Biro FM, Huster GA, et al. Acne vulgaris in premenarchal girls. An early sign of puberty associated with rising levels of dehydroepiandrosterone. Arch Dermatol 1994; 130:308–314.

32. Lucky AW, Biro FM, Huster GA, et al. Acne vulgaris in early adolescent boys. Correlations with pubertal maturation and age. Arch Dermatol 1991; 127:210–216.

33. Lucky AW, Biro FM, Simbartl LA, et al. Predictors of severity of acne vulgaris in young adolescent girls: results of a five-year longitudinal study. J Pediatr 1997; 130:30–39.

34. Mourelatos K, Eady EA, Cunliffe WJ, et al. Temporal changes in sebum excretion and propionibacterial colonization in preadolescent children with and without acne. Br J Dermatol 2007; 156:22–31.

35. Ballanger F, Baudry P, N'Guyen JM, et al. Heredity: a prognostic factor for acne. Dermatology 2006; 212:145–149.

36. Pandolfi C, Zugaro A, Lattanzio F, et al. Low birth weight and later development of insulin resistance and biochemical/clinical features of polycystic ovary syndrome. Metabolism 2008; 57:999–1004.

37. Gollnick H, Schramm M. Topical therapy in acne. J Eur Acad Dermatol 1998; 11(suppl 1):S8–S12; discussion S28–S29.

38. Leyden JJ, Wortzman M, Baldwin EK. Antibiotic-resistant *Propionibacterium acnes* suppressed by a benzoyl peroxide cleanser 6%. Cutis 2008; 82:417–421.

39. Bojar RA, Cunliffe WJ, Holland KT. The short-term treatment of acne vulgaris with benzoyl peroxide: effects on the surface and follicular cutaneous microflora. Br J Dermatol 1995; 132:204–208.

40. Krakowski AC, Eichenfield LF. Pediatric acne: clinical presentations, evaluation, and management. J Drugs Dermatol 2007; 6:589–593.

41. Mills O, Thornsberry C, Cardin CW, et al. Bacterial resistance and therapeutic outcome following three months of topical acne therapy with 2% erythromycin gel versus its vehicle. Acta Derm Venereol 2002; 82:260–265.

42. Dréno B, Bettoli V, Ochsendorf F, et al. European recommendations on the use of oral antibiotics for acne; European Expert Group on Oral Antibiotics in Acne. Eur J Dermatol 2004; 14:391–399.

43. Marqueling AL, Zane LT. Depression and suicidal behavior in acne patients treated with isotretinoin: a systematic review. Semin Cutan Med Surg 2007; 26:210–220.

44. Azoulay L, Blais L, Koren G, et al. Isotretinoin and the risk of depression in patients with acne vulgaris: a case-crossover study. J Clin Psychiatry 2008; 69:526–532.

45. Jacobs DG, Deutsch NL, Brewer M. Suicide, depression, and isotretinoin: is there a causal link? J Am Acad Dermatol 2001; 45:S168–S175.

46. Levine RM, Rasmussen JE. Intralesional corticosteroids in the treatment of nodulocystic acne. Arch Dermatol 1983; 119:480–481.

47. Zaghloul SS, Cunliffe WJ, Goodfield MJ. Objective assessment of compliance with treatments in acne. Br J Dermatol 2005; 152:1015–1021.

8.2

Treatment guidelines in adult women

Jennifer Villasenor, Diane S. Berson, and Daniela Kroshinsky

INTRODUCTION

The role of androgens is central in the pathogenesis of acne vulgaris. Androgen production leads to an increase in sebum production by sebaceous glands. Before the onset of puberty, the adrenal glands produce increasing amounts of dehydroepiandrosterone sulfate (DHEAS), which becomes metabolized in the skin to more potent hormones [e.g., testosterone and dihydrotestosterone (DHT)] by the enzymes sulfotransferase, 3β-hydroxysteroid dehydrogenase (3β-HSD), 17β-HSD, and 5α-reductase (5α-R) (1). Onset of acne lesions tends to coincide with the onset of puberty during which there is an increase in the production of androgens that results in excessive sebum production (2–6). Accumulation of sebum and keratinous material within pilosebaceous follicles blocks and dilates the follicular infundibulum resulting in the formation of microcomedones. Microcomedones provide an anaerobic, lipid-rich medium for the proliferation of *Propionibacterium acnes*. Consequently, *P. acnes* induces an inflammatory reaction by releasing chemotactic factors that attract lymphocytes and neutrophils, activating Toll-like receptors and inducing follicular keratinocyte secretion of interleukin-1 leading to keratinocyte proliferation (7,8). Interestingly, the serum levels of DHEAS correlate with the severity of comedonal acne in prepubertal females (9,10). Additionally, although still within normal limits, the serum level of circulating androgens is significantly increased in women with acne compared with women without acne (11,12). The severity of acne may also be related to the sexual maturity of males and females, which may be associated to an increase in sensitivity of the sebaceous gland to androgens (13,14). Thus, androgens play a prominent role in the pathogenesis of acne vulgaris and treatment modalities aimed at minimizing their effects may be required.

Choosing the most appropriate patient population for hormonal therapy is essential. Hormonal therapy may be the most effective option, especially in women who desire oral contraception. Additionally, women with severe seborrhea, clinically apparent androgenic alopecia, seborrhea/acne/hirsutism/alopecia (SAHA) syndrome, late-onset acne (acne tarda), and proven ovarian or adrenal hyperandrogenism may benefit from hormonal therapy (15). Although most women with acne will have androgen levels within normal limits, it is important to screen for an underlying endocrinopathy in women with (*i*) acne that is resistant to conventional therapy; (*ii*) a sudden onset of severe acne; (*iii*) acne associated with clinical signs of virilization, irregular menses, or signs of hyperandrogenism (SAHA syndrome); and (*iv*) relapsing acne lesions shortly after isotretinoin therapy (15). The most common endocrinopathies associated with acne include polycystic ovary syndrome (PCOS), late-onset adrenal hyperplasia (LOAH), or a virilizing tumor.

The clinical presentation of women who may benefit from hormonal therapy include those with varying acneiform lesions along the mandible and chin who often have flares that correlate with their menstrual cycles (16). These women usually do not have increased androgen levels above normal. However, women who present with this particular pattern of acne and other signs of virilization (e.g., hirsutism) should be screened for an underlying endocrinopathy. Signs and symptoms of androgen excess include menstrual irregularity, infertility, hirsutism, truncal obesity, polycystic ovaries detected on sonogram, recalcitrant acne, infrequent menses, female-pattern or male-pattern alopecia, deepening voice, and cliteromegaly. Women with any of these signs and women with severe acne or acne associated with hirsutism or irregular menstrual periods should be screened for an underlying endocrinopathy. Additionally, acanthosis nigricans in addition to other signs of androgen excess (e.g., HAIR-AN syndrome, hyperandrogenicity, insulin resistance, and acanthosis nigricans) should also warrant hormonal screening.

Screening tests for hyperandrogenism should be obtained in the luteal phase of the menstrual cycle and include serum DHEAS, total testosterone, free testosterone, luteinizing hormone/follicle-stimulating hormone (LH/FSH) ration, prolactin, and 17-hydroxyprogesterone (17–19). Normal total testosterone and DHEAS levels in addition to normal imaging may exclude an androgen-secreting tumor of the adrenals or ovaries. To determine whether the adrenal gland is the source of excess androgen, serum DHEAS can be measured. Serum DHEAS > 8000 ng/mL is highly suggestive of an adrenal tumor, and patients should be referred to an endocrinologist for further evaluation. Serum DHEAS levels in the range of 4000 to 8000 ng/mL may indicate congenital adrenal hyperplasia.

Elevated serum total testosterone levels may indicate an ovarian source of excess androgen. Patients with polycystic ovary disease will have irregular menstrual periods, reduced fertility, obesity, insulin resistance, hirsutism, and serum total testosterone in the range of 150 to 200 ng/dL or an increased LH/FSH (>2–3). Higher levels of serum testosterone may indicate an ovarian tumor.

HORMONAL TREATMENTS

Androgens are thought to be central to the pathogenesis of acne vulgaris because of their effects on sebum production and follicular keratosis (1,4). The effectiveness of hormonal therapy may be due to its effect on lowering circulating and local androgen levels and opposing the effect of androgens on the sebaceous gland and, possibly, on follicular keratinocytes (19,20). Specific hormonal treatments used in the treatment of acne vulgaris include antiandrogens (androgen receptor blockers) and agents used to decrease endogenous production of androgens by the ovary or adrenal gland [e.g., estrogens, combined oral contraceptives, oral glucocorticoids, and gonadotropin-releasing hormone (GnRH) agonists].

ANTIANDROGENS

Antiandrogens, or androgen receptor blockers, competitively inhibit the binding of dihydrotestosterone to its receptor (21) and include cyproterone acetate (CPA), drospirenone, spironolactone, and flutamide. Use of antiandrogens is contraindicated in men because they result in feminization and in women during pregnancy as they can feminize a male fetus (15).

CPA (10 mg, 50 mg) is a progestational antiandrogen that inhibits binding of dihydrotestosterone to its receptor. It reduces the activity of 5α-reductase, preventing the transformation of testosterone to dihydrotestosterone. It also blocks ovarian function and decreases serum androgen levels by inhibiting production of FSH and LH (15,22). Treatment with CPA should begin on the first day of the menstrual cycle. CPA is usually prescribed at doses between 2 and 100 mg daily and is often combined with ethinyl estradiol (EE) in the form of oral contraceptive (OC) Dianette/Diane-35 that is used in Europe for the treatment of acne (15). However, CPA/estrogen-containing OCs are not approved for use in the United States. CPA at a dose of 50 to 100 mg daily (with or without EE 50 µg) has been shown to result in improvement in 75% to 90% of patients treated (15,23). Reported side effects include menstrual abnormalities, breast tenderness and enlargement, nausea/vomiting, fluid retention, leg edema, headache, and melasma. Other side effects include fatigue, changes in body weight, liver dysfunction, and, rarely, blood-clotting disorders (24).

Spironolactone is an androgen receptor blocker, 5α-reductase inhibitor, and aldosterone antagonist that has been used for the treatment of hirsutism and hypertension. At doses of 50 to 100 mg twice daily, it exerts its effects by blocking androgen receptors (25) and has been shown to reduce sebum production by 30% to 50% leading to decreased acne production (15,17,22,25,26). Low doses of 25 mg twice daily or 25 mg daily may be sufficient for women with sporadic outbreaks of inflammatory lesions or isolated cysts (27). Maintenance doses range from 25 to 50 mg daily (15). Additionally, use of spironolactone in combination with an OC pill containing 30-µg EE/3-mg drospirenone has been shown to be effective and well tolerated (28).

The US Food and Drug Administration has not formally approved use of spironolactone for the treatment of acne; however, it may be used for females who have failed other therapeutic interventions. Spironolactone in low doses is generally well tolerated. However, use of spironolactone at higher doses or in females with cardiac or renal dysfunction may result in hyperkalemia. Other side effects include menstrual irregularity, breast tenderness, gynecomastia, headache, and fatigue. Spironolactone is contraindicated in women who are pregnant or at increased risk of breast cancer (29).

Flutamide is a nonsteroidal antiandrogen used for the management of prostatic hypertrophy, prostate cancer, and hirsutism. For the treatment of acne or hirsutism in females, it has been used at doses of 250 mg twice a day in combination with OCs (15,18,22). In a study comparing spironolactone and flutamide therapy in the treatment of acne, flutamide therapy was shown to have a greater effect at reducing total acne and seborrhea after three months (30). Although effective in the treatment of acne, the use of flutamide should be done with careful monitoring of liver function enzymes as cases of fatal hepatitis have been reported (31). Finasteride and other compounds with possible anti-androgenic effects (e.g., cimetidine and ketaconazole) have not been shown to be effective in the treatment of acne (32).

BLOCKING OVARIAN ANDROGEN PRODUCTION

In women who desire oral contraception and those who are concurrently being treated with isotretinoin, OCs may be an ideal choice for treatment of acne. Indications of OC treatment in acne include women with acne flare-ups before menstruation, during treatment with isotretinoin, or when oral contraception is desired; women whose acne does not respond to other therapeutic interventions; women with polycystic ovary syndrome; women with clinical signs of hyperandrogenism; women with late-onset acne; and women with proven ovarian hyperandrogenism or proven adrenal hyperandrogenism.

Estrogen in combination with a progestin (used to avoid the risk of endometrial cancer associated with unopposed estrogens) suppresses ovarian production of androgens by direct gonadotropin suppression and prevention of ovulation (9,15). Earlier generations of progestins used in OCs (e.g., estrane and gonane classes) have been reported to cross-react with androgen receptors resulting in androgenic effects and increased acne, specifically at higher doses than that which is present in newer OCs (18). Second-generation progestins such as ethynodiol diacetate, norethindrone, and levonorgestrel have the lowest androgenic activity. The third-generation progestins, including norgestimate, desogestrel, and gestodene, are more selective for the progesterone receptor and have the lowest androgenic activity since these agents are metabolized to levonorgestrel (15). Drospirenone, a progestin derived from spironolactone, has antiandrogenic and antimineralocorticoid activity and improves acne, hirsutism, and estrogen-related fluid retention associated with some OCs (33).

OCs effectively decrease acne lesions via their ability to suppress ovarian production of androgens, which reduces serum androgen levels and sebum production. The dose of estrogen required to suppress sebum production is at least 100 μg, which is greater than the dose required to suppress ovulation (32). The effect of OCs is unlikely to be local at the level of the sebaceous gland. Rather, OCs exert their effects by suppressing the secretion of pituitary gonadotropins, thereby reducing ovarian androgen production, or by increasing liver synthesis of sex hormone–binding globulin, resulting in the decrease of free serum testosterone (15,22).

The use of OCs (20 μg of EE/100 μg of levonorgestrel, 35 μg EE/norgestimate) has been shown to be effective and safe for the treatment of acne in women (10,34–36). Reduction in inflammatory lesions by 30% to 60%, improvement of acne in 50% to 90% of patients, and noninflammatory facial acne lesions have been shown following six to nine months of use (37,38). Additionally, OCs containing drospirenone have been shown to be superior to a triphasic OC containing EE/norgestimate in the treatment of acne and had comparable efficacy to Diane-35 (39).

The World Health Organization has developed a list of absolute and relative contraindications to the use of OCs (40). Absolute contraindications include pregnancy, history of thromboembolic or heart disease, liver disease, and active smoking in patients older than 35. Relative contraindications include hypertension, migraine, breast-feeding, and malignancies (29,41,42). OCs can worsen insulin resistance and are contraindicated in patients with a history of diabetes, clotting disorders, thrombophlebitis, cerebrovascular disease, and impaired liver function and in patients with increased risk of break cancer (29). A modest increase in the relative risk of developing breast cancer has also been reported in women; however, OCs may also simultaneously provide a protective effect against ovarian and endometrial cancer (43). Although the most serious side effect reported is thromboembolism, the advent of modern formulations containing reduced doses of estrogen has decreased the incidence of this particular side effect. Additionally, the reduced estrogen dose formulations have also reduced the incidence of other serious side effects, such as hypertension, in young healthy women (15). The most frequently reported side effects include metrorrhagia, nausea, vomiting, breast tenderness, headache, lower extremity edema, and weight gain. A transient flare of inflammatory acne may also occur in the beginning of OC therapy. The effectiveness of oral contraception is not reduced when used in combination with oral antibiotics, with the exception of rifampin (44,45). Specifically, studies comparing the contraceptive failure rate of patients taking OCs with antibiotics compared with patients who were not taking antibiotics found no significant difference (45–47).

BLOCKING ADRENAL ANDROGEN PRODUCTION

Low-dose glucocorticoids effectively suppresses the adrenal production of androgens and are indicated for use in patients (male or female) who have an elevated serum DHEAS, often associated with 11- or 21-hydroxylase deficiency (15). In acute flares of acne or in severe acne, glucocorticoids may be used in low doses (prednisone 2.5–5 mg or dexamethasone 0.25–0.75 mg) daily or every other day to suppress adrenal androgen production. It should be noted that patients treated with dexamethasone are at particularly higher risk for adrenal suppression (15). During treatment, patients should be followed closely for signs of adrenal suppression with ACTH (cosyntropin) stimulation tests performed two to three months after initiation of therapy. Plasma cortisol level should rise to >16 µg/dL 30 minutes after administration of cosyntropin, indicating that adrenal suppression is absent. The effectiveness of glucocorticoid therapy can be monitored by measurement of serum DHEAS, which should be decreased or normalized (18). Treatment with glucocorticoids should not exceed six months because of the risk of osteoporosis (48).

GONADOTROPIN-RELEASING HORMONE AGONISTS

GnRH agonists inhibit ovarian androgen production by blocking the cyclic release of LH and FSH from the pituitary, leading to the suppression of ovarian steroidogenesis. GnRH agonists include agents such as nafarelin, leuprolide, and buserelin, which are only available as nasal sprays or injectables (15). Thus far, only one study has demonstrated efficacy of GnRH agonists in the treatment of acne (49). In six women with acne and six women with hirsutism, treatment with Buserelin nasal spray for six months led to a decrease in ovarian steroids, LH and FSH, and acne and hirsutism. The use of GnRH agonists is limited by their expense and side effects, including ovarian estrogen suppression and the development of menopausal symptoms, headaches, and bone loss (50).

INHIBITION OF 5α-REDUCTASE

There are currently no therapies available that inhibit local androgen production within the sebaceous gland. Future research lies in designing specific inhibitors of androgen metabolizing enzymes in the skin such as 5α-reductase type 1 inhibitors. 5α-reductase inhibitors would block the local conversion of testosterone to dihydrotestosterone and are currently being developed (51–53).

EFFECTIVE HORMONAL THERAPY

Appropriate patient selection is essential when considering hormonal therapy in the treatment of acne and its success. In general, hormonal therapy in acne may be used as first-line therapy in women who desire oral contraception, have signs of hyperandrogenism, or have proven ovarian or adrenal hyperandrogenism (54,55). Hormonal therapy may also be indicated for patients with acne tarda or severe seborrhea, or when repeated courses of isotretinoin are needed to control acne. Of note, hormonal therapy works best in adult women and sexually active teens with premenstrual acne flares (18). Combined OC therapy can also be used as first-line therapy for hirsutism and acne in women with PCOS (15). Additionally, hormonal therapy can be effective in women with normal androgen levels (32).

Hormonal therapies in combination with oral antibiotics, topical retinoids, or benzoyl peroxide should be considered in patients who have recalcitrant acne. Combination therapy is the most effective treatment modality for targeting as many pathophysiologic factors as possible (27).

REFERENCES

1. Thiboutot DM, Knaggs H, Gilliland K, et al. Activity of type 1 5 alpha-reductase is greater in the follicular infrainfundibulum compared with the epidermis. Br J Dermatol 1997; 136(2):166–171.
2. Klaus W, Richard Allen J, eds. Fitzpatrick's Color Atlas and Synopsis of Clinical Dermatology. 6th ed. New York: The McGraw-Hill Companies, 2009.
3. Pochi PE, Strauss JS. Sebaceous gland response in man to the administration of testosterone, delta-4-androstenedione, and dehydroisoandrosterone. J Invest Dermatol 1969; 52(1):32–36.
4. Pochi PE, Strauss JS. Endocrinologic control of the development and activity of the human sebaceous gland. J Invest Dermatol 1974; 62(3):191–201.
5. Strauss JS, Kligman AM, Pochi PE. The effect of androgens and estrogens on human sebaceous glands. J Invest Dermatol 1962; 39:139–155.
6. Thody AJ, Shuster S. Control and function of sebaceous glands. Physiol Rev 1989; 69(2):383–416.

7. Guy R, Green MR, Kealey T. Modeling acne in vitro. J Invest Dermatol 1996; 106(1):176–182.
8. Kim J, Ochoa MT, Krutzik SR, et al. Activation of toll-like receptor 2 in acne triggers inflammatory cytokine responses. J Immunol 2002; 169(3):1535–1541.
9. Lucky AW, Biro FM, Huster GA, et al. Acne vulgaris in premenarchal girls. An early sign of puberty associated with rising levels of dehydroepiandrosterone. Arch Dermatol 1994; 130(3):308–314.
10. Lucky AW, Henderson TA, Olson WH, et al. Effectiveness of norgestimate and ethinyl estradiol in treating moderate acne vulgaris. J Am Acad Dermatol 1997; 37(5 pt 1):746–754.
11. Cibula D, Hill M, Vohradnikova O, et al. The role of androgens in determining acne severity in adult women. Br J Dermatol 2000; 143(2):399–404.
12. Thiboutot D, Gilliland K, Light J, et al. Androgen metabolism in sebaceous glands from subjects with and without acne. Arch Dermatol 1999; 135(9):1041–1045.
13. Beylot C, Doutre MS, Beylot-Barry M. Oral contraceptives and cyproterone acetate in female acne treatment. Dermatology 1998; 196(1):148–152.
14. Lucky AW, Biro FM, Huster GA, et al. Acne vulgaris in early adolescent boys. Correlations with pubertal maturation and age. Arch Dermatol 1991; 127(2): 210–216.
15. Gollnick H, Cunliffe W, Berson D, et al. Management of acne: a report from a Global Alliance to Improve Outcomes in Acne. J Am Acad Dermatol 2003; 49(1 suppl):S1–S37.
16. Olutunmbi Y, Paley K, English JC III. Adolescent female acne: etiology and management. J Pediatr Adolesc Gynecol 2008; 21(4):171–176.
17. Thiboutot D. Hormones and acne: pathophysiology, clinical evaluation, and therapies. Semin Cutan Med Surg 2001; 20(3):144–153.
18. Thiboutot DM. Endocrinological evaluation and hormonal therapy for women with difficult acne. J Eur Acad Dermatol Venereol 2001; 15(suppl 3):57–61.
19. Lucky AW. Hormonal correlates of acne and hirsutism. Am J Med 1995; 98(1A): 89S–94S.
20. Katsambas A, Papakonstantinou A. Acne: systemic treatment. Clin Dermatol 2004; 22(5):412–418.
21. Faure M, Drapier-Faure E. [Hormonal treatments of acne]. Ann Dermatol Venereol 2003; 130(1 pt 2):142–147.
22. Strauss JS, Krowchuk DP, Leyden JJ, et al. Guidelines of care for acne vulgaris management. J Am Acad Dermatol 2007; 56(4):651–663.
23. van Wayjen RG, van den Ende A. Experience in the long-term treatment of patients with hirsutism and/or acne with cyproterone acetate-containing preparations: efficacy, metabolic and endocrine effects. Exp Clin Endocrinol Diabetes 1995; 103(4): 241–251.
24. Sawaya ME, Hordinsky MK. The antiandrogens. When and how they should be used. Dermatol Clin 1993; 11(1):65–72.
25. Goodfellow A, Alaghband-Zadeh J, Carter G, et al. Oral spironolactone improves acne vulgaris and reduces sebum excretion. Br J Dermatol 1984; 111(2):209–214.

26. Akamatsu H, Zouboulis CC, Orfanos CE. Spironolactone directly inhibits proliferation of cultured human facial sebocytes and acts antagonistically to testosterone and 5 alpha-dihydrotestosterone in vitro. J Invest Dermatol 1993; 100(5):660–662.

27. Thiboutot D, Gollnick H, Bettoli V, et al. New insights into the management of acne: an update from the Global Alliance to Improve Outcomes in Acne Group. J Am Acad Dermatol 2009; 60(5 suppl 1):S1–S50.

28. Krunic A, Ciurea A, Scheman A. Efficacy and tolerance of acne treatment using both spironolactone and a combined contraceptive containing drospirenone. J Am Acad Dermatol 2008; 58(1):60–62.

29. Lowenstein EJ. Diagnosis and management of the dermatologic manifestations of the polycystic ovary syndrome. Dermatol Ther 2006; 19(4):210–223.

30. Cusan L, Dupont A, Gomez JL, et al. Comparison of flutamide and spironolactone in the treatment of hirsutism: a randomized controlled trial. Fertil Steril 1994; 61(2):281–287.

31. Wysowski DK, Freiman JP, Tourtelot JB, et al. Fatal and nonfatal hepatotoxicity associated with flutamide. Ann Intern Med 1993; 118(11):860–864.

32. Katsambas AD, Dessinioti C. Hormonal therapy for acne: why not as first line therapy? Facts and controversies. Clin Dermatol 2010; 28(1):17–23.

33. Thorneycroft IH. Evolution of progestins. Focus on the novel progestin drospirenone. J Reprod Med 2002; 47(11 suppl):975–980.

34. Redmond GP, Olson WH, Lippman JS, et al. Norgestimate and ethinyl estradiol in the treatment of acne vulgaris: a randomized, placebo-controlled trial. Obstet Gynecol 1997; 89(4):615–622.

35. Thiboutot D, Archer DF, Lemay A, et al. A randomized, controlled trial of a low-dose contraceptive containing 20 microg of ethinyl estradiol and 100 microg of levonorgestrel for acne treatment. Fertil Steril 2001; 76(3):461–468.

36. Koltun W, Lucky AW, Thiboutot D, et al. Efficacy and safety of 3 mg drospirenone/20 mcg ethinylestradiol oral contraceptive administered in 24/4 regimen in the treatment of acne vulgaris: a randomized, double-blind, placebo-controlled trial. Contraception 2008; 77(4):249–256.

37. Arowojolu AO, Gallo MF, Grimes DA, et al. Combined oral contraceptive pills for treatment of acne. Cochrane Database Syst Rev 2004; (3):CD004425.

38. James WD. Acne. N Engl J Med 2005; 352(14):1463–1472.

39. Thorneycroft H, Gollnick H, Schellschmidt I. Superiority of a combined contraceptive containing drospirenone to a triphasic preparation containing norgestimate in acne treatment. Cutis 2004; 74(2):123–130.

40. World Health Organization. Improving Access to Quality Care in Family Planning: Medical Eligibilty Criteria for Contraceptive Use. 2nd ed. Geneva, Switzerland: World Health Organization, 2003.

41. World Health Organization. Improving Access to Quality Care in Family Planning: Medical Eligibility Criteria for Contraceptive Use. 2nd ed. Geneva, Switzerland: World Health Organization, 2003.

42. Frangos JE, Alavian CN, Kimball AB. Acne and oral contraceptives: update on women's health screening guidelines. J Am Acad Dermatol 2008; 58(5):781–786.

43. Harper JC. Antiandrogen therapy for skin and hair disease. Dermatol Clin 2006; 24(2):137–143, v.
44. Baciewicz AM, Chrisman CR, Finch CK, et al. Update on rifampin and rifabutin drug interactions. Am J Med Sci 2008; 335(2):126–136.
45. Archer JS, Archer DF. Oral contraceptive efficacy and antibiotic interaction: a myth debunked. J Am Acad Dermatol 2002; 46(6):917–923.
46. Helms SE, Bredle DL, Zajic J, et al. Oral contraceptive failure rates and oral antibiotics. J Am Acad Dermatol 1997; 36(5 pt 1):705–710.
47. London BM, Lookingbill DP. Frequency of pregnancy in acne patients taking oral antibiotics and oral contraceptives. Arch Dermatol 1994; 130(3):392–393.
48. Degitz K, Placzek M, Arnold B, et al. Congenital adrenal hyperplasia and acne in male patients. Br J Dermatol 2003; 148(6):1263–1266.
49. Faloia E, Filipponi S, Mancini V, et al. Treatment with a gonadotropin-releasing hormone agonist in acne or idiopathic hirsutism. J Endocrinol Invest 1993; 16(9): 675–677.
50. Thiboutot D. Acne: hormonal concepts and therapy. Clin Dermatol 2004; 22(5): 419–428.
51. Katsambas A, Dessinioti C. New and emerging treatments in dermatology: acne. Dermatol Ther 2008; 21(2):86–95.
52. Chen W, Thiboutot D, Zouboulis CC. Cutaneous androgen metabolism: basic research and clinical perspectives. J Invest Dermatol 2002; 119(5):992–1007.
53. Thiboutot D, Jabara S, McAllister JM, et al. Human skin is a steroidogenic tissue: steroidogenic enzymes and cofactors are expressed in epidermis, normal sebocytes, and an immortalized sebocyte cell line (SEB-1). J Invest Dermatol 2003; 120(6): 905–914.
54. Zouboulis CC, Piquero-Martin J. Update and future of systemic acne treatment. Dermatology 2003; 206(1):37–53.
55. Orfanos CE, Adler YD, Zouboulis CC. The SAHA syndrome. Horm Res 2000; 54 (5–6):251–258.

9.1

Procedural treatments for acne

Whitney P. Bowe and Alan R. Shalita

INTRODUCTION

Simple physical modalities such as comedo extraction and intralesional steroid injections have been utilized in the treatment of acne for many years. Recently, new procedures including laser and light-based technologies have become available. Although many of these new modalities require more rigorous study to determine safety and efficacy, they provide a unique set of advantages for certain patient populations. These therapies provide alternative options for patients who find it difficult to adhere to traditional acne therapies, are concerned over adverse effects of systemic therapy, or for whom traditional therapies fall short in efficacy. In a climate where antibiotic resistance is increasing and isotretinoin therapy has become heavily regulated and scrutinized, such procedural treatment alternatives have become more and more desirable. This chapter will focus on procedural techniques for active acne lesions including extraction, intralesional injections, microdermabrasion, chemical peels, lasers, lights, and photodynamic therapy.

COMEDO EXTRACTION

Physical removal of individual comedones not only has been popular among dermatologists but is also a technique commonly employed by many estheticians. Comedo extraction entails the application of simple mechanical pressure using a comedo extractor (Fig. 9.1.1) to express the contents of a blocked pilosebaceous follicle. For closed comedones, it may be necessary to pierce the top of the lesion with a needle or the tip of a number 11 blade scalpel to make the extrusion less traumatic. Although the technique is widely practiced, very little has been published to date regarding its efficacy and side effect profile (1). Advantages

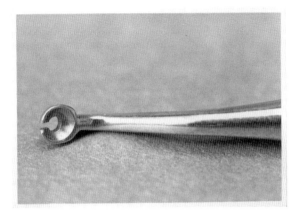

Figure 9.1.1   The Shalita comedo extractor. *Source*: Courtesy of Alan R. Shalita, M.D.

reported include a reduction in the number of future inflamed lesions and an immediate sense of improvement. However, the procedure is known to carry a risk of tissue damage, making cystic lesions worse (1) and potentially inciting inflammation by rupturing the contents of a comedo through the base of the follicle into the dermis. Open comedones reappear clinically 20 to 40 days following extraction, while closed comedones (whiteheads) reappear within 30 to 50 days. Biopsy specimens following extraction of open comedones demonstrate that it is occasionally possible to evulse the entire comedo epithelium and kernel in toto. In contrast, whiteheads, or closed comedones, cannot be completely removed with an extractor. When the entire open comedo epithelium is evulsed, new comedones do not reform. Consequently, extraction provides a temporary improvement for most noninflammatory lesions but has the potential to completely eradicate a very small percentage of open comedones (2). Care should be taken to use minimal force, as this will minimize inflammation and the risk of scarring.

INTRALESIONAL STEROID INJECTIONS

One of the most common procedures used to rapidly shrink inflammatory nodules is the use of intralesional corticosteroid injections. This modality is indicated for large, stubborn lesions or when a rapid response is desired. Concentrations of 5 mg/mL or less of triamcinolone acetonide are commonly used, and it has been demonstrated that concentrations as low as 0.63 mg/mL are just as effective as higher concentrations of 2.5 mg/mL (3). However, it is important to note that the quantity injected together with the concentration used is of paramount importance, rather than simply relying on a threshold concentration as a guide. The authors recommend injecting the smallest amount of a 2.5-mg/mL concentration with a 30-g needle directly into the lesion until the most subtle blanching is visualized. Although not studied, the authors believe that dilution with normal saline results in less stinging experienced by the patient as compared with dilution with sterile water. Following injection, nodules have been noted to flatten in 48 to 72 hours.

This procedure is not without risks and should be used judiciously in appropriate circumstances. Risks include atrophy, telangiectasias, and pigmentary alterations (4), and hypothalamic-pituitary-adrenal axis suppression has been reported with repeated injections (5,6). Although studies are lacking, most obstetricians feel comfortable with the use of occasional intralesional injections during the second and third trimesters of pregnancy so long as the total dose and frequency of injections stay within reason.

MICRODERMABRASION

Microdermabrasion is a superficial, minimally invasive technique of mechanical abrasion in which the stratum corneum is partially or completely removed. The technique is employed for mild acne scarring, aging, and pigmentary anomalies. Either a pressurized stream of abrasive particles such as aluminum oxide crystals or a roughened tip such as one made of diamond is used to physically exfoliate the skin surface. This superficial exfoliation of the stratum corneum appears to stimulate a dermal remodeling cascade similar to that seen following incisional wound healing (7). Limited data is available supporting the efficacy of microdermabrasion in acne (8), but it is generally well tolerated and requires no downtime. Proper eye protection must be worn to prevent corneal damage from stray crystals, and care must be taken to avoid aggressive treatment in areas of thin skin prone to purpura such as the eyelids. In contrast, multiple passes may be utilized over focal acne scars. The desired end point is erythema, but one may also see edema following a microdermabrasion session. Although the procedure appears to have only a very modest effect on acne scarring, it does enhance the absorption of topically applied agents (9) and thereby may increase the efficacy of a concomitant topical acne regimen. Similarly, it will likely increase the side effects from these agents including photosensitivity and dry skin. Because of its ability to facilitate penetration of topical medications, it has been used as a pretreatment for photodynamic therapy (PDT) (10).

CHEMICAL PEELS

Chemical peeling involves the application of a chemical to induce an accelerated form of exfoliation. Light peeling agents result in sloughing of cells in the stratum corneum, while deeper peeling agents create necrosis and inflammation in the epidermis or even as deep as the reticular dermis. However, even very superficial peels that remove stratum corneum only can stimulate the epidermis to thicken and can ultimately even lead to increased deposition of collagen and glycosaminoglycans in the dermis. Peeling has been used to treat active acne lesions, postinflammatory pigmentary changes from acne, as well as superficial acne scars.

Salicylic Acid

Salicylic acid is a β-hydroxy acid safe to use in all Fitzpatrick skin types and ideally suited for acne because of its keratolytic and anti-inflammatory properties (11). Even concentrations as low as 0.5% to 3% of salicylic acid have been demonstrated to speed the resolution of inflammatory acne lesions and decrease the formation of comedones (12). Salicylic acid is lipophilic and thus penetrates the pilosebaceous unit with ease.

When used in 20% to 30% concentrations as an in-office peeling agent, it is usually applied for a five-minute duration and is self-neutralizing. A pseudo-frost appears with application, and this frost becomes more apparent with more numerous passes. Side effects include erythema, dryness, burning, and crusting, which are all transient (11). Salicylism is a theoretical side effect if used over large surface areas, but this has never been reported with concentrations used to treat acne. It is contraindicated in pregnancy and in those with an aspirin allergy. Retinoids and benzoyl peroxide should be withheld one week prior to and one week following each peel to prevent uneven or erratic penetration.

Glycolic Acid

Glycolic acid is an α-hydroxy acid commonly used for conditions of abnormal keratinization (13). Reduction of comedones, papules, and pustules and overall improvement in skin texture (14) have been demonstrated in acne patients. Improvement in postinflammatory changes in black patients has also been observed (15). Furthermore, glycolic acid has been shown to increase epidermal and dermal thickness, with increased deposition of acid mucopolysaccharides, improved quality of elastic fibers, and increased density of collagen (16). Consequently, repeated peels might have a modest effect on mild acne scarring.

Glycolic acid peels produce no systemic toxicity, but disadvantages include a tendency for the acid to penetrate unevenly. There is significant variability from patient to patient with regard to reactivity and efficacy. Further complicating the standardization of this peeling agent, glycolic peels come in both free acid systems and partially neutralized systems. Consequently, a 70% free acid solution contains very close to 70% of bioavailable acid, while a 70% glycolic acid formulation from a company that uses a partially neutralized system might contain approximately 50% of biologically active acid. The depth of the peel is not related to the number of coats as is the case with salicylic acid. However, like salicylic acid peels, glycolic peels can penetrate more deeply or more unevenly in a patient who is using topical retinoids or benzoyl peroxide. Glycolic peels must be neutralized, which should be done when erythema is visualized.

LIGHT AND LASER THERAPY

The multiple pathogenic factors involved in acne provide many potential targets for light and laser therapy (17). Although well-designed studies including controls, blinding, and randomization are lacking, patients are drawn to laser and light-based technologies as a "cutting-edge" alternative to standard acne therapies.

Blue Light and Red Light

Propionibacterium acnes is an obvious target for visible light therapy as it produces photoactive compounds called porphyrins that absorb wavelengths in the visible light spectrum. Specifically, coproporphyrin III is the predominant porphyrin produced by *P. acnes*, while coproporphyrin I and protoporphyrin are produced at much lower concentrations (18). When exposed to visible light (with a maximum absorption peak at 403 nm), these photoactive compounds create reactive oxygen species that are toxic to *P. acnes*. Although the absorption of blue light is greatest, these shorter wavelengths do not penetrate as deeply into the skin as compared with red light. Thus, absorption efficiency is inversely correlated with depth of penetration. However, toxicity to *P. acnes* might not be the only mechanism of action when it comes to visible light. Blue light has been shown to reduce keratinocyte production of inflammatory cytokines including interleukin-1α, suggesting that blue light possesses anti-inflammatory properties as well as antimicrobial ones (19). Studies, although not rigorously performed, have shown benefit from both blue light therapy alone, as well as blue and red light combination therapy (20–22).

Pulsed Dye Laser

Controversial results regarding whether pulsed dye laser therapy has an effect on acne have been published (23–25). Two of the three studies fail to show a significant contribution from pulsed dye laser therapy, with one study examining the laser as monotherapy and the other as adjunctive treatment to topical therapy.

Potassium Titanyl Phosphate Laser

The use of the 532-nm potassium titanyl phosphate (KTP) laser in the treatment of acne has not been convincingly demonstrated. The largest study to date showed no significant difference between treated and control sides of the face at four weeks (26).

1450-nm Laser

Theoretically, a mid-infrared laser device would be able to penetrate to the level of the sebaceous gland, thereby heating this gland and the associated follicle and thus improve acne. A light-based treatment that could destroy sebaceous glands would have the potential to cure acne (17). Protection of the epidermis is critical to the success of such a laser treatment. A 1450-nm laser device with a cryogen cooling system was shown to cause short-term thermal alteration of sebaceous glands while preserving the epidermis in an in vivo rabbit ear model (27). Three human clinical trials have all demonstrated statistically significant reduction in acne lesion counts following 1450-nm laser treatment (27–29). Side effects were limited and transient.

Photodynamic Therapy

Although *P. acnes* is known to produce its own endogenous porphyrins in proportion to its population (30), the concept of introducing exogenous porphyrins that can then be activated by light is known as photodynamic therapy. Aminolevulinic acid (ALA) is known to be preferentially taken up by the pilosebaceous units (31). As ALA penetrates the epidermis, it enters the heme biosynthetic pathway and is converted to PpIX (32). Methyl aminolevulinate (MAL) is a lipophilic derivative of ALA. The introduction of both molecules into the skin results in higher concentrations of porphyrins, which can then be activated by red or blue light.

In 2000, a landmark study was performed demonstrating the efficacy of ALA PDT using high-fluence red light to treat acne. On the basis of measurements of sebum excretion rates, autofluorescence from follicular bacteria, as well as histological evaluation of skin biopsies, it appeared as though topical ALA PDT acted by (*i*) inhibiting sebum secretion by damaging sebaceous glands, (*ii*) sterilizing sebaceous follicles by killing *P. acnes*, and (*iii*) reducing follicular obstruction by altering keratinocyte shedding and hyperkeratosis. With the protocol used, the patients experienced severe side effects. Although subsequent studies using PDT for acne have demonstrated good clinical outcomes, the mechanism proposed following the initial study described above has since been challenged. Follow-up studies have shown clinical benefit from PDT for acne in the absence of significant changes in sebum secretion or *P. acnes* populations (33). Although PDT appears to have a clinical benefit in a number of studies (34–36), protocols have widely differed and the mechanism of action remains to be fully elucidated. The largest study to date was performed by DUSA

Pharmaceuticals, Inc. but was unfortunately never published. This multicenter randomized, controlled, investigator-blinded study was conducted on 266 patients with moderate to severe acne. Levulan in vehicle or vehicle alone was applied to the full face of participants approximately 45 minutes prior to treatment with 5 to 10 J/cm^2 of light with BLU-U (405–420 nm). Patients were treated once every three weeks for a maximum of four treatments. The results did not demonstrate a statistically significant difference between the Levulan PDT and the control group. However, both groups demonstrated a statistically significant reduction in the number of inflammatory lesions from baseline (37.5–41.7% reduction), providing further evidence that blue light alone has an effect on acne. Despite these results, there is no question that some experienced clinicians do indeed have reliably good results using PDT for acne.

Radiofrequency

The use of radiofrequency energy has recently been proposed as a nonablative treatment modality for acne. Radiofrequency currents directed at tissue cause thermal effects that depend on the electrical properties of the tissue. These thermal effects are speculated to affect sebaceous gland activity and thus have a potential effect on acne. Some preliminary studies show promise (37,38), but whether radiofrequency truly exerts a thermolytic effect on sebaceous glands remains to be determined.

Photopneumatic Therapy

A specialized device that combines negative pressure (suction) with the concomitant delivery of broadband pulsed light (400–1200 nm) has been developed for the treatment of acne. This photopneumatic device is the only laser or light-based device cleared by the Food and Drug Administration (FDA) for the treatment of comedonal and inflammatory acne. The device applies a gentle vacuum to the skin surface, thereby mechanically evacuating trapped sebum and necrotic cells. This technology also stretches the skin within the treatment tip, thereby reducing the concentration of competing chromophores such as hemoglobin and melanin so that less painful fluences of the broadband light can be moved and the light can more directly target the porphyrins in *P. acnes*. Mechanical extrusion of comedo contents and thermally injured bacteria have been observed following treatment (39). Although a number of studies have demonstrated effect on subjects suffering from mild to severe acne (40–42), none of these studies included a control group for comparison. The authors (WPB and ARS) are currently conducting the first randomized controlled trial of this technology (study underway at date of publication).

REFERENCES

1. Lowney ED, Witkowski, Simons HM, et al. Value of comedo extraction in treatment of acne vulgaris. JAMA 1964; 189:1000–1002.
2. Plewig G. Follicular keratinization. J Invest Dermatol 1974; 62(3):308–320.
3. Levine RM, Rasmussen JE. Intralesional corticosteroids in the treatment of nodulocystic acne. Arch Dermatol 1983; 119(6):480–481.
4. Callen JP. Intralesional corticosteroids. J Am Acad Dermatol 1981; 4(2):149–151.
5. Potter RA. Intralesional triamcinolone and adrenal suppression in acne vulgaris. J Invest Dermatol 1971; 57(6):364–370.
6. Zaynoun ST, Salti IS. The effect of intracutaneous glucocorticoids on plasma cortisol levels. Br J Dermatol 1973; 88(2):151–156.
7. Karimipour DJ, Rittie L, Hammerberg C, et al. Molecular analysis of aggressive microdermabrasion in photoaged skin. Arch Dermatol 2009; 145(10):1114–1122.
8. Lloyd JR. The use of microdermabrasion for acne: a pilot study. Dermatol Surg 2001; 27(4):329–331.
9. Lee WR, Shen SC, Kuo-Hsien W, et al. Lasers and microdermabrasion enhance and control topical delivery of vitamin C. J Invest Dermatol 2003; 121(5):1118–1125.
10. Nestor MS, Gold MH, Kauvar AN, et al. The use of photodynamic therapy in dermatology: results of a consensus conference. J Drugs Dermatol 2006; 5(2): 140–154.
11. Lee HS, Kim IH. Salicylic acid peels for the treatment of acne vulgaris in Asian patients. Dermatol Surg 2003; 29(12):1196–1199.
12. Shalita AR. Treatment of mild and moderate acne vulgaris with salicylic acid in an alcohol-detergent vehicle. Cutis 1981; 28(5):556–558, 561.
13. Van Scott EJ, Yu RJ. Alpha hydroxy acids: procedures for use in clinical practice. Cutis 1989; 43(3):222–228.
14. Wang CM, Huang CL, Hu CT, et al. The effect of glycolic acid on the treatment of acne in Asian skin. Dermatol Surg 1997; 23(1):23–29.
15. Burns RL, Prevost-Blank PL, Lawry MA, et al. Glycolic acid peels for post-inflammatory hyperpigmentation in black patients. A comparative study. Dermatol Surg 1997; 23(3):171–174.
16. Ditre CM, Griffin TD, Murphy GF, et al. Effects of alpha-hydroxy acids on photoaged skin: a pilot clinical, histologic, and ultrastructural study. J Am Acad Dermatol 1996; 34(2 Pt 1):187–195.
17. Webster GF. Light and laser therapy for acne: sham or science? facts and controversies. Clin Dermatol 2010; 28(1):31–33.
18. Lee WL, Shalita AR, Poh-Fitzpatrick MB. Comparative studies of porphyrin production in *Propionibacterium acnes* and *Propionibacterium granulosum*. J Bacteriol 1978; 133(2):811–815.
19. Shnitkind E, Yaping E, Geen S, et al. Anti-inflammatory properties of narrow-band blue light. J Drugs Dermatol 2006; 5(7):605–610.
20. Elman M, Slatkine M, Harth Y. The effective treatment of acne vulgaris by a high-intensity, narrow band 405-420 nm light source. J Cosmet Laser Ther 2003; 5(2):111–117.

21. Papageorgiou P, Katsambas A, Chu A. Phototherapy with blue (415 nm) and red (660 nm) light in the treatment of acne vulgaris. Br J Dermatol 2000; 142(5): 973–978.
22. Tzung TY, Wu KH, Huang ML. Blue light phototherapy in the treatment of acne. Photodermatol Photoimmunol Photomed 2004; 20(5):266–269.
23. Karsai S, Schmitt L, Raulin C. The pulsed-dye laser as an adjuvant treatment modality in acne vulgaris: a randomized controlled single-blinded trial. Br J Dermatol 2010; 15.
24. Orringer JS, Kang S, Hamilton T, et al. Treatment of acne vulgaris with a pulsed dye laser: a randomized controlled trial. JAMA 2004; 291(23):2834–2839.
25. Seaton ED, Charakida A, Mouser PE, et al. Pulsed-dye laser treatment for inflammatory acne vulgaris: randomised controlled trial. Lancet 2003; 362(9393): 1347–1352.
26. Baugh WP, Kucaba WD. Nonablative phototherapy for acne vulgaris using the KTP 532 nm laser. Dermatol Surg 2005; 31(10):1290–1296.
27. Paithankar DY, Ross EV, Saleh BA, et al. Acne treatment with a 1,450 nm wavelength laser and cryogen spray cooling. Lasers Surg Med 2002; 31(2):106–114.
28. Jih MH, Friedman PM, Goldberg LH, et al. The 1450-nm diode laser for facial inflammatory acne vulgaris: dose-response and 12-month follow-up study. J Am Acad Dermatol 2006; 55(1):80–87.
29. Wang SQ, Counters JT, Flor ME, et al. Treatment of inflammatory facial acne with the 1,450 nm diode laser alone versus microdermabrasion plus the 1,450 nm laser: a randomized, split-face trial. Dermatol Surg 2006; 32(2):249–255.
30. McGinley KJ, Webster GF, Leyden JJ. Facial follicular porphyrin fluorescence: correlation with age and density of *Propionibacterium acnes*. Br J Dermatol 1980; 102(4):437–441.
31. Divaris DX, Kennedy JC, Pottier RH. Phototoxic damage to sebaceous glands and hair follicles of mice after systemic administration of 5-aminolevulinic acid correlates with localized protoporphyrin IX fluorescence. Am J Pathol 1990; 136(4):891–897.
32. Iinuma S, Farshi SS, Ortel B, et al. A mechanistic study of cellular photodestruction with 5-aminolaevulinic acid-induced porphyrin. Br J Cancer 1994; 70(1):21–28.
33. Pollock B, Turner D, Stringer MR, et al. Topical aminolaevulinic acid-photodynamic therapy for the treatment of acne vulgaris: a study of clinical efficacy and mechanism of action. Br J Dermatol 2004; 151(3):616–622.
34. Alexiades-Armenakas M. Long-pulsed dye laser-mediated photodynamic therapy combined with topical therapy for mild to severe comedonal, inflammatory, or cystic acne. J Drugs Dermatol 2006; 5(1):45–55.
35. Goldman MP, Boyce SM. A single-center study of aminolevulinic acid and 417 NM photodynamic therapy in the treatment of moderate to severe acne vulgaris. J Drugs Dermatol 2003; 2(4):393–396.
36. Santos MA, Belo VG, Santos G. Effectiveness of photodynamic therapy with topical 5-aminolevulinic acid and intense pulsed light versus intense pulsed light alone in the treatment of acne vulgaris: comparative study. Dermatol Surg 2005; 31(8 Pt 1): 910–915.

37. Prieto VG, Zhang PS, Sadick NS. Evaluation of pulsed light and radiofrequency combined for the treatment of acne vulgaris with histologic analysis of facial skin biopsies. J Cosmet Laser Ther 2005; 7(2):63–68.

38. Ruiz-Esparza J, Gomez JB. Nonablative radiofrequency for active acne vulgaris: the use of deep dermal heat in the treatment of moderate to severe active acne vulgaris (thermotherapy): a report of 22 patients. Dermatol Surg 2003; 29(4):333–339.

39. Omi T, Munavalli GS, Kawana S, et al. Ultrastructural evidence for thermal injury to pilosebaceous units during the treatment of acne using photopneumatic (PPX) therapy. J Cosmet Laser Ther 2008; 10(1):7–11.

40. Gold MH, Biron J. Efficacy of a novel combination of pneumatic energy and broadband light for the treatment of acne. J Drugs Dermatol 2008; 7(7):639–642.

41. Shamban AT, Enokibori M, Narurkar V, et al. Photopneumatic technology for the treatment of acne vulgaris. J Drugs Dermatol 2008; 7(2):139–145.

42. Wanitphakdeedecha R, Tanzi EL, Alster TS. Photopneumatic therapy for the treatment of acne. J Drugs Dermatol 2009; 8(3):239–241.

Index

Page numbers followed by *f* and *t* indicate figures and tables, respectively.

AA. *See* Arachidonic acid (AA)
Acanthosis nigricans, 199
Acinetobacter baumannii, 158
Acne conglobata, 162
Acne eruptions
  biologics and anti–tumor necrosis
    factor-α agents, 173
  central nervous system agents,
    170–172
  chemotherapeutics, 167–168
  chloracne, 172–173
  corticosteroids, 168–169
  diagnosis of, 166–167
  hormones, 169–170
  signs and symptoms of, 167*t*
Acne fulminans (AF), 161
  clinical, 162
  differential diagnosis of, 162
  elevated blood levels of testosterone and,
    161
  frequency, 162
  imaging studies, 162
  isotretinoin and, 161
  laboratory findings, 162
  pathophysiology of, 161
Acneiform eruptions, 162, 166
Acne Intensity Score (AIS), 173
Acne lesions, procedural techniques
  chemical peeling, 210–211
  comedo extraction, 208–209
  glycolic acid, 211–212
  intralesional steroid injections, 209–210

  light and laser therapy, 212–214
  microdermabrasion, 210
  salicylic acid, 211
Acne lesions and GNF lesions
  differences between, 158
Acne medicamentosa, 166
Acne medications
  FDA Drug Risk Classification System
    for, 178*t*
Acne neonatorum, 182
Acne tarda, 199
Acne vulgaris, 162
  epidemiology, 1
  etymology, 1
  pathogenesis of, 146–147
  psychological implications, 1–2
  therapy, 55–56. *See also* Treatment
ACTH (Cortrosyn®), 192
Actinomycin-D, 168
Activator protein-1 (AP-1), 19, 47
Adapalene, 89–90, 178
  as maintenance therapy, 109
Adolescence, acne, 1, 47. *See also*
    Preadolescent acne
Adrenal hyperandrogenism, 199
Adult acne, 148–149
Aeromonas hydrophila, 158
AF. *See* Acne fulminans (AF)
African-Americans, 75. *See also* People
    of color, acne in
  sebaceous glands in, 72
Agent Orange, 172–173

AIDS, 158, 159
Alcohols, 4
All-*trans* retinoic acid (ATRA),
    19, 20
Altered bone mineralization, 140
Amineptine, 168
Aminolevulinic acid (ALA), 213
Ampicillin, 158–159
Anabolic-androgenic steroids (AAS),
    169–170
Androgen blockers, 153
Androgens, 147. *See also* Testosterone
    in comedogenesis, 32–34
    role in treatment of acne, 198
    and sebum production, 5–6
5α-Androstanedione, 60
Androstenedione, 147
Angiotensin-converting enzyme
    inhibitors, 152
Antiandrogens, 151
Antibacterial action, of sebum, 5
Antibiotics
    oral. *See* Oral antibiotics
    resistance to, 125–130
        GAS, 128–131
        S. aureus, 126–128
    topical, 95–101
    topical retinoids with, 106–107
Antimicrobial peptides, 19–20
    in sebaceous gland, 5
Antioxidants, 62–63
Anti–tumor necrosis factor (anti-TNF)-α
    therapy, 173
AP-1. *See* Activator protein-1 (AP-1)
Apert's syndrome, 8
Arachidonic acid (AA), 61
Aripipazole, 171
Arthralgias, 139
Aseptic osteolytic bone lesions, 162
ATRA. *See* All-*trans* retinoic acid
    (ATRA)
Atrophic scars, 48–49, 50*f*–52*f*. *See also*
    Scars/scarring
Azelaic acid, 95, 99, 173, 178
    for skin of color patients, 76, 79
Azithromycin, 114, 173
    efficacy of, 118
    for GI absorption, 116

Bacterial interference, 128
Benzoyl peroxide, 173, 177, 192–193, 204
    topical antibiotics with, 98–99
Biofilms, *P. acnes,* 30, 35, 36
Blood lipids
    reversible alterations in, 137–138
Bone mineral density (BMD), 140
Boxcar scars. *See also* Atrophic scars
    description of, 49, 51*f*
    punch excision/elevation for, 49
Buserelin, 153

CAH. *See* Congenital adrenal hyperplasia
    (CAH)
CA-MRSA. *See* Community-acquired
    MRSA (CA-MRSA)
Candida albicans, 186
Carbohydrates, 57–60
Cathelicidin, 5, 20
CD14, 18
CD209 macrophages, 20
Cellular retinoic acid–binding protein II
    (CRABP II), 88
Cheilitis, 137
Chemical peels, in skin of color patients, 78
Chemotactic agents, 147
Chloracne comedones, 38. *See also*
    Comedones
Cholesterol, 4
Citrus depressa, 62
Clindamycin, 177
    with adapalene gel, 106–107
    clindamycin/BPO product, 108
    for GAS infections, 129
    for reduction of *P. acnes* and
        inflammation, 75
    S. aureus and, 127
    solutions, 193
    for treatment of acne vulgaris, 95–96,
        95–100
    for treatment of noninflammatory
        lesions, 89–90
Closed comedones, 37. *See also* Come-
    dones
Cochrane database review
    of OCP, 151
    of spironolactone, 152

Combination therapy
    first-line, 106
    fixed-dose combination products,
        107–109
    overview, 105–106
    topical retinoids
        and oral antibiotics, 107
        and topical antibiotics, 106–107
    using a topical regimen, 115–116
Comedo extraction, 208–209
Comedogenesis. *See also* Comedones
    androgens in, 32–34
    cytokines in, 34
    follicular hyperkeratinization and, 29–30
    inflammation in, 30–31
    overview, 28
    P. acnes in, 35–36
    sebum lipid abnormalities in, 31–32
Comedonal acne
    preadolescent girl with, 190*f*
Comedones
    chloracne, 38
    conglobate, 38–39
    drug-induced, 38
    macrocomedones, 38
    microcomedones, 37
    nevoid, 38
    open and closed, 37
    overview, 28–29
    sand paper, 37
    submarine, 37–38
    subtypes of, 36–39
Community-acquired MRSA
    (CA-MRSA), 126
Compliance, issue of, 55–56
Congenital adrenal hyperplasia (CAH),
    147, 153, 199
Conglobate comedones, 38–39. *See also*
    Comedones
Contraceptives, 149
Corticosteroids
    for scar treatment, 49
    for skin of color patients, 77–78
Corticotropin-releasing hormone (CRH)
    and sebum production, 7–8
CRABP II. *See* Cellular retinoic
    acid–binding protein II (CRABP II)
C-reactive protein, 162

CRH. *See* Corticotropin-releasing hormone
    (CRH)
Cultural practices, 74
Cushing's disease, 192
Cutaneous immune system, 13–16. *See also*
    Innate immune system
Cyanoacrylate stripping, 109
Cyproterone acetate (CPA), 34, 153, 200
    side effects of, 200
Cytokines, 13–14
    in comedogenesis, 34
    and inflammation, 17, 18
    and *P. acnes,* 6, 18, 35
Cytotoxic agents, 147

D-alanine, 18
Dapsone, for skin of color patients, 75–76
Decontamination of loofah sponges, 157
Dehydroepiandrostenedione levels, 150
Dehydroepiandrosterone sulfate (DHEAS),
    153, 199
    production, 147, 186, 198. *See also*
        Androgens
    and sebum production, 6
Dermal fillers, for skin of color patients,
    79–80
Desogestrel, 202
Dexamethasone, 153, 203
DHA. *See* Docosahexaenoic acid (DHA)
DHEAS. *See* Dehydroepiandrosterone
    sulfate (DHEAS)
DHS. *See* Drug hypersensitivity syndrome
    (DHS)
Diane-35, 202
Dianette/Diane-35, 200
Dietary intake
    of antioxidants, 62–63
    of carbohydrates, 57–60
    of dairy, 60
    of fatty acids, 61–62
    of iodine, 64
    of vitamin A, 63–64
    of zinc, 64
Diffuse idiopathic skeletal hyperostosis
    (DISH), 140, 189
Dihydrotestosterone (DHT), 58–59, 152
Diphtheroids, 156

Docosahexaenoic acid (DHA), 61
Doxycycline
  adapalene with, 90
  administration of, 116
  recommended dosing of, 115*t*
  side effects, 119, 120
  usage, 114
Drosophila, 14
Drospirenone (Yaz), 150–151, 200, 202
Drug hypersensitivity syndrome (DHS), 120
Drug-induced comedones, 38. *See also*
  Comedones
Drug-induced hepatitis, 152
Dyspigmentation, 188

Early childhood acne, 147
EGCG. *See* Epigallocatechin-3-gallate
  (EGCG)
Endocrinopathy in women, 199
Enzymes sulfotransferase, 198
Eosinophilic pustular folliculitis, 186
Epigallocatechin-3-gallate (EGCG), 62
Erythema toxicum neonatorum, 183
Erythrocyte sedimentation rate (ESR), 162
Erythromycin, 95, 173, 177
  benzoyl peroxide with, 95–96
  and cytochrome 3A4 enzymes, 121
  estolate, 179
  oral administration, 116
  in pregnancy, 100, 121
  solutions, 193
  use of, 96
  vs. clindamycin, 96–97
Erythromycin-resistant *S. aureus,* 128
Escherichia, 157
Estrogen, 201–202
  therapy, 55
Etanercept, 173
Ethinyl estradiol, 150–151, 153
Ewing's sarcoma, 168

Fade creams. *See* Lightening agents, for
  skin of color patients
Fatty acids, 61–62
  bacterial colonization and, 13
  comedogenesis and, 31, 32, 35
  sebaceous, 3, 4

FDA Drug Risk Classification System for
  acne medications, 178*t*
FFA. *See* Free fatty acids (FFA)
FGFR. *See* Fibroblast growth factor
  receptors (FFGR)
Fibroblast growth factor receptors (FFGR),
  5, 8
Fibroblasts, in people of color, 72
Fibroplasia, 45
Filaggrin
  defined, 36
  and keratinocytes, 36
Finasteride, 201
Fixed-dose combination products, 107–109
Fluocinolone acetonide, 169
Flutamide, 152, 200, 201
Follicle-stimulating hormone (FSH), 147
Follicular hyperkeratinization, 29–30. *See
  also* Hyperkeratinization
Folliculitis, 162
Free fatty acids (FFA), 13. *See also* Fatty acids
  in sebum, 3, 4

Gemfibrozil, 138
Gestodene, 202
GH. *See* Growth hormone (GH)
GI. *See* Glycemic index (GI)
Glucocorticoids, low-dose, 203
Glucose-6-phoshate dehydrogenase
  (G6PD) deficiency, 75–76
Glycemic index (GI), 57–58
Glycolic acid, 78, 211–212. *See also*
  Chemical peels, in skin of color
  patients
GNF. *See* Gram-negative folliculitis (GNF)
Gonadotropin-releasing hormone (GnRH),
  152
G6PD. *See* Glucose-6-phoshate dehydro-
  genase (G6PD) deficiency
Gram-negative folliculitis (GNF), 156
  clinical, 157–158
  lesions and acne lesions
  differences between, 158*t*
  pathogenesis of, 156–157
  treatment of, 158–159
Granulysin, 20
Group A streptococcus (GAS)
  antibiotics, resistance to, 128–131

[Group A streptococcus]
description of, 128
β-lactam antibiotics, susceptible to, 129
in oropharynx, 128, 129
Growth hormone (GH), 58, 59

Hematuria, 162
Hirsutism, 58, 149
androgen and, 199
cyproterone acetate and, 153
flutamide and, 152
GnRH agonists and, 203
spironolactone and, 200–201
Holocrine secretion, 3
Hormonal abnormalities and acne, 148*t*
Hormonal therapy, 150–153, 204
for skin of color patients, 77
Hot-tub folliculitis, 158, 159
³H-thymidine, 29
Human β-defensins, 20
Hydrocephalus, 179
Hydroquinone, 79. *See also* Lightening
agents, for skin of color patients
2-Hydroxyflutamide, 152
17-Hydroxyprogesterone, 149, 153, 199
3β-Hydroxysteroid dehydrogenase
(3β-HSD), 198
17β-Hydroxysteroid dehydrogenase
(17β-HSD), 198
Hyperandrogenis, 199
Hyperinsulinemia, 58, 59
Hyperkeratinization, 16–18
follicular, 29–30
interleukin 1 (IL-1) in, 17
Hyperkeratosis, 29, 32
Hyperproliferation, of keratinocytes, 16,
17, 21, 29
Hypertriglyceridemia, 137
Hypertrophic scars, 48. *See also* Keloidal
scars
Hypervitaminosis A, 63, 137. *See also*
Vitamin A
Hypoxia, in wounds, 45

Ice pick scars. *See also* Atrophic scars
description of, 49, 50*f*–51*f*
punch excision for, 49

Idiopathic intracranial hypertension (IIH),
137, 138–139
adverse effects of, 137
IGF-1. *See* Insulin-like growth factor 1
(IGF-1)
IGFBP. *See* Insulin-like growth factor
binding protein 3 (IGFBP-3)
IL-1α
in comedogenesis, 30–31, 34, 35
in inflammation, 30–31
IL-1β, 18, 47
Immune system. *See* Cutaneous immune
system; Innate immune system
Immunoglobulin A, 5
Impatiens balsamina, 62
Impetigo, 128
Infantile acne, 147
in boys, 185*f,* 186
clinical presentation, 184
differential diagnosis and evaluation,
186–187
in a male infant, 185*f*
pathophysiology, 186
with pustules and nodules on the cheeks,
185*f*
treatment, 187–188
Infants
with comedonal and inflammatory acne,
184
with hormonal abnormalities, 186–187
isotretinoin in, 187–188, 187*t*
sebum production in, 186
tetracyclines in, 180
topical salicylic acid in, 179
Inflammation. *See also* Innate immune system
in comedogenesis, 30–31
hyperkeratinization and, 16–18
MMP and, 19
P. acnes in, 18–19, 35
Inflammatory bowel disease (IBD), 189–190
Innate immune system, 12–22
antimicrobial peptides and, 19–20
cutaneous, 13–16
MMP and, 19
molecular structure of, 14, 16*f*
overview, 12–13
sebum lipids and, 21–22
TLR and, 14, 15*f,* 16*f,* 18–19

Insulin-like growth factor binding protein 3 (IGFBP-3), 58
Insulin-like growth factor 1 (IGF-1), 58–59
Insulin sensitizers, 150
Intake. *See* Dietary intake
Integrin
 defined, 36
 and keratinocyte, 36
Interleukin 1 (IL-1)
 in hyperkeratinization, 17
Intralesional corticosteroids, 49, 77–78
Intralesional kenalog, 179
Intrauterine devices, 170
Iodine, 64
iPLEDGE program, 139
Isotretinoin, 63, 134
 and AF, 161
 contraindications, 136
 dosing, 136
 gastrointestinal adverse effects of, 138
 indications, 135
 in infants, 187–188, 187*t*
 mechanism of action, 135
 pharmacology, 135
 relapses, 136
 and sand paper comedones, 37
 and scar treatment, 52
 and sebum production, 6
 topical, 88–89
 for treatment of gram-negative folliculitis (GNF), 158
 in women of childbearing potential, 135

K16, 30
Keloidal scars, 48. *See also* Hypertrophic scars
Keratinocytes, 5, 8
 cytokines and, 35
 filaggrin and, 36
 hyperproliferation of, 16, 17, 21, 29. *See also* Hyperkeratinization
 of infrainfundibulum, 29, 33
 integrin and, 36
 retinoids and, 87
 tazarotene and, 89
Ketoconazole cream, 184

Ki-67, 30
Klebsiella, 157

β-Lactam antibiotics, 129
Lamotrigine, 171
Laser devices, for skin of color patients, 79
Late-onset adrenal hyperplasia (LOAH), 199
L-diaminopimelic acid, 18
Lenalidomide, 168
Leuprolide, 153
Levonorgestrel-releasing intrauterine system, 149
Levulan PDT, 214
Light and laser therapy
 blue light and red light, 212
 1450-nm laser device, 213
 photodynamic therapy, 213–214
 photopneumatic therapy, 214
 potassium titanyl phosphate (KTP) laser, 212–213
 pulsed dye laser, 212
 radiofrequency, 214
Lightening agents, for skin of color patients, 78–79
Lipid polarity, 31–32
Lipids, sebum, 3–4, 4*t*
 and comedogenesis, 31–32
 inflammatory effects, 21–22
5-Lipoxygenase (5-LOX), 21–22
Lithium, 171–172
Lupus-like syndrome, 122
Luteinizing hormone/follicle-stimulating hormone (LH/FSH), 199
Lymecycline, 173

Macrocomedones, 38. *See also* Comedones
Maintenance therapy, 109
Malassezia globosa, 183
Malassezia sympodalis, 183
Malondialdehyde (MDA), 62
Matrix metalloproteinase (MMP), 19, 45–47, 46*f*
MDA. *See* Malondialdehyde (MDA)
Melanin, 71

Melanocortins, and sebum production, 7
Melanocytes, 71–72
Melanosomes, 71–72
Menstrual cycles
hormonal acne therapy during, 199
"Metabolizing acquired dioxin-induced
skin hamartomas" (MADISH), 172
Metformin, 58, 150, 152
Methicillin-resistant *S. aureus* (MRSA),
126–127
Methyl aminolevulinate (MAL), 213
Metronidazole, 99, 178
Microcomedones, 16, 37, 198. *See also*
Comedones
histologic examination of, 29
Microdermabrasion, in skin of color
patients, 78
Mid-childhood acne
clinical presentation, 188
differential diagnosis and evaluation, 188
guide for evaluation of, 189*t*
pathophysiology of, 188
treatment, 189–190
Miliaria pustulosa, 186
Milk, comedogenicity of, 33
Minocycline, 89, 109
administration of, 116
efficacy of, 117–118
extended-release tablets, 114
recommended dosing of, 115*t*
side effects of, 120
usage, 114
MMP. *See* Matrix metalloproteinase (MMP)
Monounsaturated fatty acids (MUFA), 61
MRSA. *See* Methicillin-resistant *S. aureus*
(MRSA)
MUFA. *See* Monounsaturated fatty acids
(MUFA)
Myalgias, 139

Nafarelin, 153
Neonatal acne, 182
clinical presentation, 182
differential diagnosis and evaluation,
183–184
pathophysiology of, 183
treatment, 184

"Neonatal cephalic pustulosis" (NCP), 182
Neonatal pustular melanosis, 183
Neutrophil gelatinase–associated lipocalin
(NGAL), 6, 21
Nevoid comedones, 38. *See also* Come-
dones
NF-κB. *See* Nuclear factor κB (NF-κB)
NGAL. *See* Neutrophil gelatinase–
associated lipocalin (NGAL)
Nobiletin, 62
Norethindrone (Estrostep), 150–151
Norgestimate (Ortho Tri-Cyclen),
150–151, 202
Nuclear factor κB (NF-κB), 14, 47

OGTT. *See* Oral glucose tolerance test
(OGTT)
Open comedones, 37. *See also* Comedones
Oral antibiotics, 113–121
alternative, 118
duration of, 118–119
efficacy of, 117–118
overview, 113
rationale for, 114–115
recommended dosing of, 115–116, 115*t*
side effects of, 119–121
for skin of color patients, 76–77
topical retinoids with, 107
usage patterns with, 114
Oral contraception (OC) treatment
contraindications to the use of,
202–203
indications of, 201–202
side effects, 203
use of, 202
Oral contraceptive pills (OCP),
149, 150–151
Oral contraceptives (OC), 34, 77, 193,
201–202
Oral glucose tolerance test (OGTT), 59
Oral isotretinoin (13-*cis*-retinoic acid), 180.
See also Isotretinoin
Oral tetracycline, 169
Oropharynx, GAS in, 128, 129
Otitis externa infection, 157
Ovarian hyperandrogenism, 199
Overprescribing, 56

Patient education, for skin of color
  patients, 80
Peeling agents, light, 210–211
Penicillin-resistant *S. aureus* (PRSA),
  126
People of color, acne in, 70–80
  clinical presentation, 72–74, 73*f*
  cultural practices and, 74
  epidemiology, 70–71
  histopathology, 74
  melanin, 71–72
  pathogenesis, 71–72
  treatment
    azelaic acid, 76
    chemical peels, 78
    dapsone, 75–76
    dermal fillers, 79–80
    hormonal therapy, 77
    laser devices, 79
    lightening agents, 78–79
    microdermabrasion, 78
    oral antibiotics, 76–77
    retinoids, 74–75, 77
    topical, 74–76
Peroxisome proliferator-activated receptors
  (PPAR), 170
  in comedogenesis, 35–36
  DNA transcription and, 22
  regulation of, 22
  and sebum production, 7
Phagocytic cells, 20
Pharyngitis, 128
Photodynamic therapy (PDT), 210
Photopneumatic therapy, 214
Pituitary gonadotropins, 202
Pityrosporum, 183, 184
Plasma cortisol level, 203
PLLA. *See* Poly-L-lactic acid (PLLA)
Polycystic ovary syndrome (PCOS), 33,
  150, 153, 188, 199, 201
Poly-L-lactic acid (PLLA), 80
Pomade acne, 74
Postinflammatory hyperpigmentation
  (PIH), 70. *See also* People of color,
  acne in
  incidence of, 72
  lightening agents for, 78–79
  topical retinoids for, 75

PPAR. *See* Peroxisome proliferator–
  activated receptors (PPAR)
PPAR-γ1, 170
PpIX, 213
Preadolescent acne
  clinical presentation, 190
  differential diagnosis and evaluation,
    191–192
  pathophysiology, 191
  treatment, 192–194
Prednisone, 153
Preformed vitamin A, 63. *See also*
  Vitamin A
Pregnancy, acne during, 177
  erythromycin in, 100, 121
  systemic therapy, 179–180
  topical antibiotics in, 100
  topical antimicrobials, 177–178
  topical retinoids, 178–179
  topical salicylic acid, 179
5α-Pregnanedione, 60
Prepubertal acne, 148, 191
Progestins, 170, 201–202
Prognosis, 163
Prolactin, 147
Propionibacterium acnes, 3, 62, 147, 161,
  169, 191, 198, 213–214. *See also*
  Innate immune system
  antimicrobial response to, 19–20
  cathelicidin and, 5, 20
  description of, 18
  in inflammation, 18–19
  MMP and, 19
  TLR and, 18–19
Proteinuria, 162
Provitamin A carotenoid, 63. *See also*
  Vitamin A
PRSA. *See* Penicillin-resistant *S. aureus*
  (PRSA)
Pseudomonas aeruginosa, 158
  infection, 157
Pseudotumor cerebri, 138–139
Psoriasin, 20
Psoriasis Area and Severity Index (PASI)
  score, 173
Psychological implications, 1–2
Pubescent acne, 148
Punch excision, for scar treatment, 49

Pus, 157–158
Pyoderma faciale, 162
Pyoderma gangrenosum, 162

9-*cis* RA, 6. *See also* Retinoids, and sebum
    production
13-*cis* RA, 6, 21. *See also* Retinoids, and
    sebum production
Radiofrequency, 214
RAR. *See* Retinoic acid receptors (RAR)
Reactive oxygen species (ROS), 62–63
5α-Reductase (5α-R), 198
Retinoic acid receptors (RAR), 87, 135
    tretinoin, binding with, 88
Retinoids, 134, 173
    and scar treatment, 52
    and sebum production, 6
    for skin of color patients, 77
    topical. *See* Topical retinoids
Retinol, 63. *See also* Vitamin A
Rhabdomyosarcoma, 168
Rifampin, 203
Rolling scars. *See also* Atrophic scars
    dermal fillers for, 49
    description of, 49, 50*f*–52*f*
ROS. *See* Reactive oxygen species (ROS)
Rosacea fulminans, 162

S. aureus. See Staphylococcus aureus
    (S. aureus)
Salicylic acid, 78. *See also* Chemical peels,
    in skin of color patients
    side effects, 211
Sand paper comedones, 37. *See also*
    Comedones
Scars/scarring
    classification of, 48–49
    defined, 43
    factors influencing formation of, 47–48
    incidence of, 43
    matrix synthesis and repairing in, 47
    in people of color, 70, 72, 73*f*
        treatment, 77, 78
    study on, 44
    treatment of, 49, 52
    wound healing and, 44–45

Sebaceous glands, 43–44
    androgens and, 5–6, 32–33
    CRH and, 7–8
    factors regulating, 5–8
    FGFR and, 8
    holocrine secretion, 3
    in innate immune defense mechanism, 5,
        21–22
    lipids. *See* Lipids, sebum
    PPAR and, 7
    retinoids and, 6
Seborrhea, 186
Seborrhea/acne/hirsutism/alopecia (SAHA)
    syndrome, 199
Sebum
    in acne pathogenesis, 8
    antibacterial action, 5
    function, 4–5
    lipids, 3–4, 4*t*
        and comedogenesis, 31–32
        and immune responses, 21–22
    production, 5–8
Sebum excretion rate (SER)
    in mothers prenatally, 183
Serratia spp., 157
Serum alkaline phosphatase levels, 162
Serum total testosterone, 199–200
    and ovarian tumor, 200
Sex hormone-binding globulin (SHBG),
    150, 169
Shalita comedo extractor, 209*f*
SJS. *See* Stevens–Johnson syndrome (SJS)
Skin of color patients. *See* People of color,
    acne in
Sodium sulfacetamide, 99
Spina bifida, 179
Spironolactone, 151–152, 200–201
    side effects of, 201
Squalene, 4
Staphylococcus aureus (S. aureus), 13,
    156, 186
    antibiotics, resistance to, 126–128
    description of, 126
    erythromycin-resistant, 128
    methicillin-resistant, 126–127
    penicillin-resistant, 126
Staphylococcus epidermidis, 157
Steroid-induced acne, 168–169

Steroid rosacea, 169
Stevens–Johnson syndrome (SJS),
    120–121
Stratum corneum, 13
    hydration, 4
Streptococcus pyogenes. See Group A
    streptococcus (GAS)
Submarine comedones, 37–38. *See also*
    Comedones
Suicidal ideation, 1
Suicide attempts, 1–2
Sulfamethoxazole. *See* Trimethoprim/
    sulfamethoxazole (TMP/SMX)
Sun protection, 79

Tazarotene, 89, 179
TEN. *See* Toxic epidermal necrolysis
    (TEN)
Teratogenicity, 139
Testicular and uterine cancers, 168
Testosterone. *See also* Androgens
    and sebum production, 5–6
Testosterone and acne fulminans
    elevated blood levels of, 161
Tetracyclines, 137, 139, 179–180
    anti-inflammatory properties, 113,
        117–118
    resistance to
        GAS, 129
        S. aureus, 130
        S. pyogenes, 98
    for skin of color patients, 76–77
    tretinoin with, 107
    usage patterns with, 114
Thalidomide, 167–168
Thermolytic effect on sebaceous
    glands, 214
Thiazolidinediones, 150
TNF-α. *See* Tumor necrosis factor-alpha
    (TNF-α)
Toll-like receptors (TLR), 13, 173
    activation of, 14, 15*f*
    extracellular portion of, 14
    heterodimers, 14
    intracellular portion of, 14
    molecular structure of, 14, 16*f*
    P. acnes and, 18–19

Topical antibiotics, 95–101
    application, 96
    as combination therapy, 98–99
        with topical retinoids, 106–107
    comparison of, 96–97
    mechanism of action, 95
    overview, 95
    rationale for, 95–96
    safety considerations with, 99–101
Topical dapsone, 193
Topical retinoids, 178–179, 204
    adapalene, 89–90
    advantage of, 87
    adverse effect of, 87–88
    with antibiotics
        oral, 107
        topical, 106–107
    isotretinoin. *See* Isotretinoin
    as maintenance therapy, 88
    new developments, 90–91
    nuclear receptors and, 87
    tazarotene, 89
    tretinoin, 88
    with topical antibiotics, 106–107
Topical salicylic acid, 179
Toxic epidermal necrolysis (TEN), 120–121
Treatment, 163–164
    antibiotics for. *See specific* antibiotics
    combination therapy. *See* Combination
        therapy
    compliance issues, 55–56
    concept of, 55
    infantile acne, 187–188
    scars/scarring, 49, 52
    skin of color patients
        azelaic acid for, 76
        chemical peels for, 78
        dapsone for, 75–76
        dermal fillers for, 79–80
        hormonal therapy for, 77
        laser devices for, 79
        lightening agents for, 78–79
        microdermabrasion for, 78
        oral antibiotics for, 76–77
        retinoids for, 74–75, 77
        topical for, 74–76
    topical retinoids for. *See* Topical
        retinoids

Tretinoin, 88, 178
  with tetracycline, 107
Triamcinolone acetonide, 209–210
Triglyceride, in sebum, 3
  hydrolysis, 4
Triglyceride-induced pancreatitis, 138
Trimethoprim-sulfa, 189
Trimethoprim/sulfamethoxazole (TMP/
    SMX), 76, 114, 158–159
  side effects, 120–121
  use, 120
Tumor necrosis factor-alpha (TNF-α), 47
Type 1 5α-reductase, 32–33

Upper respiratory tract infection (URTI),
    98
  antibiotics and, 129–131
URTI. *See* Upper respiratory tract
    infection (URTI)

Valproate, 171
Virilizing tumor, 199
Vitamin A, 63–64
  daily intake of, 63
  forms of, 63
Vitamin E, 4–5

Water loss, sebum and, 4
Wax esters, 3–4

WHO
  contraindications to the use of OC, 202–203
Wilms' tumor, 168
Women, acne in
  of childbearing potential, isotretinoin in,
    135
  endocrinopathy in, 199
  history and physical examination of, 149
  laboratory examination, 149–150
  treatment
    antiandrogens, 200–201
    blocking adrenal androgen production,
      203
    blocking ovarian androgen produc-
      tion, 201–203
    clinical presentation of, 199–200
    gonadotropin-releasing hormone
      agonists, 203
    hormonal therapy, 204
    hormonal treatments, 200
    inhibition of 5α-reductase, 204
    role of androgens, 198–200
Wound healing, 44–45
  inflammatory phase of, 45
  proliferative phase of, 45
  remodeling phase of, 45

Xerophthalmia, 137

Zinc, 64
  salts, 180